Relapse Prevention with Sex Offenders

Relapse Prevention with Sex Offenders

Edited by

D. RICHARD LAWS

Florida Mental Health Institute
University of South Florida

THE GUILFORD PRESS
New York   London

© 1989 The Guilford Press
A Division of Guilford Publications, Inc.
72 Spring Street, New York, NY 10012

Printed in the United States of America

Last digit is print number: 9 8 7 6 5

Library of Congress Cataloging-in-Publication Data

Relapse prevention with sex offenders / [edited by] D. Richard Laws.
    p. cm.
  Bibliography: p.
  Includes index.
  ISBN 0-89862-381-2
  1. Sex offenders—Treatment.   2. Psychosexual disorders—Relapse—
Prevention.   I. Laws, D. Richard.
RC560.S47R45   1989
616.85'83—dc 19   88-36840
                                                                CIP

Contributors

CARMEN S. ANDERSON, M.A., Department of Law & Mental Health, Florida Mental Health Institute, University of South Florida, Tampa, Florida

KENNETH A. ANDERSON, M.A., Department of Law & Mental Health, Florida Mental Health Institute, University of South Florida, Tampa, Florida

JOHN ARMSTRONG, Burlington Probation and Parole, Burlington, Vermont

LINDA S. BEAL, M.S., Burlington Probation and Parole, Burlington, Vermont

CAROLYN H. CAREY, M.A., Child Sexual Abuse Treatment Services, Counseling Service of Addison County, Middlebury, Vermont

GEORGIA F. CUMMING, B.S., Vermont Treatment Program for Sexual Aggressors, South Burlington, Vermont

DAVID M. DAY, California State Department of Mental Health, Sacramento, California

WILLIAM H. GEORGE, Ph.D., Department of Psychology, State University of New York at Buffalo, Buffalo, New York

RODERICK L. HALL, Ph.D., Florida Department of Corrections, Tallahassee, Florida

DIANE HILDEBRAN, M.A., College Street Center for Psychotherapy, Burlington, Vermont

PAMELA JACKSON, Ph.D., Sex Offender Treatment and Evaluation Project, Atascadero State Hospital, Atascadero, California

KATURAH D. JENKINS-HALL, Ph.D., Department of Law & Mental Health, Florida Mental Health Institute, University of South Florida, Tampa, Florida

D. RICHARD LAWS, Ph.D., Department of Law & Mental Health, Florida Mental Health Institute, University of South Florida, Tampa, Florida

J. DAVID LONG, Ph.D., Rutland Mental Health Services, Rutland, Vermont

RITA K. MacDONALD, Vermont Treatment Program for Sexual Aggressors, South Burlington, Vermont

G. ALAN MARLATT, Ph.D., Department of Psychology, University of Washington, Seattle, Washington

JANICE K. MARQUES, Ph.D., California State Department of Mental Health, Sacramento, California

GARY R. MARTIN, M.S.W., College Street Center for Psychotherapy, Burlington, Vermont

ROBERT J. McGRATH, M.A., Adult Outpatient Services, Counseling Service of Addison County, Middlebury, Vermont

MICHAEL H. MINER, Ph.D., Sex Offender Treatment and Evaluation Project, Atascadero State Hospital, Atascadero, California

JOSEPH MURPHY, Sex Offender Treatment and Evaluation Project, Atascadero State Hospital, Atascadero, California

MARY K. NAFPAKTITIS, Office of the San Luis Obispo County Superintendent of Schools, San Luis Obispo, California

CRAIG NELSON, Ph.D., Sex Offender Treatment and Evaluation Project, Atascadero State Hospital, Atascadero, California

CANDICE A. OSBORN, M.A., Department of Law & Mental Health, Florida Mental Health Institute, University of South Florida, Tampa, Florida

JOHN PETTY, M.Ed., Brattleboro Center for a Safer Society, Brattleboro, Vermont

WILLIAM D. PITHERS, Ph.D., Vermont Treatment Program for Sexual Aggressors, South Burlington, Vermont

KABE RUSSEL, M.S.W., Sex Offender Treatment and Evaluation Project, Atascadero, California

GENELL G. SANDBERG, Ph.D., Parkview Psychological Services, Sioux City, Iowa

CAROL SHOCKLEY-SMITH, M.Ed., Department of Law & Mental Health, Florida Mental Health Institute, University of South Florida, Tampa, Florida

HELEN STEENMAN, Ph.D., Sex Offender Treatment and Evaluation Project, Atascadero State Hospital, Atascadero, California

V. HENLIE STURGEON, M.S., Sex Offender Treatment and Evaluation Project, Atascadero State Hospital, Atascadero, California

J. KEVIN THOMPSON, Ph.D., Department of Psychology, University of South Florida, Tampa, Florida

CARL R. VIESTI, JR., Ph.D., Sex Offender Treatment and Evaluation Project, Atascadero State Hospital, Atascadero, California

ALICIA WUESTHOFF, M.S.W., Vermont Treatment Program for Sexual Aggressors, South Burlington, Vermont

Preface

I had originally intended to write a fairly lengthy introduction to this volume. I was going to trace the origins of relapse prevention treatment, describe its history in the treatment of alcoholism and drug abuse, and describe some of its extensions to other problems, such as smoking, before arriving at the current application to sexual offending. In the course of this I planned to point out the differences between the earlier applications of RP and its use with sex offenders. However, Bill George and Alan Marlatt have relieved me of this responsibility by contributing the excellent Introduction that follows. Therefore, I will simply tell you something about this book and how it came to be the way you find it.

In 1978, a clinical psychology intern from the University of Washington named Janice Marques worked for me in the Sexual Behavior Laboratory at Atascadero State Hospital in California. During that period she showed me a prepublication manuscript by Alan Marlatt and Judith Gordon called "Determinants of Relapse." They had conceptualized a cognitive–behavioral treatment called relapse prevention, she told me, that might have application to sex offenders. In 1980, I requested a monograph from Marlatt that was one of the early statements of the rationale for the treatment. By 1981, I was at work on a grant application that incorporated many of those ideas as a central component of a proposed treatment. During these years Marques and another Atascadero intern, Bill Pithers, began formulating their own statements of this new treatment application.

When my grant application was approved in 1984, I hired Alan Marlatt and Bill George as consultants to prepare an RP treatment manual for use in the project. In the spring of 1987, Alan and Bill conducted training sessions with our therapists in Tampa. At the conclusion of these sessions I was talking to Alan and said, in what I thought was an offhand manner, "Someone ought to do a book on RP with sex offenders." He looked at me and said, "Why don't you do it?" Before I could say that I couldn't, that I had never done a book before, he scribbled a phone number on a business card and handed it to me. "Call Seymour Weingarten at Guilford," he said, "and tell him what you want to do." That's how we got here.

This is not the average edited volume. We deliberately set out to create a work that would appeal to both the specialist and the scholar, and especially to the practitioner. We decided not to prepare a volume with a small number of very long chapters on general aspects of treatment, followed by a few shorter chapters on application. This book is virtually *all* about applications. Instead we have a book of 26 chapters, 5 long ones and 21 short ones. The long ones are the Introduction, which provides an overview of RP as a treatment for sex offenders; 3 program descriptions—Marques's in California, Jenkins-Hall's in Florida, and Pithers's in Vermont; and a concluding chapter on RP outcome data. These lengthy chapters are intended to show RP in its full application within carefully conducted treatment programs. The shorter chapters deal with specific aspects of RP, the features that usually receive very brief treatment in the typical edited book. Here authors were requested to give something more than the flavor of what was done, to give the reader rather specific information on how some aspect of the treatment might be conducted. These shorter chapters deal, respectively, with sex offender problems viewed from an RP perspective, assessment of high-risk situations and coping skills, and treatment solutions to the problems in terms of both specific skills training and more global interventions.

This is intended to be a user-friendly text, but it is not a cookbook. When I was reviewing the chapters and communicating with the authors I told them: "Remember who your audience is. We're not writing this book for academic psychologists, although they will read it. We're writing primarily for the people in the hospitals, prisons, clinics, and private-practice offices who want to know how to do RP with sex offenders."

The book will not tell you specifically *how* to do RP. This is not a treatment manual. The authors are describing for you how they modified the original RP treatment to make it suitable for sex offenders. They are telling you what worked for *them* in *their* treatment setting. Those same procedures may or may not work in yours. You must remember that relapse prevention as a treatment procedure is in its infancy and that RP as applied to sex offenders is approximately postnatal.

In the Introduction George and Marlatt caution against using RP as an isolated treatment. Use that as your first principle. RP was developed as a maintenance strategy intended to preserve gains made in whatever treatment preceded it. A review of Part IV, "Programs," shows that the Marques's and Pithers's programs use RP as a sort of umbrella concept, under which a variety of activities are conducted. Jenkins-Hall's program, on the other hand, uses RP as one treatment component, then as a maintenance procedure in individual, long-term follow-up. These represent the two major uses of the treatment with sex offenders.

In order to *do* RP, I would suggest that readers closely examine all assessment and treatment procedures described in the book in order to decide which components will be best suited to your setting. Build your RP program around what will work best for you in terms of what you are already doing. Although I said that this is not a cookbook, try out what the authors say worked for them. If they did something a particular way, try it and see if it works. If they used certain words, use those phrases and see what happens. Do not be concerned about making mistakes. Be imaginative and feel free to improvise on the guidelines suggested here.

A great many procedures, techniques, inventories, forms, tests, and so forth are described in this book. We had originally intended to develop an appendix to include the most important of these with instructions for their use. It soon became apparent that space considerations would not permit this. Rather than spend time reconceptualizing, developing, testing, and validating new assessment and treatment procedures, you might wish to contact the authors and request copies of their materials. The persons working in this field are quite approachable and willing to help.

Once again, let me call your attention to a caution raised by George and Marlatt. Simply because we have gathered together a great variety of apparently face-valid procedures in a book, offered some statistical analyses, and come to optimistic, if tentative conclusions, that in no way *proves* that RP is an effective treatment for sex offenders. There is *no* definitive evidence, here or anywhere else, that RP or any other treatment is effective over the long haul with this difficult clientele. Although sex offenders have been treated for decades it has only been in very recent years that treatment has begun to be carefully documented and follow-up carefully monitored. Sadly, too few have been carefully treated, and even fewer carefully followed for long periods, to warrant excessive optimism.

In the last 10 years the focus in treatment of sex offenders has narrowed considerably. That focus is now on a central core of behavioral and cognitive–behavioral treatments, supplemented by a wide variety of other interventions. RP is solidly in the mainstream of that movement. It is my belief, and I think that this book contributes to the conclusion, that we may at last be riding a winner.

A large number of people deserve thanks for assisting me in the preparation of this volume. I first want to thank those authors that I have never met who contributed so generously to this work. Alan Marlatt and Bill George have provided information and strong support since 1984, both for our research and for this book. Special thanks are due Janice Marques, Bill Pithers, and Katurah Jenkins-Hall, the central players in this piece, who helped organize the scheme of the book, then rallied their program staff to assist in writing the chapters. Jack Zusman, Max Dertke, and Dick Swanson of the Florida Mental Health Institute were supportive throughout. And, finally, thanks go to Seymour Weingarten, Editor-in-Chief of The Guilford Press, for believing that this was the right book at the right time.

Contents

PART V. CAN RELAPSES BE PREVENTED?   311

Introduction

WILLIAM H. GEORGE
G. ALAN MARLATT

With increasing notoriety and alarm, sexual offenses (such as rape and child molestation) have come to be recognized as frequent yet underreported crimes that exact a heavy toll on the physical and psychological well-being of victims and their families. There is also growing awareness of the plight of offenders, many of whom were earlier victims themselves, and their families. Though there is uncertainty about the true incidence of offenses, it is generally acknowledged that the available statistics underestimate the problem. The more important recognition is that the gravity and durability of negative sequelae associated with sexual offenses, as well as mounting public outrage, convey a clear sense of urgency about the need for solutions that will reduce the incidence of these offenses.

Amid disagreements about the causes of sexual offenses and the utility of offender treatment, one solution that has enjoyed wide consensus is detection and punishment of the offenders. A clear benefit of this solution is that it protects society; incarcerated offenders have less access to potential victims. Similarly, registration in criminal justice monitoring systems (probation and parole) provides modest mechanisms for tracking the offender's whereabouts, restricting his/her range of travel and access to potential victims, and enforcing participation in rehabilitative endeavors. However, recidivism rates, though variable, have suggested that for some offenders punishment alone has been an inadequate solution, perhaps serving only to forestall resumption of the offense pattern. Another solution has been the application of therapeutic interventions designed to alter the offender's sexual arousal patterns related to offending. Behavioral approaches have been especially prominent in this regard. Though short-term success in modifying sexual arousal patterns has been documented, long-term posttreatment success in reducing reoffense has been disappointing (Quinsey & Marshall, 1983).

The overall picture seems to be characterized by disturbing reoffense rates for both untreated and treated sexual offenders (Furby, Weinrott, & Blackshaw, 1989; Marques & Nelson, in press). This trend may be conceptualized, in part, as a *maintenance problem*. That is, there is frequent failure to maintain non-offense patterns achieved as a consequence of adjudication, incarceration, and/ or treatment. Relapse Prevention (RP) is a treatment approach, developed within the area of addictive disorders, that is specifically designed to address maintenance problems in the changing of behavior. This Introduction describes the RP approach and its application for reducing recidivism among sex offenders. Four specific aims are encompassed: (1) to describe the origins and basic assumptions of RP, (2) to summarize the RP conceptual framework, (3) to discuss the rationale, benefits, and limitations of applying RP to sex offenders, and (4) to outline how RP treatment procedures would be applied to sex offenders.

WHAT IS RELAPSE PREVENTION?

RP is a self-control program designed to teach individuals who are trying to change their behavior how to anticipate and cope with the problem of relapse. In very general terms, relapse refers to a breakdown or failure in a person's attempt to change or modify any target behavior. The RP program focuses on enabling the person to prevent relapse and thereby to maintain the newly adopted behavior pattern. Based on social cognitive principles, RP has a psychoeducational thrust that combines behavioral skill-training procedures with cognitive intervention techniques.

Origins from the Field of Addictive Disorders

The RP model was initially developed as a maintenance program for use in the treatment of such addictive behaviors as alcohol abuse, cigarette smoking, drug abuse, and overeating (Marlatt & Gordon, 1980). For the addictions, the typical goals of treatment are either to refrain totally from performing a target behavior (e.g., to abstain from drug use) or to impose regulatory limits on the occurrence of a behavior (e.g., to diet as a means of controlling food intake). The chief emphasis in this field has generally been on getting the "addicted" person to stop engaging in the problematic behavior. However, high relapse rates in addictions treatment show that "getting stopped" gives no assurance of "remaining stopped." All too often, posttreatment changes eventually give way to a return to the pretreatment addictive pattern. It was in this context that the RP program originated as a method for maintaining long-term freedom from addiction.

Scientific and Theoretical Underpinnings
of Relapse Prevention

The underpinnings of the RP program derive from the broader social learning (Bandura, 1969, 1977a) approach to understanding human behavior, now referred to as social cognitive theory (Bandura, 1986). Based on empirical studies and hypothesis testing, the social cognitive approach has evolved from earlier behavioral theories and integrates principles from social cognition, observational learning, and behavior modification. As with other cognitive–behavioral research and treatment approaches that have been developed in recent years, the RP program combines behavioral and cognitive interventions. As a result of this heritage, the RP program makes certain critical assumptions about addictive disorders. First, addictive behavior patterns are viewed as multiply determined by past learning experiences, situational antecedent influences, prevailing reinforcement contingencies (both rewards and punishments), cognitive expectations or beliefs, and biological influences. Second, the target behavior can best be construed on a continuum between nonproblematic expression (e.g., social drinking) and addictive, or problematic, expression (e.g., alcoholism). Therefore, the same principles can be used to understand the acquisition and maintenance of nonaddictive as well as addictive behaviors. Finally, the addictive behavior can be conceptualized as a maladaptive response for coping with life stressors and dissatisfactions. An implication of this latter assumption is that more adaptive coping responses are not utilized by the individual and the addictive behavior has evolved as a habitual replacement response for this deficiency. Together, the foregoing assumptions reflect an ideology that is distinctive from the more predominant theoretical model in the addictions field, loosely known as the medical–disease model. The latter approach is predicated on the assumption that some, if not all, addictions (e.g., alcoholism) are best characterized as diseases. The RP program described here is not an outgrowth of the medical–disease model of addictions and thus does not define addictions as disease entities.

Another important feature of the RP program that stems from its social learning roots is an emphasis on self-management. As such, RP exemplifies the compensatory model of helping–coping, described by Brickman et al. (1982), in which clients are seen as responsible not for problem etiology but for problem solution. This stance eschews the traditional active-doctor/passive-patient relationship in favor of more active client collaboration and involvement. The client's resultant sense of ownership over the change process contributes to an internal locus of control and enduring behavior changes that are resistant to unsupportive environmental influences. By contrast, the medical–disease model, as described by Brickman et al. (1982), assigns the client no responsibility for either problem etiology or problem solution. Instead, the client is to accept the illness role, seek expert help, and comply with the expert's prescriptions for problem solution. According to Brickman et al., interventions that minimize client responsibility for problem solution tend to foster dependency, undermine client feelings of personal competence, and generate improvements that are attributed to external forces and only temporarily maintained.

Stages of Change in the Addictions: Treatment versus Maintenance

In the addictions field, it has become increasingly useful to conceptualize habit change as a multistage process. The significance of this strategy lies in the possibility that the relative importance and applicability of various descriptive analyses, explanatory principles, and treatment approaches may shift as an addict moves from stage to stage. Individuals may be more amenable or receptive to particular intervention strategies at different stages of change. Perhaps the most thorough and empirically cogent multistage model of habit change is the five-stage model proposed by Prochaska and DiClemente (1982, 1983) based on their work with smokers.

It is sufficient for present heuristic purposes to consider a simpler two-stage model that merely distinguishes treatment from maintenance. The treatment phase traditionally has been the predominant focus in the addictions field. Because of this disproportionate allocation of attention and energy to treatment, much more is known about cessation (getting the person to stop the addictive behavior) than about maintenance (preventing relapse). Far too often these two aims were confused because of the tacit assumption that maintenance was merely an extension of cessation. Important distinctions between initial treatment and long-range maintenance were not made clear. The fact is that very little was known about procedures designed specifically to maintain behavior change following the initial cessation, or "quit date."

Ignorance about the maintenance stage was reflected in a number of unhelpful developments. First, addicts who had undergone extensive cessation-oriented treatments were usually being discharged with few maintenance-oriented strategies beyond appeals to internal fortitude, a list of the virtues of "staying clean" (and/or the catastrophic perils of the addictive behavior), and phone numbers for an ex-addict support network. Missing were specific guidelines for how to avoid relapse. Second, open discussion of relapse was generally discouraged in treatment because it presumably could weaken commitment to cessation or, worse yet, subtly encourage relapse itself. In effect, there was no sanctioned forum in which addicts could voice fears about the maintenance stage or plan safeguards. Third, maintenance failure (relapse) was seen as indicative of treatment failure. Therefore, the overarching response to the relapse problem in the addictions field has been to strengthen initial treatment by building more comprehensive broad-spectrum or multimodel treatment packages that presumably would induce a more forceful cessation. The general idea was to create a treatment so powerful that it would be less prone to "wear off." The obvious drawback to this strategy, however, is that the addition of more techniques and procedures makes it more difficult for the client to comply with the treatment requirements (Hall, 1980). Finally, this approach included few precautionary measures reflecting the reality that, while initial treatment procedures were usually administered to the client by the therapist (e.g., aversion therapy or counseling), maintenance procedures ultimately had to be self-administered by the client. Clients were not being systematically taught to become their own therapists and to carry on the thrust of the treatment after the end of the formal therapeutic relationship.

In sum, prior to the advent of RP, there was little appreciation in the addictions field for distinguishing between the cessation and maintenance processes. Thus there was little recognition of the possibility that treatment and maintenance each might require qualitatively different analyses and intervention points. Many, if not all, of the intervention techniques were directed primarily toward initial behavior change rather than toward the long-term maintenance of this change. What was often overlooked during the treatment phase was that the maintenance of change, once it has been induced, may be governed by entirely different principles than those associated with initial cessation. RP, a system of maintenance-oriented principles and interventions, addresses this long-standing deficiency. Furthermore, since there appears to be some validity in distinguishing treatment from maintenance, another advantage of RP is that it may be applied regardless of the orientation or methods used during treatment.

Defining Relapse

The term *relapse* traditionally has been construed as an entirely negative event. Negative associations such as "treatment breakdown" and "return to addiction" reflect one of two definitions of relapse in *Webster's New Collegiate Dictionary*: "a recurrence of symptoms of a disease after a period of improvement" (1984, p. 994). This definition is clearly compatible with the medical–disease approach and thereby embodies certain implications. First, the relapse is a function of an underlying and ongoing disease entity that is internally driven by biological processes and is completely outside of the person's conscious control. Second, treatment outcome is a dichotomous all-or-none affair: One is either "cured" (or the symptoms are in remission) or one has relapsed (recidivism). Standard practice in the addictions field has been to view any return to the treated behavior (no matter how slight) after abstinence-oriented treatment as indicative of full-blown relapse. Third, relapse is viewed pessimistically as an end-state with no redeeming characteristics.

The RP approach embraces an alternative interpretation of relapse that corresponds with a second definition listed in *Webster's*: "the act or instance of backsliding, worsening, or subsiding" (1984, p. 994). This approach emphasizes that a relapse can be viewed as a single act of falling back rather than as a complete recapitulation of the pretreatment pattern. An advantageous implication of this view is that the term *lapse*, less burdened with automatically and completely negative associations, emerges as a meaningful and pivotal construct. The same dictionary defines *lapse* as "a slight error . . . a temporary deviation or fall esp. from a higher to a lower state" (1984, p. 674), for example, an isolated drink or cigarette after a period of abstinence. The mere distinction of *lapse* from *relapse* negates the usual all-or-none interpretation and permits the less pessimistic inference that lapses do not always lead to full-blown relapses. Rather than an end-state, the lapse represents a transitional state for which relapse is only one possible outcome. Other possible scenarios include return to abstinence or adoption of a moderation pattern (i.e., nonproblematic expression of the behavior, such as controlled social drinking). Thus, when viewed as a single mistake or error, the lapse can be construed as temporary, and the supposedly inevitable trajectory from lapse to relapse becomes changeable. In RP, the lapse is not viewed as an entirely negative event but as one offering the redeeming feature of representing a potentially valuable learning experience. Building a life free of former addictions is a trial-and-error process. Like mistakes in the learning of any new behavior patterns, lapses can inform the actor about unforeseen pitfalls, convey corrective feedback, and impart guidance about how one might avoid future mistakes.

Overall, definitions of *relapse* in the RP approach may be summarized as follows. Relapse is a violation of a self-imposed rule or set of rules governing the rate or pattern of a selected target behavior. This is most clearly exemplified by violations of abstinence rules in the case of substance abusers, for example, the ex-smoker who returns to smoking. Violation of a set of moderation rules also represents a relapse, as in the case of the dieter who returns to overeating. The related term, *lapse*, is used to refer to a single instance of violating the rule. For obvious reasons that will be outlined later, application of the RP model to work with sex offenders requires that these definitions be translated in a very conservative manner. With sex offenders, the term *relapse* will refer to any occurrence of a sexual offense, thus connoting full scale reestablishment of the problematic behavior. The term *lapse* will refer to any occurrence of willful and elaborate fantasizing about sexual offending or any return to sources of stimulation associated with the sexual offense pattern, but short of performance of the offense behavior.

OVERVIEW OF RP THEORETICAL CONCEPTS

The RP model and its attendant empirical support are described elsewhere (Brownell, Marlatt, Lichtenstein, & Wilson, 1986; Marlatt & George, 1984; Marlatt & Gordon, 1980, 1985). What follows is a brief overview of the overarching theoretical framework of the RP model.

The RP model consists of two primary conceptual components. The first focuses on explaining the processes that operate in certain situations to promote the occurrence of a lapse and to facilitate escalation from a lapse to a relapse. The second component focuses on explaining the operation of more subtle processes that can gradually move the recovered addict toward a set of circumstances capable of inciting a lapse. Both components are described below in general terms that are applicable to all addictive disorders. These two conceptual components are matched by two corresponding treatment components, each comprising a system of intervention strategies and procedures based on the respective conceptual components. The RP treatment interventions and their application to work with sex offenders specifically will be briefly described later in this Introduction and more extensively in subsequent chapters.

Conceptual Component 1: Determinants of Relapse

Figure 1 diagrams the descriptive and causal analysis of a relapse episode that is central to the RP approach. Beginning with the assumption that the individual has voluntarily chosen to adopt a rule or set of rules for changing the addictive behavior, the RP model postulates that he/she experiences perceived control over the behavior until a *high-risk situation* (HRS) is encountered. An HRS may be broadly defined as any situation that poses a threat to perceived control and thereby increases the probability of lapse or relapse (i.e., violation of the self-imposed rule set).

Available research findings have suggested that certain types of events prototypically represent HRSs that can predispose individuals toward relapse. For example, Cummings, Gordon, and Marlatt (1980) found that 71% of all relapses studied across various addictions were precipitated by one of three types of determinants: (1) negative emotional states (35%), or situations in which the person experienced unpleasant emotions or feelings (e.g., anger, boredom, depression) that were not occasioned by interaction with another individual; (2) interpersonal conflict (16%), or situations in which the individual recently engaged in an argument or other unpleasant interpersonal confrontation; and (3) social pressure (20%), or situations in which the individual experienced direct or indirect pressure from others to violate the rule set. Such data refuted the traditional view that relapse was determined entirely by internal physiologi-

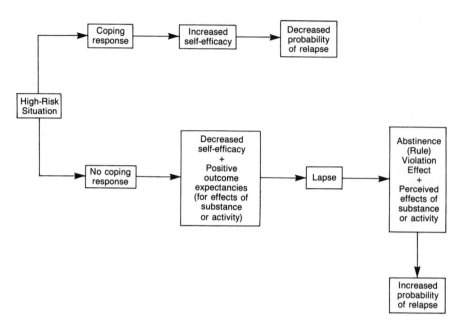

FIGURE 1. Conceptual component 1: Determinants of relapse. From "Relapse Prevention: Theoretical Rationale and Overview of the Model" by G. Alan Marlatt. In *Relapse Prevention: Maintenance Strategies in the Treatment of Addictive Behaviors* (p. 38), Eds. G. A. Marlatt and J. R. Gordon, 1985, New York: Guilford Press. Copyright 1985 by the Guilford Press. Reprinted by permission.

cal phenomena (e.g., urges), indicated that HRSs could be usefully categorized, and implicated the pivotal nature of the HRS in relapse. The RP model hypothesizes that the likelihood of a relapse depends on the person's ability to cope with HRSs. As depicted by the upper pathway in Figure 1, if the individual is able to execute an effective coping response in the HRS, the probability of relapse diminishes. This individual presumably experiences an increased sense of mastery and self-efficacy (Bandura, 1977b), that is, an expectation of successful coping in future HRSs. As more HRSs are successfully coped with, perceived control strengthens and the probability of relapse declines.

If the person instead fails to cope effectively with the HRS, then relapse becomes more probable, as outlined by the lower pathway of Figure 1. Whether the failure reflects absence of the needed coping skills or obstruction of the skills due to inhibitory anxiety or beliefs, the person perceives the situation as beyond his/her coping capacity and begins to experience feelings of helplessness and decreased self-efficacy. As the expectation of being able to cope successfully with the present and future situations declines, the person is more likely to give in to the prevailing forces. Decreased self-efficacy, the availability of the forbidden behavior, and positive expectations about that behavior (i.e., the perception that engaging in the forbidden behavior will produce some immediate gratification) will function collectively and independently to propel the person toward a lapse.

If the individual lapses, or slips, and violates his/her newly adopted rules, then a critical juncture has been reached. Will that violation remain a single isolated lapse or will it snowball into a full-blown relapse? A construct termed the "abstinence (or rule) violation effect" (AVE) has been postulated to account for how individuals react to the violation. The potency of the AVE varies with the strength and duration of the person's commitment to the new rules. The significance of the AVE lies in its capacity to facilitate the escalation of a lapse into a relapse. In its original formulation (Marlatt, 1978, 1979, 1982; Marlatt & Gordon, 1980), the AVE was hypothesized to consist of two elements. The cognitive-dissonance element refers to the conflict between one's prelapse self-image (e.g., as abstainer) and the discrepant behavior (lapse); this conflict is accompanied by feelings of discomfort and guilt. This can promote relapse because the person may continue indulgence in the forbidden behavior after the initial lapse as a way to counteract the uncomfortable emotional state or to resolve the conflict by realigning the self-image with the discrepant behavior. The personal attribution element describes the tendency to attribute the cause of the lapse to internal traits such as personal weaknesses (e.g., no willpower) or failure. This can promote relapse via a self-fulfilling prophecy, whereby expectations for continued failure will increase. The two AVE elements can operate independently or jointly to promote relapse.

Recently (Marlatt, 1985a), the AVE was reformulated to include an expanded analysis of the postlapse transition to relapse. The reformulated analysis incorporates contemporary theoretical developments in the social cognition literature, such as attribution theory and self-awareness theory. The substance of the original formulation (Marlatt & Gordon, 1980) was retained in the reformulation. However, in the reformulation, the personal attribution and cognitive-dissonance components specified initially were subsumed, respectively, by two broader constructs: cognitive attribution as to perceived cause of the lapse and affective reaction to this attribution. Thus the reformulated AVE encompasses an extended and more detailed consideration of the attributional processes and emotional reactions that hypothetically characterize the postlapse scenario.

A final postlapse contributor to relapse is the perception of gratification. Any pleasurable sensations associated with the lapse can further fuel an escalation to relapse. These sensations may include the physical reactions to the forbidden drug or activity that are subjectively experienced as positive.

The foregoing analysis explaining the path from HRS to relapse is accompanied by a corresponding system of treatment interventions that will be described later. In general, these interventions are aimed at teaching the client to anticipate and prepare for HRSs in ways designed to prevent lapses from occurring and, if they do occur, from snowballing into relapses.

Conceptual Component 2: Covert Antecedents of a Relapse Situation

The capacity for an HRS to provoke a lapse and promote relapse is rather straightforward. An important precursory question is: How does a person wind up in an HRS? Certainly, fortuitous or unavoidable events may precipitate an HRS (e.g., required attendance at a "wet" business luncheon). However, at times an HRS develops insidiously, as a result of covert antecedents.

As indicated in Figure 2, lifestyle imbalance is a key covert precursor. Intuitively, the subjective sense of feeling "stressed out" by life's routine duties and obligations (i.e., "shoulds") would appear to potentiate relapse. A preponderance of "shoulds" in one's life can lead to feelings of deprivation. Moreover, this sense of being unfairly deprived becomes especially acute if there coexists a relative shortage of self-indulgent pleasant activities (i.e., "wants"). As "shoulds" exceed "wants," a disequilibrium is created and the individual begins to feel a desire for immediate gratification that will restore balance and quell the mounting feelings of deprivation. Comments such as "I owe myself a few drinks—I deserve a break today" exemplify this experience. In addition, the newly adopted self-control program can itself be construed as a "should." Heightened desire for immediate gratification generated by an imbalanced lifestyle can

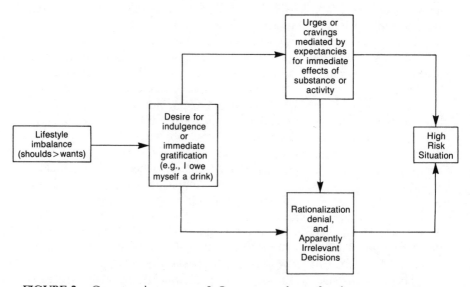

FIGURE 2.   Conceptual component 2: Covert antecedents of a relapse situation. From "Relapse Prevention: Theoretical Rationale and Overview of the Model" by G. Alan Marlatt. In *Relapse Prevention: Maintenance Strategies in the Treatment of Addictive Behaviors* (p. 48), Eds. G. A. Marlatt and J. R. Gordon, 1985, New York: Guilford Press. Copyright 1985 by The Guilford Press. Reprinted by permission.

translate into urges and cravings for indulgence in the forbidden behavior. These sensations are largely mediated by cognitive processes (e.g., expectations). In addition, conditioning processes may play a crucial role, because past stimuli associated with the addictive behavior can elicit craving. These urges and cravings can, in turn, lead the person consciously and/or unconsciously to set up an HRS that can provoke a lapse and promote relapse. Rationalizations and denial can serve to obscure or distort the true intentions that underlie a progressive series of approach behaviors masquerading as "apparently irrelevant decisions" (AIDs) (Marlatt & Gordon, 1980). For example, an ex-drinker may decide to keep a bottle of liquor in the house "in case unexpected guests drop over" or to stop in the local tavern on the way home "just to buy a pack of breath mints." While denying a desire to indulge, the addict has managed to arrive at an HRS. Then, like a lost driver trying to retrace the route, the addict cannot clearly discern how the road paved with good intentions became the road to ruin.

The foregoing analysis of covert antecedents to the HRS dictates associated treatment interventions that have a global purpose: to facilitate changes in personal habits and lifestyle so as to reduce the risk of physical disease or psychological stress. Here, the aim of the RP program is much broader in scope: to teach the individual how to achieve a balanced lifestyle and to prevent the formation of unhealthy habit patterns.

APPLICATION OF THE RP MODEL
TO UNDERSTANDING SEX OFFENDING

Parallels between sex offending and addictive disorders are easily drawn. This would seem a convincing reason to apply RP to sex offending, but it is not our predominant rationale. The applicability of the RP model for working with sex offenders is justified primarily on the grounds that recidivism can be readily conceptualized as a maintenance problem. The sex-offending-as-addiction analogy, though only a secondary and nonessential aspect of our rationale, is pertinent and plausible enough to warrant scrutiny.

Is Sex Offending an Addiction?

While there are similarities between various addictive disorders and sexual-offense patterns, the applicability of the RP approach for this population neither assumes nor necessitates adoption of a sexual-addiction construct. That is, the behavior of the pedophile or rapist need not be construed as an addiction in order to legitimize the use of RP strategies. This is in contrast to another addiction-oriented approach to sexual offending.

In a book that has become widely cited in the popular press (e.g., Chapman, 1988; Saline, 1985; Seligmann, Flowers, Gosnell, Harrison, & Nelson, 1987) as an authoritative pioneering source, Carnes (1983) argues that sexual activity can become as addictive as alcohol and other drugs. He loosely defines *sexual addiction* as a "pathological relationship to a mood-altering experience" (p. 135) and postulates three levels of sexual addiction in which sexual offending classifies as either a level-two (nuisance offenses, such as exhibitionism and voyeurism) or level-three (more serious victimizations, such as rape and child molestation) addiction. Carnes's approach stresses that sexual offending is an addiction that, like alcoholism, is best characterized as an illness. Accordingly, the treatment strategy advanced by Carnes draws very heavily on the most widely available alcoholism treatment approach, Alcoholics Anonymous (AA). The recommended treatment, in fact, is based on and guided by a direct translation of AA's "12 steps to recovery." Hence, various AA-type self-help groups have appeared: Sexual Addicts Anonymous, Sexaholics Anonymous, Sexual Abuse Anonymous, and so forth.

In our view, this sexual-addiction construct is a mixed blessing. A primary advantage of it is that, if only by the mere semantics of the phrase, it opens the door to another domain of ideas for thinking about and treating sexual paraphilias, problems that have proven to be enormously resistant to intervention. Related to this, the construct conveys an inherent legitimacy for giving priority to the therapeutic treatment of sex offenders, a population for whom even the appropriateness of treatment is routinely questioned and for whom treatment involvement, if available, is overshadowed by legal imperatives and moral indignation.

However, application of Carnes's (1983) sexual-addiction construct to sex offenders also has important disadvantages and problems, some stemming from its origins in the medical–disease model of alcoholism. For instance, with its emphases on acknowledgment of oneself as addict and admission of powerlessness, the sexual-addiction approach places the locus of responsibility for the offense pattern and for treatment outside the offender. Such an externalization of blame and treatment responsibility can backfire with offenders who are already reluctant to take any responsibility for their misdeeds and choose to view this so-called addiction as a convenient excuse before and after a reoffense. Second, acceptance of sexual offending as an addiction seems a necessary precondition for both the adoption and success of the derivative treatment approach. This is an extremely precarious contingency, given that no scientific data are provided to support the equation. Consequently, the integrity and supposed efficacy of the treatment application are dependent on an essential premise that, though perhaps intuitively credible, has limited scientific merit. More pragmatically, it is an all-or-none proposition; if the offender does not accept the critical equation, then this approach has absolutely nothing to offer him/her. Another disadvantage is the inappropriateness of the abstinence-only goal that is a hallmark of AA-type treatments. The AA approach advocates total, lifelong abstention from the mood-altering experience and has practically no provision for anything that might be considered qualified abstinence or moderated indulgence. Because the sex offender is required to abstain from only certain forms of sexual indulgence, the traditional AA approach is inherently ill equipped to guide recovery. Efforts to remedy this inherent contradiction by making exceptions to total abstinence distort the basic premise of the traditional AA philosophy and compromise the integrity of the addiction metaphor and its AA-style treatment. A final problem concerns the difficulty involved in reconciling the disease view with the punishment imperative. With alcoholics, the AA approach is not burdened with the illogical task of explaining why the disease sufferer must be punished.

From the RP perspective, whether or not sex offending is a sexual addiction may ultimately be a moot point. What matters is that sex offenders have a maintenance problem, and RP is uniquely oriented to provide treatment technologies devoted to maintenance problems. In sum, the addiction metaphor is a convenient and apt angle for introducing RP to sex offender applications, but it should not be interpreted literally or as a prerequisite condition.

Similarities between Sex Offending and Other Addictions

The sex-offending-as-addiction analogy seems so persuasive and intuitive partially because of the obvious and somewhat compelling similarities between sex offending and other addictions. Both syndromes are associated with high costs for the individual and for society. In both phenomena, there is an emphasis on immediate, short-term gratification at the expense of delayed, long-term negative consequences ("fly now, pay later" logic). As Carnes (1983) suggests, compulsive sexual activity, like various of the addictions, offers the allure of being a reliable mood-altering experience. According to anecdotal reports and superficial observations, there appears to be an impulsive, as well as a compulsive, quality to both types of activities. For example, in the case of sex offending, it has been noted that many convicted offenders report having committed many more offenses than are revealed by their official records (e.g., Abel et al., 1987). The treatment lore depicts sex offenders and addicts (especially alcoholics, gamblers, and drug addicts) as being particularly prone to denying that the target behavior is problematic and to surrounding the behavior with secrecy. No single etiological model or treatment approach exhibits clear superiority with either syndrome. As noted earlier, relapse is a persistent problem in both syndromes. It has been documented that relapse episodes for sexual offending (Pithers, Marques, Gibat, & Marlatt, 1983) and other addictions (Marlatt & Gordon, 1980) are characterized by similar types of precipitants, especially negative emotional states. Furthermore, sex offending has unique similarities to gambling, an addiction not involving ingestion of a substance, and to overeating, an addiction for which a total-abstinence treatment goal is untenable.

Differences between Sex Offending and Other Addictions

The above similarities notwithstanding, important differences exist between sex offending and addictive disorders.

Victimization

The fact that each occurrence of a sex offense involves direct and significant victimization of another individual is an extremely significant distinction. With all of the recent revelations about transgenerational negative sequelae experienced by the families of alcoholics, alcoholism and other addictions are no longer considered self-inflicted or victimless problems/crimes. Nevertheless, despite how detrimental these addictions are for sufferers and their families, the typical single occurrence of the behavior (e.g., a drink by an alcoholic) does not so devastatingly victimize another individual as does a sex offense (e.g., rape). A potential danger of adopting an addiction metaphor for sex offending is that it may tend to trivialize the grave consequences associated with *each* occurrence of the target behavior. Hence, this difference between sex offending and addictions must be emphatically drawn.

Ethical and Legal Considerations

By all accounts, the ethical and legal considerations take on much greater prominence with sex offending than with addictive disorders. The offender who reoffends has not merely relapsed but has broken the law. While it is true that for certain substance addictions relapse constitutes an illegality, the perceived severity of the infraction and the necessity of corrective legal action demand less urgency than is the case with sex offending. The ethical and legal ramifications involved when a pedophile discloses a reoffense to a therapist simply cannot be equated with those involved when an alcoholic or even a heroin addict reports a relapse.

Fantasy

Another difference between sex offending and addictions has to do with the importance of fantasy life. With all addictive disorders, the individual may dream or fantasize about engaging in the behavior. During periods of active addiction, fantasies can support the person's attachment to the addiction and can be integral links in the chain of events that precede an episode of indulgence. During periods of abstinence or controlled use, fantasies can sustain the attachment and fuel urges and cravings that may be experienced as antecedents to a lapse. Nevertheless, despite the potentially powerful function of fantasies in these processes, it seems clear that physical gratification comparable to the actual addictive activity (smoking the cigarette, having the drink, etc.) cannot be achieved through fantasy.

Fantasies play a much more potent and crucial role in the life of a sex offender (e.g., Laws & Marshall, in press). First, the discrepancy between the gratification attainable from the fantasy versus that attainable from actual indulgence in the target behavior (the sex offense) is less dramatic than with most addictions. This is true because an offender's fantasy will very likely be accompanied by genital arousal, which is typically experienced as pleasant and reinforcing in its own right. In fact, the offender can employ physical aids such as pornography to heighten the arousal achieved from the fantasies. Second, the gratification level associated with the fantasy can be readily maximized when augmented by masturbation and orgasm. Third, many sex offenders report that active and deliberate fantasizing about the offense is an integral part of the preoffense sequence. Fourth, because of the foregoing features, the offender's attachment to the offense pattern can be sustained at a very high level even during periods of externally imposed abstinence, such as incarceration.

Difficulty in Defining Lapse and Relapse

Instances of lapse and relapse are clearly discernible and definable with addictive disorders. For example, there is little equivocation about the fact that smoking a cigarette constitutes a lapse for an ex-smoker or that drinking a fifth of whiskey a day constitutes a relapse for a recovering alcoholic. With sex offenders, instances of lapse and relapse are not as unambiguously distinct as they are in addictive disorders and must therefore be defined in a more arbitrary fashion.

Translating Definitions of Lapse and Relapse

The terms lapse and relapse, so central to the RP approach, are applied to sex offending in the context of several of the foregoing concerns. Ethical and legal concerns dictate that the relapse be arbitrarily defined in a much more conservative fashion than is typical with application of RP to most addictive disorders. Any new occurrence of a sexual offense constitutes a relapse. Thus with sex offending, a single violation of the rule against performing the terminal consummatory behavior (i.e., the sex offense) connotes full scale reestablishment of the problematic behavior.

A conservative definition of a lapse highlights the importance of fantasy in sex offending. In formulating an acceptable definition of lapse, a chain of events thought to precede the typical offense has been proposed (Pithers et al., 1983) and later elaborated (George & Marlatt, 1984), hypothesizing several distinct steps: (1) an urge, fleeting thought, or dream about committing an offense (any of which may or may not be accompanied by arousal); (2) willful elaboration of fantasies about committing an offense accompanied by arousal; (3) masturbation coupled with fantasies and/or pornography related to the offense; (4) formulation of a plan of action; and (5) commission of the actual offense. This chain is a valuable heuristic tool in specifying an arbitrary point at which a lapse can be designated. In keeping with the need for conservatism, a lapse is defined early in the preoffense chain as any occurrence of willful and elaborate fantasizing about sexual offending or any sources of stimulation associated with the sexual-offense pattern. Notably, this represents the first point in the chain where the exercise of conscious control is feasible.

APPLICATION OF RP TREATMENT INTERVENTIONS TO SEX OFFENDERS

RP treatment interventions are guided by the two conceptual components, outlined earlier, that analyze how HRSs can lead to lapse and relapse and how individuals who set out to alter their behavior wind up in these situations. Based on these analyses, RP treatment procedures echo two central objectives: teaching individuals to cope effectively with HRSs and to identify and respond to the *early warning signals* that covertly steer them toward eventual HRSs. The RP intervention procedures can be organized according to these two objectives. General guidelines for how the RP interventions might be applied with sex offenders will be presented in the remainder of this Introduction. More specific guidelines are provided in subsequent chapters and elsewhere (George & Marlatt, 1984; Marques, Pithers, & Marlatt, 1984; Pithers et al., 1983).

Preconditions for RP Treatment of Sex Offenders

Motivation

An important precondition for applying RP interventions is that the offender be motivated to stop offending and to change sexual and nonsexual response patterns related to the offense pattern. As noted earlier, the RP conceptual analysis assumes that the individual has voluntarily adopted a commitment to change the problematic behavior. In many instances, but especially with sex offenders, there is substantial extrinsic pressure for the individual to change. Nonetheless, it is critical for applying RP, as well as other treatments, that the offender exhibit some appreciable recognition of the need to change and some genuine, intrinsic desire to seek change.

While the RP approach offers little promise for the unmotivated offender and cannot induce motivation, some of the RP treatment procedures to be described can be adapted to address motivation issues. For instance, *self-efficacy ratings* (Marlatt, 1985b; Merluzzi, Glass, & Genest, 1981) can be used to reflect motivation levels, and the *decision matrix* (Marlatt, 1985b) can be used to enhance recognition of the need to change. Other related techniques can be useful for working with motivational issues. For instance, straightforward *motivation ratings* (George & Marlatt, 1984) can be used to assess initial levels and monitor fluctuations across treatment. *Gestalt "hot-seat"* (Marlatt, 1985b; Perls, 1971) dialogues can be helpful in explicating and resolving ambivalence about changing; for instance, a dialogue between a client's prorelapse and antirelapse motives, or between a client and his/her sexual urges, could clarify important motivational conflicts.

Adjunctive Application

The interventions associated with both RP treatment objectives (i.e., cessation and maintenance) encompass an array of modular treatment components that can be optionally combined and idiosyncratically tailored for the particular circumstances. This versatility for compilation of modular treatment procedures is an important advantage of the RP approach. Moreover, with addictive disorders, the RP approach can either be employed as the central focus of therapy (directing both the cessation and maintenance phases of habit change) or be used adjunctively with various forms of cessation-oriented or maintenance-oriented treatment. However, with sex offenders, the RP treatment procedures are neither intended nor designed to be applied as a stand-alone intervention.

When used with sex offenders, the RP approach should be paired with a cessation-oriented intervention. Incarceration alone, though it prevents occurrence of offenses in the free community, should not be considered an adequate cessation intervention for three notable reasons. First, incarceration is an externally imposed stoppage that does not require from the offender any motivation for voluntary commitment to changing the offense pattern. Second, as outlined earlier, the offender can maintain attachment to the offense pattern through fantasy. Finally, depending on the nature of the offense pattern (e.g., homosexual pedophilia or exhibitionism), it is conceivable that the offender could continue actively engaging in some semblance of the offense pattern while incarcerated.

An acceptable cessation-oriented program with which RP could be paired should, at the very least, involve traditional talk therapy, or counseling. More stringent cessation intervention might involve arousal–reduction procedures aimed at curtailing the degree of sexual arousal the offender experiences in response to stimuli associated with the offense pattern. Behavior-modification techniques, including various forms of aversive conditioning and orgasmic reconditioning, have been successfully used for modifying offender arousal patterns (Quinsey & Marshall, 1983). Biological interventions, such as use of the drug Depo-Provera, have been employed to achieve nonspecific reductions in sexual arousal (Berlin, 1983). The RP approach can be integrated or combined with any of these cessation-oriented procedures in the context of various treatment formats, including inpatient or outpatient therapy and group or individual therapy. Moreover, because sex offenders frequently suffer from other primary or secondary mental health disorders, it is advantageous that RP is sufficiently versatile to be applied adjunctively with treatment for other problems.

Treatment Component 1:
Specific Intervention Techniques for HRSs

The primary goal of these techniques is to teach the offender to better handle an HRS that would otherwise potentiate a lapse. A combination of behavioral and cognitive skills are taught that will enable the offender to react more competently and confidently to HRSs. Figure 3 shows how the HRS analysis (Conceptual Component 1) permits multiple sites for intervention.

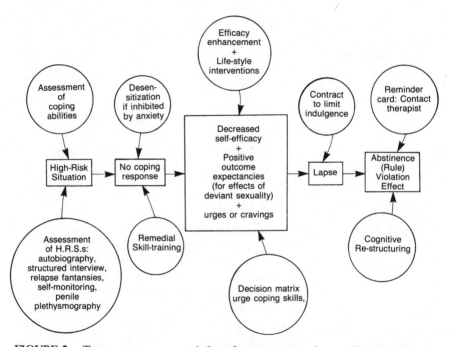

FIGURE 3. Treatment component 1: Specific interventions for sex offender high-risk situations. From "Relapse Prevention: Theoretical Rationale and Overview of the Model" by G. Alan Marlatt. In *Relapse Prevention: Maintenance Strategies in the Treatment of Addictive Behaviors* (p. 54), Eds. G. A. Marlatt and J. R. Gordon, 1985, New York: Guilford Press. Copyright 1985 by The Guilford Press. Adapted by permission.

Assessment

At the start of RP treatment, assessment is a prominent intervention activity. The prominence and focus of assessment activity fluctuate and shift as the treatment unfolds; however, assessment remains an ongoing and integral part of the entire treatment process. At the earliest points in RP treatment, assessment procedures are organized primarily around two main aims: HRSs and skills assessment.

Assessment of HRSs

An essential aspect of teaching offenders to handle HRSs in constructive and adaptive ways is first enabling them to identify and anticipate these situations. Earlier we discussed prototypic kinds of HRSs. However, ultimately each client has a unique profile of HRSs and consequently the identification of his/her HRSs must be an individualized process. Various idiographic assessment procedures can be applied for this purpose.

Some procedures are especially appropriate for collecting background information. For instance, instructing the offender to prepare an *autobiography* of life as a sexual deviate can provide a rich source of information on the forces that shaped the person's current pattern of sexual gratification and offending. The instructions should be worded to tap into the positive and negative aspects of the person's self-image as a sexual deviate. A *structured interview* can also be useful in gathering detailed but more systematic information about the person's past and present patterns of sexual deviance. In *relapse fantasies*, the offender is asked to describe dreams or imagined scenarios that might lead to reoffending. Together, techniques such as these provide ample material for formulating informed speculations about the specific types of HRSs that are most likely to challenge the specific offender's efforts at long-term behavior change.

Another technique for assessing HRSs, *self-monitoring*, offers an effective method for identifying current forces related to sexual offending. Self-monitoring requires that clients keep a record of each episode in which they experience an urge to engage in deviant sexuality. An ongoing record of the offender's urges will reveal both the emotional and environmental events that may serve as cues for urges and lapses. The record should include a subjective rating of urge intensity (e.g., on a scale of 1 to 10) and a description of the circumstances (time of day, location, presence or absence of others, and activities). To assess less obvious internal correlates, offenders should be asked to report thoughts and to describe and numerically rate mood states experienced before, during, and after the episodes. Urge data from self-monitoring can be transposed onto line or bar graphs that visually highlight the patterns of situational influences that depict their unique profiles of HRSs.

A final technique for assessing HRSs with sex offenders is direct observation of sexual arousal via *penile plethysmography*. Briefly, this laboratory procedure involves presenting the offender with various audio and/or visual depictions of erotic stimuli while measuring penile tumescence (Laws & Osborn, 1983). This objective data can reveal particular types of activities and victim characteristics that are likely to threaten the offender's perceived control and restraint. This methodology is also useful in assessing the effectiveness of arousal–reduction procedures.

Assessment of Preexisting Coping Abilities

Determining the adequacy of preexisting coping abilities is a critical assessment target. The *Situational Competency Test* was devised to measure ability to cope with situational temptations. Though originally based on work with alcoholics (Chaney, O'Leary, & Marlatt, 1978), this technique can be adapted for sex offenders as well as for other addicts (see Miner, Day, & Nafpaktitis, Chapter 10, this volume). The procedure involves presenting a series of written or audio-taped descriptions of potential lapse and relapse situations. Each description ends with a prompt for a response from the offender. The responses are scored on a number of dimensions, including response duration and latency, degree of compliance, and specification of alternative behaviors. With a pedophile, for example, the situations might include invitations to spend time alone with a child, and the subject's responses may reveal deficient assertion skills. In a similar technique, *self-efficacy ratings* (Marlatt, 1985b), a list of potential lapse or relapse situations is presented and the offender uses a 7-point scale to rate subjective expectation of successfully coping with each situation. Ratings across a wide range of situations enable the individual to identify both problematic situations and skill deficits in need of remedial training. Results from these types of assessment can later dictate the focus of skill-training procedures.

Alternative Specific Skill Training

After HRSs and skill deficits have been assessed, the RP approach begins to concentrate on teaching the offender alternative ways of coping with these situations. The alternative coping skills are intended to counteract the habitual tendency to cope by indulging in deviant sexuality.

Risk Recognition

A first step in skill training is learning to recognize HRSs ahead of time. Through such recognition, anticipated HRSs come to function as warning signs that signal the need for behavior change in the same way that road signs signal the need for alternative action. Recognition of an upcoming HRS then becomes a choice point at which the individual can opt to simply avoid or take a detour around a risky situation, such as a video arcade for a pedophile. However, in many cases routine avoidance of particular HRSs is unrealistic. Therefore, coping skills that enable the individual to get through unavoidable HRSs must be acquired.

Remedial Skill Training and Self-Efficacy Enhancement

Remedial skill training, a cornerstone of RP treatment, seeks to rectify the deficiencies in coping skills. The specific content of the skill-training program is variable and will depend on the needs of the individual. Possible content areas include assertiveness, stress management, relaxation training, anger management, communication skills, and general social and/or dating skills. The RP approach routinely includes training in more general problem-solving skills (see Goldfried & Davison, 1976), which are flexible enough to be generalizable across different situations and problem areas. Actual methods for teaching new skills include many standard behavior-therapy techniques (e.g., McFall, 1976), such as behavior rehearsal, instruction, coaching, evaluative feedback, modeling, and role-playing. Cognitively oriented methods, such as cognitive self-instruction (e.g., Meichenbaum, 1977), are also employed for teaching constructive self-statements that parallel and bolster the new behaviors. Eventually, the offender begins to apply the new skills to real-life situations. When it is not practical to rehearse the new coping skills in real-life situations, *relapse rehearsal* is an especially pertinent technique in which the offender is instructed to imagine being in an actual HRS and performing more adaptive behaviors and thinking more adaptive thoughts. Regular *homework assignments* are an essential aspect of RP treatment. Homework is important for troubleshooting and consolidating the newly acquired skills and for facilitating transfer of the new repertoire to the real world. A universal and pervasive thrust with all RP treatment techniques is *self-efficacy enhancement*. To promote the offender's self-efficacy, employment of the various training techniques is accompanied by instructions to imagine that the rehearsed experience is accompanied by mounting feelings of competence and confidence. As a consequence, the person experiences heightened expectations of successful coping in future real-life situations, thereby reducing the probability of relapse.

To summarize, implementation of a specific skill-training program will be dictated by the offender's unique profile of HRSs. If the offender typically engages in pedophilic masturbatory fantasies and cruises schoolyards after arguments with a spouse or significant other, then what might be most indicated are communication or anger-management skills for coping with those interactions more constructively. In working with pedophiles, it is sometimes useful to distinguish between coping skills applicable to interpersonal HRSs involving adults versus those involving children. If a rapist's risky encounters cluster around work stress, then relaxation training and/or stress-management training would be indicated. If an offender experiences frequent and intense urges when lonely or bored, then perhaps training in dating and social skills is called for. If intrapersonal HRSs characterized by depression are problematic, then perhaps cognitive therapy for depression should be applied adjunctively with RP.

Decision Matrix

To counteract positive expectancies of gratification from the deviant sexuality, the *decision matrix* is an effective technique for forcing the offender to consider simultaneously both positive and negative potential outcomes. The decision matrix is an eight-cell table organized according to three bilevel variables (thus a 2 × 2 × 2 organizational arrangement). The three variables are (1) behavioral choice (indulgence in deviant sexuality versus adherence to the self-control program), (2) time frame (immediate versus delayed effects), and (3) valence (positive versus negative effects). For each cell of the table, the offender is instructed to supply all the expected outcomes that he/she associates with that specific triangulation of variables. For example, one of the eight cells would require enumeration of all immediate negative effects associated with returning to the pattern of deviant sexual indulgence, while another would encompass the delayed positive effects of adherence to the self-control program and so on. When placed on a 3 × 5 index card, the decision matrix becomes a convenient and easily accessible aid for handling temptation situations. Examination of the decision matrix whenever confronted with an HRS helps to combat exaggerated positive expectancies by forcing the offender to actively undertake a fuller consideration of the consequences of his choices.

Urge Coping

Cravings (subjective desires for immediate gratification) and urges (behavioral intentions) to indulge in the forbidden sexual activity can be directly triggered by external cues, such as the sight of people who resemble former victims, or can occur as a consequence of covert antecedents (as outlined earlier under Conceptual Component 2). Sex offenders must be prepared for the high probability that urges (used subsequently as a catchall phrase for both desires and intentions) will occasionally occur. Cessation-oriented treatment programs can inadvertently convey the unreasonable expectation that treatment will eliminate all desire for deviant sexual indulgence. Arousal–reduction treatments, whether behaviorally or biologically based, may be especially problematic in this regard, particularly if the therapy produces a rapid impact and fosters an illusion of "cure." This expectation is unfortunate because urges are practically inevitable, and when they do occur the treated offender has little guidance about how to cope with them. In fact, treated offenders who believe that urges have been eliminated may interpret urges as signifying treatment failure and as confirming their status as inveterate sexual deviates. Akin to the abstinence violation effect hypothesized to follow a lapse, such an interpretation of an urge can promote relapse, as in a self-fulfilling prophecy (Pithers et al., 1983). Thus it is important that the offender be equipped with urge coping skills.

The discomfort created by urges is largely internal, so *cognitive urge coping skills* have obvious utility. Cognitive strategies are employed to combat problematic perceptions of urges. One strategy involves instructing offenders not to view urges as signifying treatment failure but instead as representing conditioned automatic reactions to the external or internal cues of an HRS. Another strategy warns against viewing an urge as characterized by a linear and indeterminate rise in discomfort. Instead, it is stressed that urges are curvilinear and determinant; that is, they are triggered by HRS cues, and they rise in intensity, reach a peak, and then subside. From this perspective, the offender's task is to wait out the urge, to endure the moments of peak urge discomfort, and to look forward to the downside. In evoking the *urge surfing* analogy, urges are likened to ocean waves (they rise, crest, and fall) and the offender's task is metaphorically likened to that of the surfer learning to "ride out" the urge-wave and to maintain balance without "wiping out." In a final cognitive strategy, the offender is instructed to view the urge with detachment as an approaching external entity that can be fended off. A useful metaphor here is that of the samurai warrior, whose task is to become skilled at recognizing an urge and fending it off until it eventually subsides.

Behavioral urge coping skills are useful for both preventing and managing urges. The frequency of externally triggered urges can be reduced through simple *stimulus-control* techniques aimed at minimizing exposure to these cues. This could mean removing paraphernalia associated with the offense pattern, such as a pornography collection. *Avoidance strategies* are also helpful in reducing the frequency of externally triggered urges. Certain events or situations associated with the offense pattern simply have to be avoided temporarily while the offender develops more effective skills for coping with HRSs. Possibly, particular events may permanently drop from the offender's life. Generally, avoidance strategies can often come in handy for dealing with unexpected HRSs that emerge. Another behavioral technique for coping with urges is to label the urge verbally as soon as it registers in consciousness. This can take the form of a barely audible self-statement (e.g., "oops, here it comes"). A final behavioral technique requires that the offender perform an action that serves momentarily to *break the continuity of the urge*. The onset of an urge and the speed of its ascent often unfold as an automatic, habitual sequence interwoven with familiar environmental forces. A simple behavioral maneuver that disrupts this sequence can readily defuse the urge. The actual behavior can be as minor as changing one's seating arrangement or as major as escaping the situation by going for a walk.

Coping with a Lapse

The possibility that the offender will experience a slip by indulging a deviant masturbatory fantasy or formulating a loose plan for sexual victimization must be anticipated. The postslip reaction is a pivotal intervention point in the RP model, because it determines the degree of escalation from a single isolated slip to a relapse. The first step in anticipating and dealing with this reaction is to formulate with the client an explicit *therapeutic contract* to limit the extent of indulgence if a slip occurs and to renew the commitment for changing. The fundamental method of intervention after a slip is the use of *cognitive restructuring* to counteract the cognitive and affective components of the AVE. The main objective here is to enable the offender to construe the slip as a unique occurrence, a mistake. The offender who views the slip as an irreversible failure or as evidence that the cessation achieved through treatment (or incarceration) has totally collapsed may succumb to the conflict, guilt, and personal attribution that characterize the AVE and, in turn, promote relapse.

A useful method here is to have the offender carry a wallet-sized *reminder card* with instructions to read and follow in the event of a slip. The text of the card should include information for contacting a therapist, treatment center, or specific support person. Most importantly, the text should also include a cognitive restructuring antidote to the AVE that incorporates the following principles:

1. The occurrence of a single slip does not indicate treatment failure and inevitable relapse.

2. The slip should be viewed as a reasonable mistake in learning how to maintain a self-control program, and it should be evaluated for how it can contribute constructively to the learning process.

3. Overemphasis on the postslip feelings of guilt and conflict (cognitive-dissonance component of the AVE) can precipitate further indulgence. Instead, those feelings should be viewed as natural reactions of disappointment that accompany momentarily unfulfilled aspirations; that is, feelings that will run their course and subside if not actively intensified and nurtured.

4. Blaming the slip on personal weakness (personal-attribution component of the AVE) can create a self-fulfilling prophecy that promotes further indulgence. Instead, responsibility should be distributed across both external situational forces that prevail in the HRS and internal deficits in coping skills. Notably, this type of internal attribution optimistically emphasizes modifiable skills rather than more stable trait-like characteristics (e.g., lack of will power) that yield pessimistic prospects for change.

Treatment Component 2:
Global Lifestyle Intervention Techniques

As outlined earlier (under Conceptual Component II), an imbalanced lifestyle characterized by more "shoulds" (obligations and duties) than "wants" (indulgence in gratifying activities) can pave the way for relapse by producing a chronic sense of deprivation, which in turn, produces a desire for immediate gratification. Previously, the offense sequence and elements of it had been the immediate gratification that potently restored a sense of balance and empowerment to a lifestyle experienced by the offender as "unfairly" imbalanced and powerless. After cessation of deviate sexual endeavors, chronically unmet desires for indulgence can manifest as urges, cravings, and distortions that lead the offender to meander "unintentionally" closer to the brink of relapse while at the same time disavowing any conscious desire to reoffend.

The final thrust in the RP program is teaching the offender to achieve and maintain a balanced lifestyle that will "inoculate" him/her against the covert antecedents to relapse and will promote mental and physical well-being. These strategies and their optimal intervention points in the covert approach to HRSs (Conceptual Analysis 2, see Figure 2) are schematically represented in Figure 4.

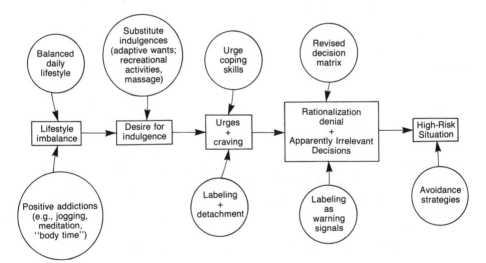

FIGURE 4. Treatment component 2: Global lifestyle interventions. From "Relapse Prevention: Theoretical Rationale and Overview of the Model" by G. A. Marlatt. In *Relapse Prevention: Maintenance Strategies in the Treatment of Addictive Behaviors* (p. 61), Eds. G. A. Marlatt and J. R. Gordon, 1985, New York: Guilford Press. Copyright 1985 by The Guilford Press. Reprinted by permission.

Recognition of Lifestyle Imbalance

The first step in preempting the steady, subtle progression from lifestyle imbal-ance to relapse is to raise the offender's consciousness about these processes. An effective way to start is by having the offender employ self-monitoring tech-niques to inventory the "wants" and "shoulds" that prevail in his/her life. By keeping a daily record of duties and obligations on one hand and indulgences on the other, the offender can become acutely aware of the discrepancy between these "shoulds" and "wants."

Restoring Lifestyle Balance

As the offender comes to recognize and appreciate the contribution of lifestyle imbalance to chronic feelings of deprivation and ultimately to relapse prospects, various methods for restoring balance will be taught. These methods involve development of and regular participation in constructive indulgences that function as "wants."

Positive Addictions

In contrast with negative addictions, such as deviant sexual indulgence, that initially feel good but produce long-term harm, positive addictions (e.g., jog-ging) produce short-term discomfort while yielding long-range benefits (Glasser, 1976). After short-term discomfort has been surmounted, a positively addicting activity comes to be perceived as a "want," contributes to long-term health and well-being, and provides an adaptive coping response for life stressors. Activities having potential for positive addiction include meditation, relaxation induc-tions, jogging, and other forms of regular exercise. It is important, at least in the beginning, that the activity be structured in a way that minimizes perception of it as simply another "should" in the offender's life. For example, the "should-ness" created by adoption of a rigorous exercise routine could be circumvented by instead adopting the more flexible *bodytime concept.* Here, the emphasis is on a regular commitment to engaging in a stimulating nonsexual physical activity. The way the time is spent should vary across a range of options, such as physical exercise, hot-tubbing, saunas, yoga, manicures, dance, and so forth. Other strategies for reducing initial disincentives of positive addictions include making it an easily learnable and readily available activity and arranging for it to be done with others as an enjoyable social activity. As the offender becomes accustomed to the reinforcing bodily sensations inherent in the activity, the activity becomes a method for achieving a constructive "high" that can sup-plant the former tendency to obtain pleasant indulgences through deviant sexuality or other destructive habits.

Substitute Indulgences

Another strategy for restoring "wants" to an unbalanced lifestyle is adoption of substitute indulgences. These activities need to be immediately enjoyable and may or may not contribute to tangible, long-term benefits. Examples include attending concerts or movies, cooking gourmet meals, gardening, playing a musical instrument, pursuing hobbies or other creative tasks, playing cards or board games, taking scenic drives, reading novels, and so forth. For clients with a greater sense of adventure, riskier activities, such as motorcycling, sailboarding, skydiving, skiing, rock climbing, or hang gliding, might be appropriate. Many aficionados of these sports report that the exhilaration and risk involved generates an addicting "high." Overall, the key is to add activities to the person's life that are perceived as "wants" and not as additional "shoulds." One caution is that these must not be activities that were previously linked with the offense pattern.

Recognition of Urges and Apparently Irrelevant Decisions

As noted earlier, urges to indulge in deviant sexuality will inevitably occur, and it is important that the offender receive training in how to cope with them. Recall that when urges develop as a consequence of covert antecedents to relapse, they may become masked by cognitive distortions and defense mechanisms. Recognition is the obvious first step in coping with urges that do not operate at a conscious level. Once such urges are recognized, the cognitive and behavioral *urge coping skills* outlined earlier can be implemented by the offender. Unrecognized urges can exert a potent influence by allowing for "apparently irrelevant decisions" (AIDs) that inch the offender closer to relapse.

To counteract this process, the offender must receive training in how to "see through" the distortion and denial. The offender must instead learn to recognize AIDs as representing unacknowledged urges and disavowed pursuit of relapse. This recognition begins with consciousness raising and education about the role of these AIDs as covert relapse antecedents. Explicit self-talk can be helpful here. By acknowledging to oneself that certain minidecisions actually represent urges (e.g., a pedophile who chooses to take walks that reliably meander by neighborhood pools, parks, or schoolyards at times when they are predictably crowded with children), the offender becomes able to use these experiences as *early warning signals*. When viewed in this way, such events can come to be seen as cues for deploying urge coping skills and/or lifestyle balancing techniques. The *relapse roadmap* enables the offender to envision the maintenance phase metaphorically as a journey from initial cessation to prolonged abstinence. In preparing an individualized roadmap, the offender identifies AIDs that might possibly lead to HRSs and ultimately to relapse.

SUMMARY AND CONCLUSIONS

In this Introduction, we have described the origins, basic assumptions, and definitions that characterize the RP model. The RP conceptual framework outlining the role of both acute and chronic processes in potentiating relapse across various addictions was also described. The RP approach remains a relatively new development in the addictions field. Although various component aspects of the model enjoy empirical support in the addictions field (Brownell et al., 1986; Curry, Marlatt, & Gordon, 1987; Marlatt & Gordon, 1985), neither the complete conceptual model nor the system of interventions has been subjected to a definitive test. A number of independent research groups are engaged in efforts to evaluate the validity of the RP model and the efficacy of its treatment techniques with various addictive disorders.

Comparatively speaking, application of the RP model to sex offenders is an even newer development. This application, as we have indicated, does not require that sex offending be viewed as an addiction. We have noted that, while sex offending shares striking similarities with addictions, there are important differences between the two phenomena. Nonetheless, we believe that RP conceptual analyses and the derivative treatment techniques offer a highly promising approach for preventing recidivism among sex offenders. The intervention procedures outlined in this Introduction and detailed in subsequent chapters are oriented toward teaching offenders how (1) to maintain termination of the offense pattern and of indulgence in deviant sexuality and (2) to build a balanced lifestyle that is resistant to psychological stress and unhealthy habit patterns and is characterized by a harmonious interplay between work and play activities.

The confidence and optimism we feel about the application of RP to sex offending are quite strong. However, this enthusiasm remains tempered by various precautionary concerns. First, RP is not a magical solution. It is simply a new addition to the already available strategies for dealing with this complicated societal problem. Second, an adequate application of RP requires an offender who is motivated to change, adjunctive cessation treatment (preferably including arousal–reduction techniques), and very diligent work by both the offender and the therapist in implementing the RP procedures. Third, the stakes are very high. Sex offending is an emotionally charged and increasingly visible problem in America. A publicized relapse by an offender treated with RP could have unfortunate repercussions for the continuing viability of the RP application in this domain. Finally, our confidence in the utility of applying RP to sex offending is without empirical support. We have been encouraged by the enthusiastic reception RP has received from treatment personnel and by anecdotal reports of successful RP application with offenders. Multiple programs applying RP with sex offenders are now in existence, three of which are described in Chapters 22, 23, and 24. Ultimately, the wisdom of using RP to treat sex offenders will be determined by data collected in these initial programs and future clinical investigations.

ACKNOWLEDGMENTS

Preparation of this chapter was supported in part by funds from the National Institute on Alcohol Abuse and Alcoholism by way of a New Investigator Research Award (AA06776) to William H. George. Gratitude is expressed to R. Lorraine Collins for reviewing an earlier draft of this paper and to Alexandra Atrubin for her assistance with library work. Insightful remarks from Ron Nelson and Mary Schohn about maintaining offense patterns during incarceration are gratefully acknowledged.

REFERENCES

Abel, G. G., Becker, J. V., Mittelman, M., Cunningham-Rather, J., Rouleau, J. L., & Murphy, W. D. (1987). Self-reported sex crimes of non-incarcerated paraphiliacs. *Journal of Interpersonal Violence, 2*, 3–25.

Bandura, A. (1969). *Principles of behavior modification.* New York: Holt, Rinehart & Winston.

Bandura, A. (1977a). *Social learning theory.* Englewood Cliffs, NJ: Prentice-Hall.

Bandura, A. (1977b). Self-efficacy: Toward a unifying theory of behavior change. *Psychological Review, 84*, 191–215.

Bandura, A. (1986). *Social foundations of thought and action: A social cognitive theory.* Englewood Cliffs, NJ: Prentice-Hall.

Berlin, F. S. (1983). Sex offenders: A biomedical perspective and a status report on biomedical treatment. In J. G. Greer & I. R. Stuart (Ed.), *The sexual aggressor* (pp. 83–123). New York: Van Nostrand Reinhold.

Brickman, P., Rabinowitz, V. C., Karuza, J., Coates, D., Cohn, E., & Kidder, L. (1982). Models of helping and coping. *American Psychologist, 37*, 368–384.

Brownell, K. D., Marlatt, G. A., Lichtenstein, E., & Wilson, G. T. (1986). Understanding and preventing relapse. *American Psychologist, 41*, 765–782.

Carnes, P. (1983). *Out of the shadows: Understanding sexual addiction.* Minneapolis: CompCare Publications.

Chaney, E. F., O'Leary, M. R., & Marlatt, G. A. (1978). Skill training with alcoholics. *Journal of Consulting and Clinical Psychology, 46*, 1092–1104.

Chapman, R. S. (1988, May 31). There's help for sex addicts. *The Buffalo News,* p. C-2.

Cummings, C., Gordon, J. R., & Marlatt, G. A. (1980). Relapse: Strategies of prevention and prediction. In W. R. Miller (Ed.), *The addictive behaviors* (pp. 291–321). Oxford, UK: Pergamon.

Curry, S., Marlatt, G. A., & Gordon, J. R. (1987). Abstinence Violation Effect: Validation of an attributional construct with smoking cessation. *Journal of Consulting and Clinical Psychology, 55,* 145–149.

Furby, L., Weinrott, M. R., & Blackshaw, L. (1989). Sex offender recidivism: A review. *Psychological Bulletin, 105*(1), 3–30.

George, W. H., & Marlatt, G. A. (1984). *Relapse prevention with sexual offenders: A treatment manual.* (Available from Florida Mental Health Institute, 13301 Bruce B. Downs Blvd., Tampa, FL 33612-3899)

Glasser, W. (1976). *Positive addiction.* New York: Harper & Row.

Goldfried, M. R., & Davison, G. C. (1976). *Clinical behavior therapy.* New York: Holt, Rinehart & Winston.

Hall, S. (1980). Self-management and therapeutic maintenance: Theory and research. In P. Karoly & J. J. Steffen (Eds.), *Toward a psychology of therapeutic maintenance: Widening perspectives* (pp. 263–300). New York: Gardner.

Laws, D. R., & Marshall, W. L. (in press). A conditioning theory of the etiology and maintenance of deviant sexual preference and behavior. In W. L. Marshall, D. R. Laws, & H. E. Barabaree (Eds.), *Handbook of sexual assault.* New York: Plenum.

Laws, D. R., & Osborn, C. A. (1983). How to build and operate a behavioral laboratory to evaluate and treat sexual deviance. In J. G. Greer & I. R. Stuart (Eds.), *The sexual aggressor* (pp. 293–335). New York: Van Nostrand Reinhold.

Marlatt, G. A. (1978). Craving for alcohol, loss of control, and relapse: A cognitive-behavioral analysis. In P. E. Nathan, G. A. Marlatt, & T. Loberg (Eds.), *Alcoholism: New directions in behavioral research and treatment* (pp. 271–314). New York: Plenum.

Marlatt, G. A. (1979). Alcohol use and problem drinking: A cognitive–behavioral analysis. In P. C. Kendall & S. D. Hollon (Eds.), *Cognitive-behavioral interventions: Theory, research, and procedures* (pp. 319–355). New York: Academic.

Marlatt, G. A. (1982). Relapse prevention: A self-control program for the treatment of addictive behaviors. In R. B. Stuart (Ed.), *Adherence, compliance and generalization in behavioral medicine* (pp. 329–378). New York: Brunner/Mazel.

Marlatt, G. A. (1985a). Cognitive factors in the relapse process. In G. A. Marlatt & J. R. Gordon (Eds.), *Relapse prevention: Maintenance strategies in the treatment of addictive behaviors* (pp. 128–200). New York: Guilford.

Marlatt, G. A. (1985b). Cognitive assessment and intervention procedures for relapse prevention. In G. A. Marlatt & J. R. Gordon (Eds.), *Relapse prevention: Maintenance strategies in the treatment of addictive behaviors* (pp. 201–279). New York: Guilford.

Marlatt, G. A., & George, W. H. (1984). Relapse prevention: Introduction and overview of the model. *British Journal of Addiction, 79,* 261–273.

Marlatt, G. A., & Gordon, J. R. (1980). Determinants of relapse: Implications for the maintenance of behavior change. In P. O. Davidson & S. M. Davidson (Eds.), *Behavioral medicine: Changing health lifestyles* (pp. 410–452). New York: Brunner/Mazel.

Marlatt, G. A., & Gordon, J. R. (Eds.) (1985). *Relapse prevention: Maintenance strategies in the treatment of addictive behaviors.* New York: Guilford.

Marques, J. K., & Nelson, C. (in press). Understanding and preventing relapse in sex offenders. In M. Gossop (Ed.), *Relapse and addictive behavior*. Beckenham, Kent, UK: Croom Helm.

Marques, J. K., Pithers, W. D., & Marlatt, G. A. (1984). Relapse prevention: A self-control program for sex offenders. Appendix to: Marques, J. K. *An innovative treatment program for sex offenders: Report to the legislature*. Sacramento: California Department of Mental Health.

McFall, R. M. (1976). *Behavioral training: A skill-acquisition approach to clinical problems*. Morristown, NJ: General Learning Press.

Meichenbaum, D. (1977). *Cognitive–behavior modification*. New York: Plenum.

Merluzzi, T. V., Glass, C. R., & Genest, M. (Eds.). (1981). *Cognitive assessment*. New York: Guilford.

Perls, F. (1971). *Gestalt therapy verbatim*. New York: Bantam.

Pithers, W. D., Marques, J. K., Gibat, C. C., & Marlatt, G. A. (1983). Relapse prevention with sexual aggressives. In J. G. Greer & I. R. Stuart (Eds.), *The sexual aggressor* (pp. 214–239). New York: Van Nostrand Reinhold.

Prochaska, J. O., & DiClemente, C. C. (1982). Transtheoretical therapy: Toward a more integrative model of change. *Psychotherapy: Theory, Research, and Practice, 19,* 276–288.

Prochaska, J. O., & DiClemente, C. C. (1983). Stages and processes of self-change of smoking: Toward an integrative model of change. *Journal of Consulting and Clinical Psychology, 51,* 390–395.

Quinsey, V. L., & Marshall, W. L. (1983). Procedures for reducing inappropriate sexual arousal: An evaluation review. In J. G. Greer & I. R. Stuart (Eds.), *The sexual aggressor* (pp. 267–289). New York: Van Nostrand Reinhold.

Saline, C. (1985, February). Indecent obsession. *Philadelphia,* pp. 101–110.

Seligmann, J., Flowers, C., Gosnell, M., Harrison, J., & Nelson, M. (1987, July 20). Taking life one night at a time: 'Sex addicts' seek help. *Newsweek,* pp. 48–49.

Webster's new collegiate dictionary (9th ed.). (1984). Springfield, MA: Merriam-Webster.

I

PROBLEMS

In this section we begin examination of typical problems encountered in the daily lives of sex offenders. While these do not include all possible problems, they represent central ones that can promote lapses into deviant behavior and, ultimately, relapse to the sexually deviant lifestyle.

Initially, Marques and Nelson discuss some of the common risk factors seen in sex offenders. Their focus is on the interaction of environmental and personal elements of high-risk situations. Environmental risk elements are the situational or behavioral events (e.g., availability of a victim, weapon, alcohol, or drugs) that increase the likelihood of a sex offense. Personal elements include global (e.g., sociopathic personality) or specific factors (e.g., deviant cognitions) that also increase the probability of offending. They conclude that a thorough analysis of these elements and their interaction is essential to treatment planning and preventing relapse.

Jenkins-Hall and Marlatt discuss one of the central concepts of the original RP model, apparently irrelevant decisions (AIDs) in the lives of sex offenders. The point they make about AIDs is that the more frequently the offender puts himself in harm's way (e.g., a pedophile who "happens" to pass by a schoolyard, a rapist driving around with no destination in mind), the more likely a sex offense is to occur. They recommend using the AID as a cue for initiating a coping response rather than as a cue for engaging in lapse behavior.

Marlatt discusses the very serious problem of immediate gratification (the PIG), another concept from the original RP. The PIG wants what he wants when he wants it, and this poses a very high risk for sex offenders in situations in which urges are strong and craving for deviant sexual activity is high. One way to control this problem is to detach oneself from the urges and craving and view them objectively as the external phenomena they are. Once you feed the PIG, he warns, the more you will have to feed him.

In a major departure from traditional RP, Russell, Sturgeon, Miner, and Nelson discuss the abstinence violation effect (AVE) in sex offenders. In its original conception, the AVE was triggered by a return to the proscribed behavior, that is, a lapse that involved drinking alcohol, drug abuse, smoking, and so forth. In sex offending, however, a return to the behavior means commission of another crime and victimization of another person. Thus, AVE as a risk problem for sex offenders has been redefined as conscious, deliberate deviant fantasizing that often promotes masturbating to deviant fantasy or deliberate offense planning, thus increasing the probability of reoffense. The authors recommend use of the AVE to enhance the offender's perception of risk and as a cue to initiate coping responses.

1

Elements of High-Risk Situations for Sex Offenders

JANICE K. MARQUES
CRAIG NELSON

According to the relapse prevention (RP) model, a critical point in the relapse process is the high-risk situation, broadly defined as a set of circumstances that threatens the individual's sense of self-control. If one faces and fails to cope effectively with a high-risk situation, the likelihood of lapse and relapse increases. In contrast, if an individual encounters and copes successfully with the threatening situation, self-control is reestablished and the relapse process is stopped.

For the sex offender, high-risk situations may be defined as conditions that jeopardize the offender's sense of control over his illicit sexual behavior and, therefore, increase his chances of slipping back into deviant thoughts, urges, or actions. Given the importance of this link in the chain of events leading to relapse, examination and analysis of the high-risk situations faced by sex offenders are critical to our understanding of the relapse process. In this chapter, we will describe some common elements found in the high-risk situations reported by child molesters and rapists and will discuss how these elements may interact to encourage relapse.

The literature on addictive behaviors includes a number of studies that have analyzed the relapse process and have proposed a consistent nosology for high-risk situations (Brownell, Marlatt, Lichtenstein, & Wilson, 1986; Marlatt & Gordon, 1985). In general, situations are categorized as either interpersonal or intrapersonal and as either positive or negative. The system used by Chaney and Roszell (1985), for example, proposed three intrapersonal risk situations (negative emotional states, negative physical states, and testing control), two interpersonal situations (conflict and social pressure), and one combination (enhancement of intra- or interpersonal positive emotional states.)

A number of authors have noted the similarities between these relapse situations and those described for rapists and child molesters and have found that the classification systems developed for addictive behaviors could be applied with these offenders (see Miner, Day, & Nafpaktitis, Chapter 10, this volume). At this time, however, our understanding of the relapse process in sex offenders is quite limited. Unlike studies of drinkers or dieters, follow-up studies in the area of sexual aggression typically report only rearrest figures; they do not analyze the processes and events that lead to relapse or to successful maintenance (continued abstinence). Retrospective interview data and case studies have suggested that there are some common high-risk situations for these offenders, such as negative emotional states, substance abuse, and deviant sexual arousal (Marques & Nelson, in press; Pithers, Marques, Gibat, & Marlatt, 1983). On the other hand, the heterogeneity of the sex offender population is well documented (Knopp, 1984), and offense patterns are often highly individual and idiosyncratic. Taken together, these findings suggest that, while there are certainly some common risk factors for sex offenders, the prediction of a given offender's high-risk situations requires a thorough analysis of the individual's unique characteristics and environment.

In our program, California's Sex Offender Treatment and Evaluation Project, the analysis of high-risk situations involves breaking down the situation into distinct elements, factors, or conditions, each of which plays a part in promoting relapse. The peril inherent in any risk situation is directly related to the number, strength, and interaction of the risk elements represented. In addition to helping the offender understand and predict dangerous situations, this analysis is used to prescribe specific coping skills for the prevention of relapse.

Consistent with social learning theory (Bandura, 1977; Mischel, 1968, 1973), our analysis of high-risk situations does not focus exclusively on personality factors but recognizes that sex offenses are determined by multiple contextual and personal variables. In this view, the degree to which stimulus conditions, such as external cues and expected consequences, appear similar across situations determines, in part, the stability of an individual's behavior. On the other hand, variations in the relevant stimulus conditions may lead to markedly discrepant behavior in that same individual. Thus it has become axiomatic that the best predictor of future behavior is past behavior of the same individual in a similar context.

While recognizing the importance of these situational determinants, our analyses also emphasize that the ongoing behavior of an individual constantly changes the environment. As the person responds and interacts with the situation, the external cues and contingencies shift and accommodate. In this fashion, the interaction between the individual and the environment may be constantly altering the determinants of behavior. From a social learning perspective, then, behavior is a function of personal variables, situational variables, and their interaction. To the degree that the relevant personal factors, the important environmental elements, and the manner in which they interact can be determined, one's prediction of future behavior will be enhanced. Using such a model, recommendations for improving the predictive process for violent and dangerous behavior have been described (Megargee, 1976; Monahan, 1981). In an RP program for sex offenders, the essential predictive question becomes: What will cause this individual to reoffend? The extent to which future high-risk situations are accurately anticipated determines the degree to which relevant coping strategies can be developed. If the prediction of future high-risk situations is inaccurate, either irrelevant or inadequate coping strategies may be prescribed.

In the following discussion, two broad categories of high-risk elements will be presented, generally corresponding to the domains of environmental variables and personal variables. Analysis of high-risk situations into relevant environmental elements, personal elements, and their interaction is a highly complex process. It can be likened to that of putting together the pieces of a jigsaw puzzle. The appropriate pieces must first be selected and then joined together in the correct position in order for the complete picture to emerge. Although tedious and often difficult, it is a necessary process for each offender if he is to develop relevant and effective coping strategies.

ENVIRONMENTAL ELEMENTS

Environmental high-risk elements are situational or behavioral events that increase the chances of a sexual offense. They serve as the cues and contingencies for illicit sexual behavior. According to social learning theory (Mischel, 1973), the important external or situational variables are those that provide information influencing an individual's expectations, constructions, motivations, evaluations of stimuli, or ability to generate responses. In the present context, the most relevant environmental high-risk elements are those variables shown to increase the risk of relapse. For purposes of illustration, several types of situational elements that could carry such influence will be considered.

One of the most obvious environmental elements is the presence of a potential victim. It is, of course, impossible to commit a sexual crime without gaining access to a victim. For instance, a child molester will not be at risk to reoffend while he is in prison, just as an alcoholic will be unlikely to get drunk in the detoxification unit. On the other hand, someone sexually attracted to boys will certainly introduce a major factor if he becomes a Boy Scout leader. This risk is similar to that encountered by the abstinent drinker who continues to frequent taverns or maintains a well-stocked liquor cabinet at home or the gambler who visits Nevada on vacation, creating the "downtown Reno effect" (Marlatt & Gordon, 1985).

Although it can be argued (and often is by offenders) that there is no way to totally avoid contact with individuals who might be victimized, the failure to carefully manage exposure to potential victims often represents an important ingredient in the recipe for a high-risk situation. A recent study of the situations that resulted in offenses among sex offenders at Atascadero State Hospital revealed that over half of the 27 child molesters surveyed reported that their victims lived in their own households (Day, Miner, Nafpaktitis, & Murphy, 1987). Such proximity to victims served as a risk element in the high-risk situations that eventually led to the offenses.

Previous reviews of high-risk contexts for violent offenses (e.g., Monahan, 1981) have noted that the availability of a weapon can be an important element in these crimes, as can be access to alcohol or other disinhibitors. Obviously, as in the case with all environmental factors, the level of risk associated with weapons or alcohol will depend on a number of personal elements (such as presence of a drinking problem or experience of negative emotional states). The substance-abuse component will be explored further in the section below on personal elements.

Interpersonal conflict has been recognized as a risk factor in the relapses of individuals with a variety of problem behaviors, such as drinking, smoking, drug abuse, gambling, and overeating (Cummings, Gordon, & Marlatt, 1980). Similarly, interpersonal stressors—such as marital discord; disagreements with significant others, coworkers, or superiors; and social isolation—have also been described as precipitants of sexual crimes (Gebhard, Gagnon, Pomeroy, & Christenson, 1965). Such conflicts may give rise to the negative emotional states (personal elements such as anger, frustration, loneliness, and impaired self-esteem) that often precede sex crimes (Groth, 1979, Pithers et al., 1983; Queen's Bench Foundation, 1976). They may also establish a sense of deprivation that, in turn, the offender may use to justify his illicit sexual behavior.

Although our analyses of high-risk situations emphasize the elements close to the crime, a number of more global elements and early antecedents (Marques, Pithers, & Marlatt, 1984) are also considered as risk factors. For example, lifestyle factors may serve to increase the probability of relapse. Gebhard et al. (1965) reported that 87% of their large sample of sexual offenders had been convicted of some crime other than a sex offense prior to the age of 26. A criminal lifestyle in which financial existence was largely dependent on illegal activities (e.g., drug dealing, welfare fraud, prostitution, burglary) was recently reported by nearly 30% of a sample of sex offenders (Day et al., 1987). Such a criminal lifestyle can promote the belief that the offender does not need to follow the rules of society or be subject to its sanctions. Similar disinhibiting beliefs are likely to result from a lifestyle that involves spending time with other sexually deviant individuals.

In some cases, early antecedents, such as the offender's own physical or sexual abuse as a child, may continue to serve as elements with which the offender must be prepared to cope. More often, such distant precursors are included in our analyses as contributing factors to current personal variables, such as attitudes, cognitive distortions, or affective elements.

An exhaustive review of environmental risk factors is beyond the purpose of the present discussion. As this brief review indicates, a wide range of possible situational variables must be considered and their relevance for a given offender determined by analysis of the conditions surrounding his particular crime(s). Although many offenders are acquainted with or live in close proximity to their victims, this is not true for all, and victim availability does not explain the behavior of the rapist or child molester who actively "cruises" in search of victims. Similarly, a criminal lifestyle is a relevant high-risk factor for some offenders but is clearly not so for the molester who is a middle-class school teacher. Environmental factors are highly individualized and never provide a complete picture of the high-risk situations that will be confronted by an offender.

PERSONAL ELEMENTS

In addition to environmental factors, other pieces of the high-risk situations puzzle are personal variables or internal risks that the offender must be prepared to control effectively. As was the case with environmental variables, personal elements include both global factors (such as personality attributes) and specific factors (such as thoughts) that enhance the probability of slipping back into the offense pattern. From a social learning perspective (Mischel, 1973), these variables include what an individual knows and can do, how information is encoded and construed, expectancies associated with certain behaviors in particular stimulus situations, incentives and aversions produced by subjective stimulus values, and self-regulatory systems and rules that are used to evaluate one's own performance.

From an RP viewpoint, one of the major internal states associated with successful abstinence from a forbidden behavior is a sense of self-control (Marlatt & Gordon, 1985). By definition, a high-risk situation increases the risk of reoffense by threatening one's sense of self-efficacy over the indulgent behavior. It is not surprising, therefore, that 31 of 38 sexual offenders interviewed by Day et al. (1987) regarding the circumstances leading up to their crimes reported a perceived loss of such control. To the extent that an offender's expectancy is that he will not be able to control his own actions, in particular his sexual behavior, the risk of relapse increases.

A deviant sexual arousal pattern, characterized by significant arousal to or even a preference for inappropriate partners or violent acts, may be one of the most important risk elements for child molesters and rapists. Through the use of penile plethysmography (Earls & Marshall, 1983), deviant patterns of arousal have been documented in both child molesters (e.g., Freund, 1967; Quinsey, 1977) and rapists (e.g., Abel, Barlow, Blanchard, & Guild, 1977; Barbaree, Marshall, & Lanthier, 1979). Initial psychophysiological assessments of 67 participants in the Sex Offender Treatment and Evaluation Project found that 66% showed evidence of deviant sexual arousal (significant arousal to either stimuli of children or themes of aggression against women). While these assessments also found that 13% of the offenders showed a nondeviant arousal pattern and that 21% did not respond to the laboratory stimuli, they do suggest that for many offenders sexual aggression against women or sex with children may hold high stimulus value and serve as an incentive or motivator for illicit sexual behavior.

As described in the previous section, the environmental elements of interpersonal conflict and stress are likely to produce negative affective states. Anger, frustration, depression, or rejection have long been recognized as important contributors to the commission of sexual crimes (Groth, 1979). The Queen's Bench Foundation (1976) found that nearly 77% of the rapists in their study reported such feelings prior to their attacks. Similarly, Pithers et al. (1983) reported that 75% of the sex offenders they sampled experienced a negative emotional state immediately prior to their crimes. Day et al. (1987) found that 17 of the 38 offenders they questioned reported feelings of anger at the time of their offenses. This affect was most prominent among rapists, three-quarters of whom described such feelings. In contrast, less than a third of the child molesters described feelings of anger, and approximately half of them reported some type of positive emotional state immediately preceding their crimes. Frequently, this was defined as a feeling of affinity with or closeness to the victim.

Again, as was the case for environmental factors, the heterogeneity of the sex offender population in terms of specific personal elements is evident. In some cases, negative affective states serve as signals or motivators for sexual misconduct; for example, frustration and anger may incite the offender to regain a sense of power and control, "get back" at one who has delivered a perceived slight, or simply attempt to feel better by engaging in the prohibited sexual behavior. In other cases, positive emotional states may motivate the offender to enhance these pleasurable feelings through sexual gratification. An analysis of each offender's emotional precursors and their intensity is necessary to specify and evaluate their role in his high-risk situations.

As was mentioned in the previous section, the availability and consumption of alcohol and other disinhibiting substances can be an important risk element for sex offenders. High rates of alcoholism and alcohol abuse at the time of the crime have previously been detected among rapists (Rada, 1975) and child molesters (Frisbie, 1969). Of 168 sex offenders in prison who were interviewed after volunteering for the Sex Offender Treatment and Evaluation Project, 60% reported a significant history of alcohol or drug abuse during their lives. Seventy percent of these offenders reported being under the influence of drugs or alcohol at the time of their crimes. This element was most common for rapists, with 87% describing a history of substance-abuse problems and 89% reporting substance abuse at the time of their offenses. It was least common among child molesters who had male victims, 60% of whom had a history of substance abuse and 42% of whom reported being under the influence at the time of their crimes. Although the accuracy of such figures may be questioned, given the offenders' propensity to use intoxication as a justification or rationalization for their deviant behavior, the use of drugs and alcohol has definitely helped set the stage for many sexual offenses. Clearly, this element can serve as a disinhibitor of urges and fantasies regarding illicit sexual behavior that may be harbored by offenders. Its interaction with other risk elements will be considered in greater detail in a later section.

Other personal variables that may promote offense and reoffense among some child molesters and rapists are rationalizations, justifications, and cognitive distortions. Such statements as "she was being seductive," "I wasn't hurting him," "I was teaching the child about sex," or "she deserved what she got" have been encountered by most clinicians who treat sex offenders.

The Multiphasic Sex Inventory (MSI; Nichols & Molinder, 1984) scores of participants in the Sex Offender Treatment and Evaluation Project provide information on the extent and variation of these rationalizations and justifications. The Cognitive Distortion and Immaturity Scale of the MSI is designed to examine the degree to which the offender blames others for his predicament and views himself as a victim. Items on this scale include, for example, "In some ways I was used by the person who reported me" and "I have never believed my sexual contact with a child was a crime because I did not have intercourse or penetration with him/her." Of the 72 offenders administered this inventory when they began treatment, 14% were classified in the range of having great difficulty accepting responsibility for their actions, 22% were categorized as having distortions that reflected a victim stance, and 39% scored in the range of having cognitive distortions that reflected immaturity. Only 25% were classified as accepting accountability for their crimes. The Justification Scale of the MSI also attempts to tap cognitive variables that offenders may use to excuse their behavior (e.g., "My sexual problem is not as serious as that of others"). Using the cutoff scores suggested by the authors of the inventory, 43% of the offenders were classified as showing at least a "marked" degree of justification of their sexually deviant behavior.

These types of cognitive distortions reflect the self-regulatory systems and rules that govern and activate the behavior of the individual. That is, if an offender views his deviant behavior as rational and justified in a given situation, deviant actions under like circumstances in the future will also be congruent with these beliefs and therefore will be more likely to occur.

Although the RP model typically distinguishes between high-risk situations and the skills required to cope with the various situations, it also recognizes that a given situation will be high risk only to the extent that an individual has difficulty coping with it. One set of skill deficits frequently reported as a risk factor for sex offenders is in the area of social skills (Abel, Blanchard, & Becker, 1978). Both homosocial and heterosocial skills deficits have been detected in rapists (Fisher & Rivlin, 1971) and child molesters (Frisbie, 1969; Gebhard et al., 1965; Langevin, 1983), and social-skills training is often included in treatment programs for sex offenders (e.g., Abel, Becker, & Skinner, 1985). While social incompetence is certainly not a sufficient causative factor for sexual crimes, it may work in concert with other factors (Quinsey, 1984). Such deficits, if present, may serve as examples of the deficiencies in knowledge and response capabilities that interact with environmental elements to promote illicit sexual behavior.

Personal elements, like their situational counterparts, are a subset of the pieces of the jigsaw puzzle that compose high-risk situations. Again, an exhaustive catalogue of internal risk elements is beyond the scope of this chapter. Additional risk elements in this category might include specific factors, such as sexual dysfunctions and lack of sexual knowledge, as well as more global factors, such as attitudes toward women, empathy deficits, and impaired self-esteem. The relevance of any given element is highly individual. The data do not support generalizations that all offenders necessarily have deviant sexual arousal patterns, lose their sense of control over their lives, experience negative emotional states before offending, or lack social skills. Rather, the data suggest the wide variability of relevance for each of these elements.

INTERACTION OF ENVIRONMENTAL
AND PERSONAL ELEMENTS

Extending the metaphor of putting together a jigsaw puzzle, the interaction of the environmental and personal elements represents the process by which these pieces fit together to form a high-risk situation. From our social learning perspective, only environmental elements that differentially affect personal factors, such as one's expectations, motivations, constructs, or ability to generate response patterns, are considered relevant in defining high-risk situations. For example, it was noted earlier that the presence of a potential victim is an important environmental risk factor for the commission of a sexual offense. Although this element may be a necessary component on the chain leading to sexual crimes, it is obviously not a sufficient factor. Add a personal element of a deviant sexual arousal pattern, however, and an image of a potential offense begins to emerge. The risk inherent in the combination of these factors is greater than either element alone. If the offender is also experiencing interpersonal stress that generates a negative affective state, abuses drugs or alcohol, and maintains a belief that the potential victim may not be harmed by the crime, a high-risk situation emerges in clear focus, and the individual's self-control is threatened.

Unfortunately, few high-risk situations are as clear and neatly arranged as that posed above. Consider, for example, that the element of a deviant sexual arousal pattern is absent. As was noted above, not all offenders generate deviant sexual arousal patterns in psychophysiological assessments. How is it that such offenders committed their sexual crimes? One could hypothesize that the pattern has been modified through the aversive consequences of arrest and incarceration. This is a less than parsimonious explanation in the absence of specific reconditioning procedures designed to modify sexual interests (Quinsey & Marshall, 1983). Another possible explanation is that deviant sexual interest may be aroused only under certain specific conditions. There is some laboratory data to suggest that this may, in fact, be the case. For example, it has been reported that nonoffender males who falsely believed they had ingested alcohol responded with greater sexual arousal to stimuli depicting rape and nonsexual violence against women than did similar subjects who had not been deceived in this manner (Briddel et al., 1978). Thus the simple expectation of the disinhibiting effect of alcohol may grant one "permission" for responses to sexual stimuli that would otherwise be inhibited.

Disinhibitors of sexual arousal to deviant stimuli may also include the cognitive factors described earlier. For example, distorted beliefs that the victim will not be injured or may even enjoy the illicit sexual act could be a requisite for arousal to the external cue. Research on nonoffenders supports this possibility. Malamuth and Check (1983) found undergraduate males to be more sexually aroused by rape stimuli when the victim was described as sexually aroused than when the victim displayed disgust. These authors (1980) also found that college subjects became more aroused by rape audiotapes after being exposed to similar stimuli that depicted the victim as becoming sexually aroused than after hearing depictions in which the victim continued to abhor the assault.

Affective elements may also serve to facilitate deviant sexual interest and its expression. Yates, Barbaree, and Marshall (1984) reported that an experimental manipulation to provoke anger toward a woman immediately prior to exposure to sexual stimuli significantly enhanced arousal to verbal descriptions of rape among a sample of nonoffender males. Similarly, in a laboratory analogue, Marques (1981) found that rapists were most likely to report an urge to rape when they were both angry and sexually aroused.

In addition to disinhibiting deviant sexual arousal, high-risk elements may blur the distinction between permitted and prohibited sexual behavior, enhancing the risk of committing the illicit sexual act. Barbaree, Marshall, Lightfoot, and Yates (1983), for instance, found that alcohol significantly impaired discrimination between rape and mutually consenting sexual scenes among nonoffender males.

Although more research on offenders is needed in order to analyze the offense-potentiating interactions of high-risk elements, it is clear that the elements in combination can produce quite different effects than their simple addition would predict. The assembled jigsaw puzzle creates a very different picture than it does when the pieces are askew. If offenders are to prepare coping strategies for high-risk situations, the correct risk elements must be individually identified and placed in a configuration that is specific to them. Elements and connections that are irrelevant will only confuse the picture and leave the offender ill prepared to maintain control.

Although it is perhaps naive to expect a complete picture of why a high-risk situation poses a threat of reoffense to a particular rapist or child molester, the thorough analysis of the offender's personal and environmental elements and their interaction is an important part of preventing relapse. In the Sex Offender Treatment and Evaluation Project, a variety of assessment tools are used to accomplish this goal. Nelson and Jackson (Chapter 14, this volume) have described one analytic technique, the construction of cognitive–behavioral offense chains, which is used to identify the target configuration of high-risk elements for an offender's individualized RP program.

REFERENCES

Abel, G. G., Barlow, D. H., Blanchard, E. B., & Guild, D. (1977). The components of rapists' sexual arousal. *Archives of General Psychiatry, 34*, 895–903.

Abel, G. G., Becker, J. V., & Skinner, L. J. (1985). Behavioral approaches to treatment of the violent sex offender. In L. H. Roth (Ed.), *Clinical treatment of the violent person* (pp. 100–123) (DHHS Publication No. ADM 85-1425). Rockville, MD: National Institute of Mental Health.

Abel, G. G., Blanchard, E. B., & Becker, J. V. (1978). An integrated treatment program for rapists. In R. Rada (Ed.), *Clinical aspects of the rapist* (pp. 161–214). New York: Grune & Stratton.

Bandura, A. (1977). Self-efficacy: Toward a unifying theory of behavioral change. *Psychological Review, 84*, 191–215.

Barbaree, H., Marshall, W., & Lanthier, R. (1979). Deviant sexual arousal in rapists. *Behaviour Research and Therapy, 17*, 215–222.

Barbaree, H. E., Marshall, W. L., Lightfoot, L. W., & Yates, E. (1983). Alcohol intoxication and deviant sexual arousal in male social drinkers. *Behaviour Research and Therapy, 21*, 365–373.

Briddell, D. W., Rimm, D. C., Caddy, G. R., Krawitz, G., Sholis, D., & Wunderlin, R. J. (1978). Effects of alcohol and cognitive set on sexual arousal to deviant stimuli. *Journal of Abnormal Psychology, 87*, 418–430.

Brownell, K. D., Marlatt, G. A., Lichtenstein, E., & Wilson, G. T. (1986). Understanding and preventing relapse. *American Psychologist, 41*, 765–782.

Chaney, E. F., & Roszell, D. K. (1985). Coping in opiate addicts maintained on methadone. In S. Shiffman & T. A. Willis (Eds.), *Coping and substance use* (pp. 297–293). New York: Academic.

Cummings, C., Gordon, J., & Marlatt, G. A. (1980). Relapse: Prevention and prediction. In W. R. Miller (Ed.), *The addictive behaviors* (pp. 291–321). Oxford, UK: Pergamon.

Day, D. M., Miner, M. H., Nafpaktitis, M. K., & Murphy, J. F. (1987). *Development of a situational competency test for sex offenders*. Unpublished manuscript.

Earls, C. M., & Marshall, W. L. (1983). The current state of the technology in the laboratory assessment of sexual arousal patterns. In J. G. Greer & I. R. Stuart (Eds.), *The sexual aggressor: Current perspectives on treatment* (pp. 336–362). New York: Van Nostrand Reinhold.

Fisher, G., & Rivlin, E. (1971). Psychological needs of rapists. *British Journal of Criminology, 11*, 182–185.

Freund, K. (1967). Erotic preference in pedophilia. *Behaviour Research and Therapy, 5*, 339–348.

Frisbie, L. (1969). *Another look at sex offenders in California* (Research Monograph No. 12). Sacramento: California Department of Mental Hygiene.

Gebhard, P., Gagnon, J., Pomeroy, W., & Christenson, C. (1965). *Sex offenders: An analysis of types*. New York: Harper & Row.

Groth, A. N. (1979). *Men who rape: The psychology of the offender*. New York: Plenum.

Knopp, F. H. (1984). *Retraining adult sex offenders: Methods and models*. Syracuse, NY: Safer Society Press.

Langevin, R. (1983). *Sexual strands: Understanding and treating sexual anomalies in men*. Hillsdale, NJ: Erlbaum.

Malamuth, N. M., & Check, J. V. P. (1980). Penile tumescene and perceptual responses to rape as a function of victim's perceived reaction. *Journal of Applied Social Psychology, 10*, 528–547.

Malamuth, N. M., & Check, J. V. P. (1983). Sexual arousal to rape depictions: Individual differences. *Journal of Abnormal Psychology, 92*, 55–67.

Marlatt, G. A., & Gordon, J. R. (Eds.). (1985). *Relapse prevention: Maintenance strategies in the treatment of addictive behavior*. New York: Guilford.

Marques, J. K. (1981). Effects of victim resistance strategies on the sexual arousal and attitudes of violent rapists. In R. B. Stuart (Ed.), *Violent behavior: Social learning approaches to prediction, management and treatment* (pp. 138–172). New York: Brunner/Mazel.

Marques, J. K., & Nelson, C. (in press). Understanding and preventing relapse in sex offenders. In M. Gossop (Ed.), *Relapse and addictive behaviour*. Beckenham, Kent, UK: Croom Helm.

Marques, J. K., Pithers, W. D., & Marlatt, G. A. (1984). Relapse prevention: A self-control program for sex offenders. Appendix to: Marques, J. K. *An innovative treatment program for sex offenders: Report to the legislature*. Sacramento: California Department of Mental Health.

Megargee, E. (1976). The prediction of dangerous behavior. *Criminal Justice and Behavior, 3*, 3–21.

Mischel, W. (1968). *Personality and assessment*. New York: Wiley.

Mischel, W. (1973). Toward a cognitive social learning reconceptualization of personality. *Psychological Review, 80*, 252–283.

Monahan, J. (1981). *The clinical prediction of violent behavior* (DHHS Publication No. ADM 81-921). Rockville, MD: National Institute of Mental Health.

Nichols, H. R., & Molinder, I. (1984). *The multiphasic sex inventory manual* (Available from Nichols and Molinder, 437 Bowes Drive, Tacoma WA 98466)

Pithers, W. D., Marques, J. K., Gibat, C. C., & Marlatt, G. A. (1983). Relapse prevention with sexual aggressives: A self-control model of treatment and maintenance of change. In J. G. Greer & I. R. Stuart (Eds.), *The sexual aggressor: Current perspectives on treatment* (pp. 214–239). New York: Van Nostrand Reinhold.

Queen's Bench Foundation. (1976). *Rape: Prevention and resistance.* San Francisco: Author.

Quinsey, V. L. (1977). The assessment and treatment of child molesters: A review. *Canadian Psychological Review, 18,* 204–220.

Quinsey, V. L. (1984). Sexual aggression: Studies of offenders against women. In D. Weisstub (Ed.), *Law and mental health: International perspectives* (Vol. 1) (pp. 84–123). New York: Pergamon.

Quinsey, V. L., & Marshall, W. L. (1983). Procedures for reducing inappropriate sexual arousal: An evaluation review. In J. G. Greer & I. R. Stuart (Eds.), *The sexual aggressor: Current perspectives on treatment* (pp. 267–289). New York: Van Nostrand Reinhold.

Rada, R. T. (1975). Alcoholism and forcible rape. *American Journal of Psychiatry, 132,* 444–446.

Yates, E., Barbaree, H. E., & Marshall, W. L. (1984). Anger and deviant sexual arousal. *Behavior Therapy, 15,* 287–294.

2

Apparently Irrelevant Decisions in the Relapse Process

KATURAH D. JENKINS-HALL
G. ALAN MARLATT

DEFINITION OF CONCEPT

The relapse process for different types of sex offenders has similar precursors. Most sexual offenses are precipitated by a negative emotional state, followed first by deviant sexual fantasies and then by a conscious plan, which ultimately leads to the relapse behavior (Pithers, Marques, Gibat, & Marlatt, 1983). It is the planning stage of the relapse process that is of interest here.

Although planning may at times be covert, based on unconscious defense mechanisms, sexual offenses occur mainly as a result of conscious planning. For example, many pedophiles set out in advance to win a child's trust by establishing a friendship, buying gifts, and granting favors in order to gradually introduce the inappropriate sexual behavior. Once the child's friendship is won, the offender may then plan ways to be alone with the child in order to insure privacy. After he has arranged for privacy, he may then set out to systematically progress from appropriate to inappropriate touching so as not to raise the child's suspicion. Similarly, the act of rape has usually been planned down to the last detail prior to its execution. Paraphernalia have been purchased (masks, gloves, weapons, etc.), escape routes thought out, and times calculated well in advance of the offense. Many women have been examined and discarded as possible victims prior to selecting the right one. Rapists have often stalked their victims, once selected, for days or weeks in order to execute the act.

The conscious planning of offenses occurs prior to the offender's experiencing sufficient personal and/or psychological distress over the offending behavior and prior to his attempting to gain control over it. Once the offender begins the attempt to control his deviancy, but before he has gained adequate control, he is usually presented with approach–avoidance conflicts. On the one hand, he realizes the severity of his problem, the likely consequences of his behaviors, and the need for control. At the same time, he feels driven to carry out the deviant sexual behavior. These approach–avoidance conflicts, coupled with his lack of appropriate coping responses, may cause the offender to engage in covert–unconscious planning of the sexually deviant behavior. This process of covert planning is referred to as "apparently irrelevant decisions" (AIDs) and is carried out in this manner to minimize the negative reactions of self and others to the deviant behavior (Marlatt, 1985a). An alternative acronym to AID is SUBTLE (seemingly unimportant behaviors that lead to errors).

Prior to involvement in situations that may decrease perceived control over the sexually deviant behavior (high-risk situations), the offender often makes a series of rationalized decisions, or AIDs, during which he has little or no awareness of their relationship to the relapse behavior. Once in the high-risk situation, he convinces himself that the situational cues are so strong and compelling that the initial lapse is inevitable (Marlatt, 1985a). An example of an AID made by a pedophile is described by Pithers et al. (1983) as follows:

> Imagine a pedophile who emerges from the front door of his home to take a walk along the tree-lined street of his suburban residence. Nearing the sidewalk he decides to turn left. After a brief excursion, he notices a school playground brimming with gleefully playing children. . . . Since the individual was familiar with his neighborhood, he would have been cognizant that going left would take him by the school, whereas turning right would have led him away from the high risk area . . . the decision to walk left was an apparently irrelevant one. (p. 225)

The pedophile in the above example might go on to justify his behavior by saying he saw a particular child who looked lonely or distressed and decided it would be the humane thing to be friendly to the child. Thus begins the process of relapse.

Psychological Defenses and Apparently Irrelevant Decisions

Sex offenders use a variety of psychological defenses in order to carry out the relapse process. Among the most salient are denial, projection, and rationalization. Several researchers have described these defenses as prominent characteristics of the personality profile of sex offenders (e.g., Hall, 1988). Understanding these defenses is crucial to understanding the concept of AIDs and the process by which AIDs should be handled in therapy.

Denial is an unconscious defense mechanism that allows the individual to completely inhibit or ignore external reality and consequent internal anxiety (Nace, 1987). In sex offenders, it serves to block an accurate appraisal of the severity of the deviant behavior, its impact on the victims, and its potential consequences to the offender. Rationalization is the process by which unacceptable thoughts and behaviors are justified by convincing oneself of their social acceptability (Gatchel & Mears, 1982). Projection is the process of attributing unacceptable impulses (e.g., sexual urges) to others (Gatchel & Mears, 1982). More simply, denial ignores, rationalization justifies, and projection blames. It is quite common to hear offenders deny that their behavior toward victims was harmful. They rationalize that the victim deserved the sexual aggression or needed the "affection," and they see the victim as the aggressor, projecting seductive, promiscuous behavior onto him/her. One often hears how the child "wanted it" or the rape victim was "asking for it." Consider the following scenario:

> A pedophile in outpatient treatment described how he had a hectic day at work and was asked at the last minute to run an errand for his boss. This made him increasingly anxious about being late for dinner at his mother's, so anxious that he decided to take an alternate route because it would be faster. This route took him near an area of town where he had offended in the past. However, he would save about 10 minutes. As he drove through the area, he saw a child he knew from his neighborhood who looked exhausted and was carrying a heavy load. He was unaware of any sexual interest in the child, only that the child needed his assistance. The client took the time to stop and ask the child if he needed a lift. The child accepted the ride and was taken directly to his home. The child spontaneously gave the client a hug upon exiting the car. After dinner, the offender remembered the child's hug and how good it felt to receive a child's affection again. Hours later, he "found himself" experiencing deviant urges and masturbated to sexual fantasies of a child who looked similar to the boy he had assisted, but he failed to see the relationship.

In this example, the offender made a series of AIDs through the use of rationalization, denial, and projection. He began by rationalizing his taking of an alternative route (it would save him time). The decision to take the alternative route was his first AID. Next, the offender rationalized that the child needed his help. The decision to stop to assist the child was his second AID. The offender allowed the child to get into his car but denied that the child's being there had any significant impact on his sexual urges. The decision to give the child a ride was his third AID. The offender then allowed the child to give him a hug, again denying the impact of this behavior and viewing it as something the child really wanted to do (projection). The decision allow the child to hug him was the fourth AID. The client later found himself thinking how good the hug felt, experienced urges, and made a conscious decision to masturbate to a fantasy involving a male child. He denied the relationship of the earlier events of the day to the deviant masturbation (lapse) until it was pointed out to him in therapy.

The above scenario demonstrates how deeply embedded AIDs can be in psychological defenses, especially rationalization. Marlatt (1985b) described the process of AIDs as follows:

> In the covert planning of a relapse set-up, the individual engages in a series of mini-decisions to set the stage for the ostensibly justifiable initial lapse. Each mini-decision must be *justified by an "explanation"* [rationalization] that satisfies the self and others and which does not "blow the cover" on the covert nature of the operation. (p. 271; emphasis added)

Consequently, the offender often describes how he "finds himself" in high-risk situations and vehemently denies the covert planning.

APPARENTLY IRRELEVANT DECISIONS
AND PEDOPHILES

Many of the decisions made by pedophiles can, in retrospect, be considered AIDs. These decisions may range from those immediately tied to the offense pattern (e.g., the decision to babysit) to those that seem further removed and unrelated to a given offense (e.g., the decision to take a certain job.) Following are some areas of daily living in which AIDs are commonly made.

Vocational and Avocational Decisions

A large number of pedophiles seek employment in occupations that will put them in direct contact with children. It is not uncommon to find pedophiles who have become youth ministers, Boy Scout leaders, youth athletic coaches, or grade school teachers. When questioned about their choice of employment, most clients will attribute their selection to benevolent reasons, such as their love for, commitment to, and desire to help children. Many report having worked with children all their lives and cannot foresee pursuing a vocation that does not afford some contact with children. Unfortunately, a self-perpetuating pattern exists whereby the offender has learned to find comfort only in the presence of children (i.e., he feels grossly inadequate with adults) and has sought this involvement in the work setting to meet his needs for affiliation. When challenged in therapy to view the selection of an occupation or hobby involving children as an AID, the majority of pedophiles will point out that their initial motivation was not sexual and will seek to persuade the therapist that their motives were entirely altruistic. One Little League coach who had molested more than 200 children felt extremely depressed because no one recognized how much good he had done for the low-income boys on his team. It took almost 6 months in active therapy before he would begin to entertain the notion that his motivation for coaching was partly sexual.

Pedophiles also choose hobbies and recreational activities that will bring them in contact with children. Several report being interested in comic books, electronic games, electric trains, and other children's toys. They purchase these items and set up a "gameroom heaven" for unsuspecting children. Each decision to visit the toy store could be considered an AID.

Relationship Decisions

Some pedophiles choose relationships that afford them automatic, intimate access to children. They become involved with women with children of the age and sex they desire as victims. They may even convince themselves of their love for the woman, without readily acknowledging the sexual attraction to her child. They set up dating situations that will involve "family activities," during which more time is spent with the child than with the woman. Some incest offenders who are pedophiles move from family to family, repeating the same pattern of molestation until they are discovered. When questioned about his choice of mates, one offender rationalized that "it's hard to find a woman my age without children these days."

A more subtle pattern of decision making about relationships occurs when the offender chooses an adult partner who looks or behaves like an adolescent. It is difficult for the offender to see how what appears to be an "appropriate" adaptive behavior may promote his sexual deviancy.

Decisions to Frequent High-Risk Places

It is quite common for pedophiles to make AIDs regarding places they go and the time of their arrival. Many will choose to take a walk in a park near a schoolyard just as school is letting out. They choose strategic times to go into public restrooms, usually after a child has entered (blaming it on "the call of nature"). They frequent video arcades during early evening hours (because they are "fascinated by electronics"). They choose G-rated movies on weekends and frequent shopping malls during high-volume shopping times, both places where children are likely to be found unsupervised.

Some of the places cited above readily lend themselves to "legitimate" excuses for being there (e.g., the restroom, the shopping mall). Others require more ingenuity and imagination to develop rationalizations to justify the decision making process leading to the high-risk behavior. Consider the decision-making process of one offender who had difficulty controlling his compulsion to frequent public restrooms, where he masturbated to deviant fantasies while reading graffiti:

He was told by his therapist to keep a journal. He had gone to several nearby drugstores, but they didn't have the type of notebook he was interested in. He was running late but was afraid to come to the session without the journal. He had contracted specifically not to go near a K-Mart (his greatest high-risk area). However, that was his only choice; he knew they would have what he was looking for. After purchasing the notebook, he began to feel "sick" because of his anxiety about being late for the session. He had no choice but to use the restroom. After being seated in the restroom, he began to have sexual urges.

Decisions to Assist and Befriend

Perhaps the most commonly used rationalization and subsequent AID leading to high-risk situations is the decision to assist and/or befriend a child who is "in need." Many pedophiles have an affinity for those children who appear lonely, neglected and/or poor, or in need of guidance and supervision. For example, Finkelhor (1984) found that a child's low socioeconomic status and loneliness are two important risk factors for sexual victimization. One might speculate as to why the above characteristics might be attractive. Is the offender prone to altruism? Does he identify with something missing from his own childhood? Or is such a child an easier mark, more susceptible to his ingratiating behaviors and less likely to report his inappropriate behavior?

Once the pedophile befriends a child, he usually convinces himself that he loves the child and has his/her best interests at heart. He strongly believes that establishing a sexual relationship has little or nothing to do with his decision to assist/befriend. In fact, the offender usually lavishes the child with nonsexual attention, gives the child appropriate guidance in other areas of his/her life, and attempts to teach the child moralistic behaviors. For these reasons, the pedophile often becomes offended when confronted with his apparent sexual motives for befriending the child he loves.

APPARENTLY IRRELEVANT DECISIONS
AND RAPISTS

Working through apparently irrelevant decisions made by rapists is a much more challenging task than with pedophiles. The decision-making process of the rapist is different from that of the pedophile, and consequently AIDs are more difficult to pinpoint and identify with rapists. The reason for this difficulty is that the rapist's motives are generally more apparent and his intentions are less well defended than the pedophile's. As stated earlier in this chapter, AIDs are generally motivated by a need to minimize the negative reactions of the self and others (Marlatt, 1985a). Implicit in this statement is that the one who engages in covert planning has some deep-felt concern about the impressions he makes on others and perhaps is concerned about the integrity of his own self-esteem. This type of concern appears to be more congruent with the personality style of many pedophiles than it is with that of the majority of rapists. While the personality style of pedophiles appears to be more passive–dependent, that of rapists seem to be more aggressive–narcissistic (Hall, 1988). The personality style of rapists lends itself to feelings of entitlement and inflated self-esteem. Thus, when a rapist makes the decision to rape, it is often a conscious one, not precipitated by a chain of AIDs, because he has little or no concern about the impact of his behavior on others and there are no immediate threats to his self-esteem.

Moreover, when a pedophile makes a conscious or unconscious decision to be sexually involved with a child, his goal is usually to gain the child's consent and approval. Rapists, on the other hand, by definition expect to engage the victim without consent. Therefore, the approach to the two behaviors is different. The pedophile woos the child and must be covert. In contrast, the rapist takes what he wants; the very nature of his mission is more overt.

This is not to say that rapists never engage in covert planning of sexual offenses. Some clinicians might view such decisions as taking an isolated route home, leaving the house in the early morning hours to jog, or deciding to carry a weapon when there is no apparent threat as apparently irrelevant decisions. In our experience in challenging these types of decisions, we have found that offenders readily acknowledge them as relevant. In fact, if prompted, most rapists will generally admit to some conscious planning prior to carrying out the rape.

However, in situations in which the issue of consent can be disputed (e.g., date or acquaintance rape), the offender may use a host of psychological defenses and a series of AIDs to justify the rape behavior. Consider, for example, a young man who had been convicted of a more brutal rape in the past and who was currently in treatment for a date-rape conviction:

> He had been drinking beer all day and was in a partying mood. He met a girl at a service station where he had gone to get his car washed. He had dated this girl in the past and had engaged in kissing and fondling with her on prior dates. The girl agreed to party with the client. The client decided to drive to a secluded spot in an isolated area, where he provided as much cocaine and beer as his date wanted. He began to approach his date for sex, at which time, by his account, "she said no, but meant yes." He made a joke about her having to walk home, and thereafter the date appeared to give in to the sexual encounter. He was too high to remember the exact details but did not remember her physically resisting his advances.

In the above example, the client made several decisions that might be considered AIDs. He decided to get high (lowering his inhibitions); he decided to provide drugs for his date (lowering her inhibitions and capacity to defend herself or to give consent); he decided to drive to the isolated spot; he decided to interpret her "no" as "yes" and proceed with the sexual act.

In general, relapse prevention strategies are more difficult to apply with those sex offenders for whom an established pattern of offense is unclear. Many rapists who come to the attention of clinicians will have offended only once (that they will acknowledge). The multiple, ritualistic rapist is more often locked away in a correctional facility. Several first-time rapists are actually more accurately diagnosed as having antisocial personality disorders with a history of other criminal behavior, the last of which was the rape. In these cases, much of the work in identifying AIDs has to do with examining the decisions to engage in the precursive antisocial behavior (e.g., burglary, armed robbery). Consider the following example:

> A client described how he was high and feeling bored. For excitement, he decided to burglarize an apartment, something he had done on several prior occasions. He chose an apartment in the same complex where he had just left a party. After breaking into the apartment and looking for something to steal, he spotted a woman and man sleeping in their bedroom. He thought it would be exciting to steal an intimate kiss while the woman slept. He proceeded to kiss the woman's genitalia. The woman, of course, awoke with a start, waking her husband, who accosted and restrained the client until the police arrived.

In the above example, it is clear that the client's decision-making process was more antisocial and went beyond making decisions that were apparently irrelevant. Although one could examine the relevance of his decision to get high or to burglarize to the subsequent rape behavior, the level of intervention needed to challenge this client's thinking goes beyond the scope of relapse prevention. The criminal thinking in this case, what Yochelson and Samenow (1976) refer to as "superoptimism," interacts with all decision-making processes and warrants more attention to global thinking rather than AIDs. For this reason, most clinicians who use relapse prevention as an approach usually avoid treating rapists with extensive criminal histories or adopt other therapeutic approaches in addition to relapse prevention.

INTERVENING IN THE AIDS PROCESS

As stated earlier, unconscious defense mechanisms allow an individual to hide from himself the true motives for his actions for the protection of the ego. Because making AIDs is inextricably tied to one's underlying defensive structure, this type of decision making also serves to protect the ego. With this protective function of AIDs in mind, it becomes clear how difficult the task of *appropriately* challenging AIDs is for the therapist and how difficult acknowledging AIDs is for the client. Therapists can expect to meet resistance when confronting a client with the fact that he has made an AID. It is crucial that a good working relationship be established with the client prior to this confrontation. It is also useful if the client is familiar with the conceptual framework of relapse prevention and is already able to identify those crucial points in his cognitive–behavioral chain that led to relapse. If a client has an accurate assessment of what his high-risk situations are, he is usually willing to examine the decisions he has made to get himself there. The work in therapy involves pointing out the rationalizations he has used in making the decisions that lead to the given high-risk situation. Clients who are at the working stage of therapy will eventually come to accept their motives as related to their sexual deviancy, when this is pointed out in a therapeutic manner. The problem, of course, is that the AID is usually acknowledged after the fact (i.e., after the client has engaged in high-risk behavior). The goal of therapy, then, is to get the client to be in tune with his decision making, so that he catches himself making AIDs and identifies them as early warning signals, or cues, to initiate adaptive coping responses. The client may then use cognitive restructuring (see Jenkins-Hall, Chapter 18, this volume) to change these decisions to more rational ones.

REFERENCES

Finkelhor, D. (1984). *Child sexual abuse: New theory and research.* New York: Free Press.

Gatchel, R. J., & Mears, F. G. (1982). *Personality, theory, assessment, and research.* New York: St. Martin's.

Hall, R. L. (1988). Assessment and diagnosis. In G. W. Barnard, A. K. Fuller, Lynn Robbins, & T. Shaw. *The child molester: An integrative approach to evaluation and treatment* (pp. 48–56). New York: Brunner/Mazel.

Marlatt, G. A. (1985a). Relapse prevention: Theoretical rationale and overview of the model. In G. A. Marlatt & J. R. Gordon (Eds.), *Relapse prevention: Maintenance strategies in the treatment of addictive behaviors* (pp. 3–70). New York: Guilford.

Marlatt, G. A. (1985b). Cognitive assessment and intervention procedures for relapse prevention. In G. A. Marlatt & J. R. Gordon (Eds.), *Relapse prevention: Maintenance strategies in the treatment of addictive behaviors* (pp. 201–279). New York: Guilford.

Nace, E. P. (1987). *The treatment of alcoholism.* New York: Brunner/Mazel.

Pithers, W. D., Marques, J. K., Gibat, C., & Marlatt, G. A. (1983). Relapse prevention with sexual aggressives: A self-control model of treatment and maintenance of change. In J. G. Greer & I. R. Stuart (Eds.), *The sexual aggressor* (pp. 214–239). New York: Van Nostrand Reinhold.

Yochelson, S., & Samenow, S. E. (1976). *The criminal personality: A profile for change* (Vol. 1). New York: Aronson.

3

Feeding the PIG: The Problem of Immediate Gratification

G. ALAN MARLATT

URGES AND CRAVING: A CASE HISTORY

During a recent visit to Atascadero State Hospital in California, I interviewed a group of sex offenders about the circumstances leading up to their most recent arrests and incarcerations. One of the men, Bob X, was reluctant at first to talk. "There's not much to say," Bob said slowly. "I picked up a girl at a playground near my house and sexually molested her. I was caught and sent back here." The hospital records showed Bob was a repeat offender and had committed the act that led to his most recent arrest just 90 days after his previous discharge from Atascadero. After repeated questioning from members of the group, Bob gradually revealed the following scenario concerning the events that day that led up to his offense.

Bob thought he was getting along okay after his previous release from the treatment program. He was attending outpatient aftercare meetings and had his old job back. He told the group that a relapse was the furthest thing from his mind when he awoke that Saturday morning, the day of his offense. His therapist had encouraged him to establish new contacts with women, and he was encouraged by a friendly conversation he had had the day before with an attractive female clerk at a convenience store near his home. He had spent the evening and the next morning thinking about how he might ask her out for a date. Around noon, he drove over to the store and struck up a conversation with the clerk. Although he felt the same old anxiety and shyness he usually felt with adult women, he mustered up his courage and asked if she wanted to go to a movie with him on Friday night. "She turned me down cold," Bob remembered bitterly, "told me she already had a boyfriend and wasn't interested, period." Chagrined and dejected, Bob left the store and drove back home.

Once back in his apartment, Bob was feeling both depressed and angry. He felt victimized by the clerk and wanted to get back at her in some way. In an attempt to calm his nerves, he smoked a joint and put some loud rock music on his stereo. The music and marijuana blunted his anger, and his thoughts began to ramble. The stereo blared with Madonna's "Material Girl." Bob remembered that Suzie, one of his "special friends," was a big Madonna fan; he had bought her a copy of the same album when he first began courting her for eventual sexual favors. Spurred on by this memory, Bob began reminiscing about Suzie and her sensual young body. He particularly liked the way she looked the day he had first touched her; she had on a white halter top, cute pink shorts, and pink running shoes to match. She was quite a little flirt, Bob mused, with her suntanned legs and ponytail. Soon he was filled with electric sexual excitement as he recalled the time he had forced Suzie to have sex with him. It had happened right there in his apartment; he had felt so strong, virile, and powerful when Suzie succumbed to his sexual advances. As his mind filled with the images of this sexual conquest, Bob became physically aroused. He paced back and forth, his body filled with lust and sexual craving combined with a sense of personal power and magnetic appeal. He felt trapped inside his apartment, alone with no plans for the day. On an impulse, he decided to go out for a pack of cigarettes.

As it turned out, Bob never did buy his smokes. He decided to take the "long way" and drive to a store on the other side of town. He did not want to go back to the same convenience store he had visited a few hours before. On the drive across town, Bob found himself driving by a park and playground frequented by what Bob called "lots of young Lolitas"—one of his favorite haunts. At first, things in the playground looked pretty dead, so Bob continued on his drive. He was still feeling the high of the marijuana and the sexual tingling in his loins. Suddenly, he spotted her, playing with a group of kids on the edge of the park. She looked a lot like Suzie, slender and innocent. He parked his car at the side of the road to get a better look. He then put a Madonna cassette on his car stereo and rolled down the windows. It was a warm, clear afternoon under blue California skies. Bob took out the binoculars from the glove compartment and focused them on the young girl. So inviting, so young, so helpless, Bob mused as he watched her doing somersaults on the green park lawn. He felt his sexual arousal grow stronger. She looked 11, maybe 12, about the same age as Suzie and just as exciting.

Bob turned up his stereo, opened the door, and strolled over to the girl, who was drinking from the water fountain, apart from her friends. He felt a strange kind of confidence and control as he approached her; he had done this before, he knew his lines. "Excuse me, miss, can you help me? I'm lost, I'm new in town, and I'm trying to find the Eastside Shopping Mall. Do you know where it is?" She smiled and told him she knew where it was—that she hung out there a lot with her buddies. Bob asked her what her name was. "OK, Sally, can you come down to my car and point the way? Or maybe you could show me by getting in, and I could give you a lift over there?" As they approached his car, Sally could hear the car stereo. "Sounds like Madonna," she said. "Is that her latest album?" Bob told her that she could hear it much better inside his car. He gave her a pat on the buttocks as she got in the passenger's seat. "It's just down here a few blocks and then we turn right," Sally said. Bob turned up the stereo even louder as they drove off. He could hardly wait until he turned his fantasies into reality once again. He was in charge, in control of the situation.

Afterward, Bob felt terrible; in fact, he began to feel bad almost immediately after he climaxed in the tryst with Sally. He made no attempt to conceal his identity, although he threatened her with more physical harm if she told her parents or the police what he had done to her. His earlier excitement was gone. Instead, as he drove home, he felt a heavy dullness come over him, a gray wave of depression and guilt. He had gone over the line, as he had many times before.

The next morning Bob was arrested. Apparently Sally had remembered his license plate number.

Bob's relapse episode was a product of multiple determinants. Although other factors, such as the nature of Bob's treatment program, his personality structure, and his lack of a stable social relationship may have played contributing roles, in this chapter we focus on the motivational constructs associated with his offense: his experience of sexual cravings and urges. Taken together, the experience of strong sexual craving and the urge to relieve this craving through sexual acting out constitute what we have called the "problem of immediate gratification," or the "PIG" effect (Marlatt & Gordon, 1985). A review of Bob's case may help us understand the nature of the beast—how the PIG operates and how it contributes to a sexual relapse.

Bob's sexual desire and urge to engage in illicit sexual activity did not just materialize out of thin air. His sexual yearnings were provoked by a number of interlocking events and emotional reactions. Bob's problems began that day with his unsuccessful attempt to make a date with the convenience store clerk. His intentions were good ones; after all, he was following the advice of his therapist by attempting to establish an adult dating relationship. The fact that he was turned down was not unusual, given the circumstances. Rather than taking this rejection in stride, perhaps by planning an alternative method of meeting women, Bob felt personally rejected by the episode. In his mind, the clerk in the store was "one up," and he felt "put down" by what happened. Feeling dejected, he began brooding about what had occurred and felt more and more upset and angry. Such negative emotional states are breeding grounds for the PIG.

In an attempt to cope with his negative feelings back in his apartment, Bob did two things that increased the probability of relapse. First, he smoked marijuana. Although the pot may have tranquilized his depression and anger to some extent (it made him feel a "buzz" that distracted him from his negative affect), it also put him in a frame of mind in which sensual fantasies and associated sexual urges were enhanced. Second, he put on a phonograph record that triggered associative memories linked with past sexual exploits. Suddenly, he was besieged by fond thoughts about Suzie and her charms. He relived an experience in his imagination in which he had molested Suzie. It is important here to note that in his fantasy, as he later related it to the group at the hospital, he was the powerful seducer; his virility and sexual prowess were no match for the prepubescent Suzie. On a psychological level, Bob compensated for feeling "one down" after his failed attempt to make a date; he was now "one up" and back in control, back in power. Unfortunately this compensatory shift was accompanied by a marked increase in his sexual craving and urges. He switched from being "turned off" to "turned on." Thoughts of turning his fantasy into reality primed the PIG effect; Bob was hungry for some real action to satisfy his sexual and aggressive desires. In the framework of relapse prevention as outlined in this book, Bob had already experienced a lapse: fantasies of illicit sexual activity coupled with physical arousal.

While experiencing this sexual restlessness and arousal, Bob made an "apparently irrelevant decision" (AID) to leave his apartment on an ostensible quest for cigarettes. He actually drove himself directly into a high-risk situation for relapse when he "decided" to go by the playground on his way to the store. By doing so, he set the stage for what happened next. Although the sight of Sally appeared to be the precipitating element in the relapse episode, his prior emotional state and associated sexual fantasies were critical predisposing factors in the chain of events leading up to the sexual assault. These latter factors provided a background, highlighting the salience and attractiveness of Sally as a sexual cue. Bob experienced a kind of tunnel vision at this point, as all his thoughts and energies focused on Sally as a means of resolving his sexual tension. His goal was almost at hand; the PIG loomed large in his mind and actions.

Bob's craving for the gratification of his tension and arousal reached a peak in the sexual assault itself. Once again, he experienced a strong surge of power and control as he began his overt seduction. These feelings crested at the moment of his orgasm. He felt the acute pleasure and release of sexual tensions wash over him like a wave breaking on the shore. This intensely reinforcing experience represents the essence of the PIG. The reward is immediate and intensely gratifying, not unlike the rush, or high, of cocaine or other drugs. The experience of this immediate gratification is the core reinforcement in the addiction process. The intensity of the PIG may be enhanced if both sexual and aggressive drives are gratified in the act of release, as is often the case with sex offenders like Bob.

The reinforcing consequences of this release are often short lived, however. In Bob's case, he experienced a sudden shift of emotional reactions almost immediately after the consummation of his sexually aggressive act. The craving and excitement, once gratified, were immediately replaced by feelings of depression and guilt. The sudden letdown was in marked contrast to the intense pleasure of the sexual release. It was as though the wave of excitement he had been riding suddenly crested and he was dumped unceremoniously on the beach of reality. For many offenders, the low that follows the high of the sexual act sets the stage for the pattern to be repeated. Since, from Bob's perspective, the negative reactions and decreased self-esteem that followed on the heels of the sexual acting-out could be canceled out or transformed only by another sexual encounter, the probability of his repeating this pattern of activities increases. The intensity of the PIG effect increases to the extent that the individual is experiencing prior negative emotions; the *contrast* between the low and the high is the essential element here. The high of the sexual reinforcement is accentuated by the depth and intensity of the low that precedes the act of release.

THE SOURCES OF URGES AND CRAVING

Some authors, myself included, have made a distinction between the terms *craving* and *urge*, whereas others have used the terms interchangeably. When a distinction has been made, "craving" refers to the subjective desire or need to experience the effects of a consummatory response, be it sex, drug taking, eating, and so forth. An "urge" is defined as a compulsive intention to engage in a specific behavior that will satisfy or reduce the craving. Whereas craving is a global state of intense arousal or desire, it is often diffuse and may not be related to a specific object of gratification (craving may be gratified by several outlets). An urge, on the other hand, is directed toward a particular object or target. Bob's sexual craving was elicited by several overlapping determinants (e.g., interpersonal rejection, marijuana and music, memories of a previous sexual encounter with Suzie), all of which later focused into his urge to sexually molest Sally. As such, the craving–urge construct has been defined by some addiction experts as the final common pathway of complex motivational forces determining the overt addictive behavior (Baker, Morse, & Sherman, 1987; Cox & Klinger, 1988).

Clients are often overwhelmed by craving and urges, partly because they have mistaken beliefs about the cause (source) of these experiences. After discharge from an inpatient treatment center (or period of incarceration), clients may suddenly experience strong urges as they return to their usual environment. Often they attribute these intense desires to internal, endogenous factors, such as erosion of willpower or the eruption of an underlying disease process. Others conclude that treatment was ineffective or that the effects of the program have worn off, thereby rendering them vulnerable to craving. Such attributions are likely to increase the probability of relapse, to the extent that the individual feels helpless in the face of powerful internal or external forces that are perceived to be beyond personal control.

To counter such self-defeating attributions, clients need to be taught that most craving–urge experiences are responses that are triggered by external cues and discriminative stimuli. According to some addiction theorists (e.g., Ludwig & Wikler, 1974), craving is elicited by conditioned stimuli that have been previously associated with the addictive behavior. From this perspective, craving can be conceptualized as a conditioned response, an automatic response not unlike the salivation of Pavlov's dogs produced by a cue (the sound of a bell). In Bob's case, the conditioned stimulus was the music of the Madonna record that elicited associative memories of his sexual exploits with Suzie. Smoking marijuana augmented the somatic and emotional impact of this craving response and facilitated his sexual urges. By driving by the playground on his way to buy cigarettes, Bob subjected himself to discriminative stimuli (park and playground cues) that signaled the availability of sexual targets. As such, the physical setting often enhances craving to the extent that it is associated with past sexual experiences. When Bob spotted Sally, once again he was under the influence of powerful external cues, augmented by Sally's similarity in appearance to Suzie (stimulus generalization).

In addition to the influence of these conditioned and discriminative stimuli, Bob's craving was potentiated by his experience of rejection when he attempted to make a date with the convenience store clerk. His feeling "put down" by the woman set the stage for sexual fantasies in which he imagined himself in the dominant "one up" role vis à vis his sexual victim. The anticipated contrast between his feelings of being victimized by the store clerk and his subsequent sexual victimization of Sally increased his sexual craving and desire. Craving is enhanced by the experience of prior deprivation. Just as hunger grows in strength as a function of prolonged food deprivation, sexual craving is enhanced by prior sexual deprivation or rejection. Stated in another way, Bob suffered a blow to his self-efficacy when he was turned down for a date; his desire for sexual control and gratification was correspondingly increased. In the theoretical model of relapse prevention outlined by Marlatt and Gordon (1985), positive outcome expectancies (the desire or craving for gratification) associated with the addictive behavior are heightened when the individual's self-efficacy (perceived coping ability) in the situation is low. In Bob's case, the locus of his personal power (self-efficacy) switched from within himself to the addictive target. In other words, he needed to act out his sexual impulses against Sally to restore his sense of power and strength—much like alcoholics who rely on alcohol as an external crutch to fortify their own illusory sense of power and control.

The restorative power of drugs or sexual activity is fleeting and short lived, however. Once the craving has been gratified by the consummatory act, the individual is plunged into a contrasting emotional state, characterized by negative emotions (e.g., guilt, remorse, decreased self-esteem), often enhanced by the reactions of others. Once again, the seeds of craving grow in this soil of discomfort and decreased self-efficacy, and the cycle is set to repeat itself. As in any addiction cycle, the quick fix of the PIG is followed by a downside that sets the stage for another bout of craving and indulgence (Solomon, 1977). The "cure" for craving is also the "cause" of the next cycle of craving. This cycle of oscillating emotional states (from down to up and down again) illustrates the biphasic nature of the PIG process. Once fed, the PIG becomes immediately hungry for more. The more one feeds the PIG in the short run, the hungrier it gets in the long run.

REFERENCES

Baker, T. B., Morse, E., & Sherman, J. E. (1987). The motivation to use drugs: A psychobiological analysis of urges. In P. C. Rivers (Ed.), *Alcohol and addictive behaviors* (pp. 257–323). Lincoln: University of Nebraska Press.

Cox, W. M., & Klinger, E. (1988). A motivational model of alcohol use. *Journal of Abnormal Psychology, 97*, 168–180.

Ludwig, A. M., & Wikler, A. (1974). "Craving" and relapse to drink. *Quarterly Journal of Studies on Alcohol, 35*, 108–130.

Marlatt, G. A., & Gordon, J. R. (Eds.) (1985). *Relapse prevention: Maintenance strategies in the treatment of addictive behaviors.* New York: Guilford.

Solomon, R. L. (1977). An opponent-process theory of acquired motivation: IV. The affective dynamics of addiction. In J. J. Maser & M. E. P. Seligman (Eds.), *Psychopathology: Experimental models* (pp. 66–103). San Francisco: Freeman.

4

Determinants of the Abstinence Violation Effect in Sexual Fantasies

KABE RUSSELL
V. HENLIE STURGEON
MICHAEL H. MINER
CRAIG NELSON

A major step in the process leading to relapse, from a relapse prevention (RP) perspective, is the response that accompanies an initial slip, or lapse, in one's pledge of abstinence. This pattern of reactions, referred to as the "abstinence violation effect" (AVE); (Marlatt & Gordon, 1980, 1985), represents the cognitive and affective responses that propel an individual into a full-blown relapse. Ex-smokers, for example, who light up a single cigarette may return to habitual smoking if this slip leads them to redefine themselves as smokers. Similarly, ex-alcoholics may greatly enhance the chances of a return to the former drinking pattern if a slip is reinforced by being perceived as a coping response to feelings of being helpless or powerless. As with the addictive behaviors, how sex offenders react to lapses (i.e., deviant sexual urges, thoughts, or fantasies) may determine whether they regain their commitment to abstinence or relapse by perpetrating a new sex crime (Marques & Nelson, in press; Marques, Pithers, & Marlatt, 1984; Nelson, Miner, Marques, Russell, & Achterkirchen, 1988; Pithers, Marques, Gibat, & Marlatt, 1983). For sex offenders, the AVE is characterized by a lowered sense of self-esteem, a perception of impaired self-control, and an expectation of failure. This chapter will examine the AVE as it has been manifested and observed in participants in an inpatient treatment program for sex offenders. The important determinants of the AVE will be characterized, and situations that have been observed to precipitate lapses and their concomitant AVEs will be described. Three case examples, which demonstrate how the determinants of the AVE affected its manifestation during the course of treatment, will be presented. Finally, conclusions regarding the broader implications of examining the AVE in sex offenders will be tentatively offered.

63

DETERMINANTS OF THE AVE

The cognitive and affective aspects of the AVE are dimensional phenomena. They vary in intensity depending on a variety of factors, such as the nature of the prohibited behavior, the nature and strength of the commitment to abstinence, the degree to which one can rationalize or justify the lapse as caused by external sources, the length of abstinence preceding the lapse, the effort or cost expended in previously maintaining abstinence, and the presence of significant others. An AVE is believed to be relatively intense if the lapse is attributed to stable, global factors that are believed to be out of one's control (e.g., lack of willpower, a personality defect, a result of a disease). On the other hand, an AVE is thought to be less intense if the lapse is attributed to external, unstable, or specific factors that are perceived to be under one's influence and control (e.g., a momentary failure to avoid or escape a high-risk situation). It is hypothesized that an AVE's intensity, and therefore its influence in precipitating a single lapse into a full relapse, is determined by both the cognitive dissonance aroused by the lapse and the attribution of blame, or fault, to oneself for its commission (Marlatt & Gordon, 1980, 1985).

For the sex offender, a lapse presents a conflict between the offender's self-image as an abstainer from illicit sexual behavior and the recent experience of the prohibited deviant thought or urge. Such self-statements as "If I am no longer a molester, why am I getting turned on to fantasies of a child?" or "Why am I suddenly thinking about forcing this woman to have sex if I'm no longer a rapist?" represent this state of internal conflict. Cognitive dissonance (Festinger, 1957), aroused by the discrepancy between the offender's self-image as an abstainer from the deviant sexual behavior and the occurrence of an incongruent behavior or thought, is characteristic of the AVE. An attempt to alleviate the cognitive dissonance and its discomfort by altering the self-image to conform with the experience of the lapse is one mechanism by which the AVE may engender relapse. A self-statement such as "I must still be a sex offender" reduces the dissonance and its discomfort. Such statements also promote the return to the illicit sexual behavior, since it is now concordant with the offender's beliefs about himself.

A second cognitive reaction to the lapse that is characteristic of the AVE is self-attribution. To the degree that the slip cannot be attributed to a unique and unusual set of circumstances, the offender is likely to ascribe the lapse to his own deficiencies. A lack of willpower, internal weakness, a deficit in character, or a lack of effort in treatment may all be ways in which an offender attributes self-blame (Nelson, in press). The extent to which the lapse is construed as a personal failure is directly related to one's expectation of continued failure (Abramson, Seligman, & Teasdale, 1978). The previously abstinent offender's self-efficacy (Bandura, 1977) diminishes, and his resistance to future lapses decreases.

PRECIPITATING THE AVE

California's Sex Offender Treatment and Evaluation Project is described later in this book (Marques, Day, Nelson, & Miner, Chapter 22, this volume). The incarcerated child molesters and rapists who participate in this program receive treatment modeled on the RP approach in an environment that, by design, minimizes their chances of lapsing into deviant sexual thoughts and urges. The environment isolates them from many of the conditions and potential victims that constituted the high-risk situations that precipitated their crimes. The offenders enter treatment after several years of forced abstinence through incarceration. Typically, the combined effect of this period of abstinence and the aversive nature of prison results in a degree of confidence that they will never reoffend. They frequently view themselves as "cured," and they fail to appreciate the importance of controlling and coping with risk factors in order to maintain their abstinence when released to the less restrictive environment of the community.

Preparing an offender to cope with the lapses and their concomitant AVEs that can be anticipated in the future is an integral part of treatment from an RP perspective. Although the hospital environment tends to minimize the chances that lapses into deviant sexual urges, thoughts, and fantasies will occur in response to external cues, participants in the project have reported a wide range of situations that have stimulated such lapses. Seeing appealing children in the hospital's visiting room or on television, becoming angry with a female staff member, or experiencing frustration within the hospital are instances reported by a few offenders that have prompted lapses followed by the sense of a loss of self-control and self-esteem indicative of an AVE.

All offenders in the project participate in an assessment of their sexual arousal patterns through the use of penile plethysmography. Briefly, assessment procedures involve exposing the offender to a series of both deviant and nondeviant sexual stimuli in the form of slides, audiotapes, and videotapes while their penile erection responses are electronically measured and recorded (Laws & Osborn, 1983). This evaluation permits an identification of deviant sexual objects that can then be targeted for treatment.

During this assessment, offenders frequently lapse by generating sexual arousal to deviant themes. Although two-thirds of the project participants have generated significant responses to deviant stimuli during this evaluation at the time of their admission, few have reported signs of an associated AVE. This is a curious result, as many of the determinants of an AVE are present. The offenders have made a commitment to abstinence, they have several years of forced abstinence behind them prior to the lapse, many expressed confidence in their ability to refrain from deviant sexual fantasies and acts in the future, and their lapse was recognized by significant others in the form of their therapists, who review the data. Yet the deviant sexual arousal generated in the laboratory provokes few signs of the sense of impaired self-control or lowered self-esteem that would be expected of an AVE. Upon further consideration of the data with the offenders, they often discounted the arousal as a result of an unusual or atypical situation that was irrelevant to their chances of offending. These offenders indicated that they were simply responding in the manner requested of them in the assessment procedures. They attributed the arousal to the demands of the situation and external sources. Thus the self-attribution necessary for an AVE was absent.

The treatment component that has been most frequently observed to elicit an AVE is the task of developing a pool of individualized sexual stimuli for subsequent use in olfactory aversion treatment (Laws, Myer, & Holmen, 1978; Maletzky, 1977). These stimuli consist of slides and audiotaped descriptions of explicit sexual activity prepared by the offender that are paired with a noxious odor (ammonia) in treatment sessions to reduce their stimulus value. These descriptions typically include past actual sexual contacts, favorite former masturbatory fantasies, or new fantasies developed while looking at the slides. It is in this process of preparing explicit deviant sexual fantasies that some offenders clearly exhibit the characteristics of an AVE. In this situation, because the fantasies are internally generated, the arousal is attributed to the offender and cannot be blamed on external sources.

In effect, the process of writing deviant sexual fantasies creates a "programmed lapse." This induces a return of the offender's forbidden arousal and its attendant AVE under the guidance and supervision of the therapist (Marlatt & Gordon, 1985; Marques, 1984; Pithers, 1983). Once the AVE is experienced by the offender, its power and potency often can be more readily appreciated and appropriate coping responses to neutralize its relapse-engendering effects can be developed.

In order to demonstrate the AVE as it occurs in this situation, three case studies are presented below. These cases represent a sample in the variety of manifestations of the AVE that have been observed in the process of preparing stimuli for olfactory aversion treatment in the Sex Offender Treatment and Evaluation Project.

The Case of Scott: The Experience of the Classic AVE

Scott is a 40-year-old, married man with a lifelong history of molesting female children. He was raised in an incestuous family and was physically abused as a child. Scott had committed incest with a natural daughter for more than a decade, and he had also molested victims outside his immediate family. He had made a commitment to abstain from molesting prior to his arrest, and he claimed that he had been able to adhere to this vow of abstinence for the 2 years prior to being sentenced and sent to prison. As a result of this period of abstinence, he believed that he was "cured." He no longer considered himself to be a child molester, and he thought he would never again have sexual fantasies about underaged girls. In short, Scott's beliefs about his abstinence had many of the characteristics that set the stage for a relatively intense AVE should he ever lapse into deviant sexual fantasies.

The initial assessment of his sexual arousal pattern in the sexual behavior laboratory revealed arousal to female adults as well as a deviant arousal pattern oriented toward prepubescent girls. The arousal he evidenced during the assessment procedures, although mildly upsetting to him, was not experienced as a lapse, because he attributed it to the demands of the situation rather than to any weakness within himself. Thus no discernable AVE was noted.

Based on these assessment results, a course of olfactory aversion treatment to decrease his sexual arousal to female children was recommended. Scott began constructing 12 sexually explicit fantasies to be used in this treatment procedure. He was instructed to make the fantasies as sexually potent as possible and to use specific details from his prior victims.

After he started writing the fantasies, he became sexually aroused while looking at a magazine with pictures of prepubescent girls. He perceived the little girls as posing in a provocative manner yet realized that he had not interpreted such pictures as provocative or sexually arousing for years. He recognized that "This is just like having a lapse." Later that night, he became sexually aroused and masturbated while recalling the fantasies and memories of his prior victims. He was shocked by the intensity of his arousal and by the clarity of the memories with which he was flooded. He was both excited and frightened. This lapse, the deviant sexual fantasy, precipitated an AVE, that is, his sexual arousal was quickly followed by intense feelings of guilt and failure. He became depressed and ruminated over such thoughts as "I was sure I was cured, but this proves I've been a molester all along" and "I'll always be just like my father."

Although highly embarrassed, Scott related this information to his therapist, who first helped him to label his experience as an AVE. He was reassured that this was a typical response to experiencing a slip after a period of abstinence. Secondly, the therapist helped him examine and confront some of his cognitive distortions, such as "Since I lapsed again, I'll never change." These thoughts resulted in lowered self-esteem, an expectation of failure, an impaired sense of self-control, and a belief that treatment had failed. Next, Scott and the therapist collaborated in developing several positive self-statements to cope with the AVE, such as "I've just lapsed, but I can stop myself before I relapse." Finally, the therapist instructed Scott to substitute images of adult partners if he ever again had fantasies that involved minors. He was instructed to stop masturbating if he was unsuccessful in redirecting the fantasy.

Following the crisis precipitated by the lapse and its AVE, Scott completed a course of olfactory aversion, which reduced his deviant arousal to insignificant levels. Regular follow-up evaluations prior to his parole to outpatient treatment indicated that the reduction of the deviant arousal to insignificant levels was sustained. These techniques enabled Scott to regain a sense of self-control over his behavior and thoughts, and his expectation shifted back to a belief that he would be able to maintain abstinence from his propensity to molest young girls. In addition, it was believed that by experiencing the "programmed lapse" and its concomitant AVE in a controlled setting, he was prepared to cope more effectively with future lapses when he returned to the community.

The Case of Mark: An Attempt to Anticipate the AVE

Mark is a 36-year-old, single homosexual who was first arrested for a sex crime as an adolescent. He had previously received treatment to control his interest in molesting boys. Mark reported a 2-year period of abstinence prior to his last offense, and he had been in prison for 1 year before entering treatment this time. Although he had broken his commitment to abstinence by his last offense, he discounted its significance by describing it as an isolated incident that resulted from a unique set of circumstances. He was confident that he would be able to remain abstinent in the future because such a unique situation would never recur. As with Scott, his strong commitment to abstinence, his confidence in his self-control, and his rationalization that his offense was due to external causes created an environment ripe for a strong AVE should he ever lapse.

His initial physiological assessment revealed significant arousal to adolescent as well as adult males. Based on his assessment results, olfactory aversion was recommended, and Mark began preparing deviant sexual fantasies to be used in the treatment procedure. In an attempt to minimize the AVE he might experience in preparing the fantasies, the reactions of other participants were reviewed with him. Specifically, he was informed that previous participants had experienced some arousal when preparing these fantasies that led them to become frustrated and discouraged and to feel a loss of control over their sexual urges. He was assured that this was a programmed lapse and that he would benefit from learning to cope with it.

Irrespective of these discussions, Mark reported feeling depressed (the AVE) when he lapsed during the preparation of the fantasies. His depression emanated from a series of cognitive distortions, such as "I've only been fooling myself. I thought I'd changed, but I'll never have enough control of myself to not get excited." With the assistance of his therapist, he was able to develop positive self-statements to cope with the AVE, such as "I may experience a lapse from time to time, but I can be in control of how I react to the lapse. I may experience sexual thoughts involving boys, but I can lessen their recurrence by not masturbating to them. I can stay in control by doing this." These self-statements increased his self-efficacy and diminished the frequency with which he had thoughts of having failed in treatment. The increased sense of self-control also resulted in an increase in self-esteem that renewed his expectation of being able to maintain abstinence.

Mark successfully completed a course of olfactory aversion treatment, which resulted in a decline of his measured sexual arousal to adolescent males to insignificant levels. This pattern was sustained in follow-up assessments prior to his parole to outpatient treatment.

As with Scott, Mark's experience with a significant programmed lapse and its consequent AVE in a controlled setting under the supervision of his therapist permitted a more realistic alignment of expectations for future lapses and an opportunity to develop strategies to cope successfully with the AVE in the community. The attempt by the therapist to prepare Mark for the expected AVE, however, did not appear to be successful. It seemed that the actual experience of the loss of control and failure represented by the AVE was required in order for him to appreciate its impact fully.

The Case of Stephen: A Failure to Elicit the AVE

Stephen is a 41-year-old divorced father with a lengthy history of molesting both male and female children. He was raised in an alcoholic family, and he had previously received treatment in several programs for his own drug-abuse problems. His first conviction for child molestation had resulted in his discharge from military service 10 years prior to his present offense, which involved sexually molesting two nieces and a nephew over a period of several months.

Stephen described himself as having a strong sex drive that resulted in his masturbating, often to fantasies involving children, two or three times per day. He verbalized a commitment to abstinence, but he perceived his fantasy life as a separate issue. He did not view his deviant sexual thoughts as necessarily a violation of his vow of abstinence. Stephen believed that it was permissible to maintain his fantasies about boys as long as he did not act on them. Thus he did not identify his deviant sexual urges or thoughts as lapses. Instead, he tended to define lapses as actions he would take to try to seduce potential victims (e.g., offering them alcohol, inviting them to stay over at his house for the night).

It was not surprising that Stephen's initial assessment in the sexual behavior laboratory revealed significant arousal to male children. Following orgasmic reconditioning treatment (Marquis, 1970) to increase and stabilize his arousal to mutually consenting sex with adult males, olfactory aversion to diminish his arousal to boys was initiated. In preparation for this treatment, Stephen was assigned the task of developing sexual fantasies to be utilized as stimuli. Unlike most participants completing this procedure, Stephen quickly completed the task and failed to exhibit any signs of an AVE. He felt in control, satisfied with his cooperation in the assigned task, and hopeful that treatment would be successful in preventing him from reoffending.

Stephen had made a vow of abstinence and perceived no violation of that pledge resulting from having sexual fantasies about children. Consequently, the sexual arousal elicited in the process of preparing his deviant fantasies was not experienced as a programmed lapse, as in the two previous cases. His self-image as an abstainer included an evaluation that his sexual urges and thoughts about children were acceptable, provided he did not act on them. Therefore, the responses aroused by the task were consistent with this self-image. Without the perception of a lapse, it was consistent that no cognitive dissonance was engendered nor self-blame aroused to evoke the AVE. The project staff perceived such thoughts as risky, and once Stephen's thinking came to light it became a treatment issue to confront.

It has been our experience that the failure to observe an AVE in other offenders during the process of writing deviant sexual fantasies could also be traced to the failure to elicit the requisite lapse. For some, like Stephen, it was a sign that their dedication to abstinence did not include an expectation to refrain from deviant sexual fantasies. For others, the deviant fantasies they prepared failed to elicit any significant sexual arousal. In short, the presence of an AVE depends on the offender's perceiving his experience as a lapse. This perception, in turn, is tied to the nature of the commitment to abstinence.

DISCUSSION AND SUMMARY

This chapter has focused on the characteristics of the AVE and the differences in how offenders may manifest this phenomenon. The AVE is a complex of cognitive and affective factors that follows the experience of a lapse, or slip, into deviant sexual thoughts, fantasies, or urges. The salient characteristics appear to be a decline in self-esteem, a feeling of loss of control over one's illicit sexual behavior, and an expectation of failure. As one can see, this phenomenon can set the stage for a full-blown relapse if the patient has not learned an adequate set of coping responses.

In this chapter, we have explored the cases of three individuals who varied in how they experienced or failed to experience an AVE during a treatment procedure. It has been hypothesized that the experience of sexual arousal to deviant themes following a commitment to and a period of abstinence would result in an AVE. In an inpatient setting, we have found that offenders who routinely exhibited significant deviant sexual arousal (a lapse) in the context of a physiological assessment have not experienced a concomitant AVE. We have found, however, that many patients have experienced the AVE when they have been asked to write their own fantasies as part of olfactory aversion treatment. When the characteristics of these two situations are explored, the necessary and sufficient precursors to the AVE become clearer. Apparently, two factors must be present in order for an individual to experience an AVE following arousal to a deviant theme: (1) The individual must experience the arousal as a lapse, and then (2) he must attribute the cause of that lapse to himself.

The assessment procedure in the sexual behavior laboratory does not appear to precipitate an AVE, because the offender is more likely to perceive the cause of his arousal as due to the artificial nature of the laboratory and the assessment instructions. This lack of self-attribution also appears present in the case of Stephen, who did not experience an AVE during fantasy writing. He perceived the assignment as a treatment program requirement to engage in deviant sexual fantasies. Therefore, his fantasy writing had the same characteristics as the initial assessment procedures and could be viewed as an acceptable part of therapy, not something for which he took responsibility.

The second necessary factor is that the arousal must be viewed as a lapse. In the first two case studies, the offenders viewed their sexual arousal to fantasies of children as lapses. Scott, in fact, overtly labeled his experience as a lapse. The identification of a lapse and its atribution to internal factors led both Scott and Mark to experience cognitive dissonance. This dissonance was clearly not present in the case of Stephen. He did not experience his arousal to fantasies of children as a lapse, since his initial commitment to abstinence did not include a commitment to eschew fantasies. Lapses to Stephen involved overt behavior aimed at procuring sex with a child.

Sex offenders often enter treatment with the expectation that they will be "cured" and will never again have to confront the deviant sexual urges or arousal that contributed to their crimes. These beliefs may be reinforced by periods of abstinence promoted by incarceration or the trauma and public humiliation of being arrested and convicted. For many offenders, both situations may temporarily disrupt any pattern of deviant sexual thoughts or urges they may have harbored. Others believe they will be able to maintain abstinence by willpower and their personal conviction never to reoffend. Still other offenders may externalize the blame for their crimes to atypical life circumstances that are unlikely to be repeated. All three stances may promote unrealistic expectations of success in maintaining abstinence from deviant sexual behavior, expectations that exacerbate the risk that a lapse may progress to a relapse. While in a period of abstinence, such offenders may dismiss the personal relevance of the lapse and the subsequent thoughts and feelings it may engender that are represented in the AVE. Although they may quickly grasp an intellectual understanding of the potential danger of experiencing an AVE, they minimize its importance and pertinence to themselves. Precipitating a programmed lapse under the supervision and direction of a therapist in a controlled setting permits an examination of the relevance of the AVE to the offender. Therapists in both inpatient and outpatient settings can precipitate the AVE in a controlled, supervised fashion by assigning offenders the task of developing personal deviant fantasies. The benefit of developing coping skills through a programmed lapse appears to provide a potency unobtainable in a theoretical discussion of the AVE. Once the importance of this effect is appreciated, expectations about future success can be more realistically aligned and appropriate coping strategies can be developed to combat the relapse-promoting characteristics of the AVE.

REFERENCES

Abramson, L. Y., Seligman, M. E. P., & Teasdale, J. D. (1978). Learned helplessness in humans: Critique and reformulation. *Journal of Abnormal Psychology, 87*, 49–74.

Bandura, A. (1977). Self-efficacy: Toward a unifying theory of behavioral change. *Psychological Review, 84*, 191–215.

Festinger, L. (1957). *A theory of cognitive dissonance*. Palo Alto, CA: Stanford University Press.

Laws, D. R., Myer, J., & Holmen, M. L. (1978). Reduction of sadistic sexual arousal by olfactory aversion: A case study. *Behaviour Research and Therapy, 16*, 281–285.

Laws, D. R., & Osborn, C. A. (1983). How to build and operate a behavioral laboratory to evaluate and treat sexual deviance. In J. G. Greer & I. R. Stuart (Eds.), *The sexual aggressor: Current perspectives on treatment* (pp. 293–335). New York: Van Nostrand Reinhold.

Maletzky, B. M. (1977). Booster sessions in aversion therapy: The permanency of treatment. *Behavior Therapy, 8*, 460–463.

Marlatt, G. A., & Gordon, J. R. (1980). Determinants of relapse: Implications for the maintenance of behavior change. In P. Davidson & S. Davidson (Eds.), *Behavioral medicine: Changing health lifestyles* (pp. 410–452). New York: Brunner/Mazel.

Marlatt, G. A., & Gordon, J. R. (Eds.) (1985). *Relapse prevention: Maintenance strategies in the treatment of addictive behaviors*. New York: Guilford.

Marques, J. K., & Nelson, C. (in press). Understanding and preventing relapse in sex offenders. In M. Gossop (Ed.), *Relapse and addictive behavior*. Beckenham, Kent, UK: Croom Helm.

Marques, J. K., Pithers, W. D., & Marlatt, G. A. (1984). Relapse prevention: A self-control program for sex offenders. Appendix to: Marques, J. K. *An innovative treatment program for sex offenders: Report to the legislature*. Sacramento: California Department of Mental Health.

Marquis, J. N. (1970). Orgasmic reconditioning: Changing sexual object choice through controlling masturbation fantasies. *Journal of Behavior Therapy and Experimental Psychiatry, 1*, 263–271.

Nelson, C., Miner, M., Marques, J., Russell, K., & Achterkirchen, J. (1988). Relapse prevention: A cognitive–behavioral model for treatment of the rapist and child molester. *Journal of Social Work and Human Sexuality, 7*, 125–143.

Pithers, W. D., Marques, J. K., Gibat, C. C., & Marlatt, G. A. (1983). Relapse prevention with sexual aggressives: A self-control model of treatment and maintenance of change. In J. G. Greer & I. R. Stuart (Eds.), *The sexual aggressor: Current perspectives on treatment* (pp. 214–239). New York: Van Nostrand Reinhold.

II

SOLUTIONS: ASSESSMENT

This section considers solutions to some of the problems facing sex offenders. We emphasize solutions through a variety of assessment procedures, first the assessment of high-risk situations and then of coping skills.

HIGH-RISK SITUATIONS

Many clinicians who work with criminals show considerable disdain for the reputed unreliability of official records. Pithers, Beal, Armstrong, and Petty show that careful analysis of existing clinical and criminal records greatly strengthens the clinician's position when first meeting a sex offender. Especially interesting is their systematic identification of immediate and early precursors to sexual aggression.

Long, Wuesthoff, and Pithers demonstrate the utility of creating a new clinical record by having the offender produce an autobiography. They found that this device requires the client to reflect upon his own life, identifying important life events. In terms of treatment procedures, the autobiography offers the therapist a view of the client's phenomenological world.

MacDonald and Pithers discuss the use of self-monitoring in the identification of high-risk situations. The system they describe is quite elaborate, involving systematic daily journal keeping. Although not applicable to every treatment situation, their method provides the offender with a powerful tool for monitoring his emotional and cognitive processes on a continuous basis.

In my own contribution to this section I describe the use of penile plethysmography to monitor deviant and nondeviant sexual arousal throughout an entire course of treatment for a single individual. In demonstrating the use of the procedure I chose a particularly difficult case of a resistant client who seemed finally to comply with treatment and gain some benefit, but who was eventually terminated at his own request. In the absence of the penile measures, this would have been considered a marginal case. The penile measures, however, showed throughout that treatment failed to have an impact on the client's deviant cognitions, which became more, rather than less, deviant. The client remained at very high risk.

The contribution by Day, Miner, Sturgeon, and Murphy is an exceptionally careful piece of work demonstrating the intercorrelation of penile and self-report measures in the determination of high risk. They formed composite scores from data obtained from a plethysmographic assessment and from the Multiphasic Sex Inventory and compared their discriminative ability. They found, as we have in our research, that simple self-report items will often classify sex offenders as well as the sophisticated plethysmographic examination.

COPING SKILLS

The development of a situational competency test was one of the procedures of the original RP approach. Miner, Day, and Nafpaktitis describe the adaptation of the procedure to sex offenders. The purpose of the situational competency test is to identify those situations in which the offender lacks the ability to cope, thus identifying a major target for treatment. The procedures may also be used as an outcome measure of the extent to which clients have developed the requisite coping skills.

Self-efficacy ratings, like the Situational Competency Test, give indications of existing coping skills in that the client reveals information about his expectancies for success in a particular situation. Although he is skeptical of their utility with rapists, Hall notes that they may be useful in identifying clients at risk for relapse, revealing high-risk situations and anticipating a client's reaction to an initial lapse.

Sandberg and Marlatt discuss another modified technique from the original RP approach, relapse fantasies. These guided relapse scenarios also give indications of an offender's strengths and weaknesses in coping skills. These free-form fantasies, emitted by the client in the presence of the therapist, can yield information that might be missed in the more structured self-efficacy ratings and the situational competency test.

A · HIGH-RISK SITUATIONS

5

Identification of Risk Factors through Clinical Interviews and Analysis of Records

WILLIAM D. PITHERS
LINDA S. BEAL
JOHN ARMSTRONG
JOHN PETTY

Clinical interviewing is both a scientific and an artistic endeavor. The *science* of clinical interviewing entails researching available information about the client prior to meeting him so that the interaction may be as goal oriented and productive as possible. While reviewing background information, a clinician generates hypotheses that may be investigated during the subsequent interview. This scientific process strongly influences one's preparedness for the interview and the accuracy of the information derived from it.

Although most relapse prevention assessment techniques require the client's active participation, analyses of clinical and criminal records permit preliminary assessment of his high-risk situations before he has entered the therapist's office. Research has demonstrated that a wide range of offense precursors can be reliably identified through analyses of criminal and clinical records (Pithers, Buell, Kashima, Cumming, & Beal, 1987; Pithers, Cumming, Beal, Young, & Turner, 1989; Pithers, Kashima, Cumming, Beal, & Buell, 1987, 1988). Since sexual aggressors tend to deny, minimize, and distort self-reported information, acquiring as much information as possible about the client and his offenses prior to the psychological evaluation is essential to an adequate interview. To the extent that offense precursors are identified beforehand, the clinical interview can be conducted more efficiently, focusing on the thought processes that enabled the client to abuse and on other factors relevant to his treatment (e.g, degree of empathy for victims).

The clinician's ability to depart from a structured format for an interview, following up on intuitive hunches with a carefully timed and phrased question, represents the *artistic* element of interviewing. An artistically performed interview yields information beyond that available from one that is overstructured and controlled. In this chapter, we provide information that will permit scientific preparation for artistic interviews of sexual aggressors in order that the offender's risk factors may be discerned.

REVIEWING CLINICAL AND CRIMINAL RECORDS

Prior to meeting the client, the clinician should obtain and carefully review the following documents: (1) police affidavit, (2) victim's statement, (3) offender's statement, (4) affidavits of witnesses, (5) a computerized check of criminal history, (6) presentence investigation reports, (7) psychological evaluations, and (8) a developmental history. These sources provide considerable information about the offender's family background, developmental history, sexual experience, academic attainment, prior criminal acts, ability to enter into and maintain intimate relationships, substance-use pattern, vocational history, and recreational habits.

Identification of Precursors through Record Reviews

Pithers, Kashima, Cumming, Beal, and Buell (1988) analyzed randomly selected case records of 200 convicted sexual offenders, consisting of 136 pedophiles and 64 rapists. In reviewing each subject's data, the authors attempted to identify offense precursors, or risk factors, that appeared to predispose toward or precipitate sexual victimization.

Precursors to offenses determined to have occurred within 6 months of the subjects' offenses are presented in Table 5.1. Risk factors noted to have occurred at least 6 months prior to the offense, and which generally predisposed toward deviant behavior, are contained in Table 5.2.

Table 5.1 shows several differences in immediate precursors to rape and pedophilic acts. A greater percentage of rapists than pedophiles experienced generalized anger (88% of rapists; 32% of pedophiles), displayed anger toward women (77% vs. 26%), acted suddenly and opportunistically rather than grooming the victim (58% vs. 19%), and used alcohol or another drug prior to offending (56% vs. 30%).

In contrast, depression was observed more commonly among pedophiles (38%) than rapists (3%), and pedophiles were more likely than rapists to acknowledge having planned the exact circumstances of their offenses (73% vs. 28%). During clinical interviews, a greater proportion of pedophiles (51%) than rapists (17%) revealed a preference for fantasies of abusive, rather than consenting adult, sexual acts.

TABLE 5.1. Immediate Precursors to Sexual Aggression[b]

Precursor	Rapists[a]	Pedophiles[a]
Anger		
Generalized, global	88	32
Toward women	77	26
Anxiety	27	46
Assertive-skills deficit	42	23
Boredom	45	28
Cognitive distortions	72	65
Depression	3	38
Abusive sexual fantasies	17	51
Disordered sexual arousal pattern	69	57
Driving car alone without destination	17	1
Emotionally inhibited/overcontrolled	58	51
Interpersonal dependence	30	48
Low self-esteem	56	61
Low victim empathy	61	71
Opportunity (e.g., a hitchhiker)	58	19
Personality disorder	61	35
Planning of sexual offense	28	73
Sexual-knowledge deficit	45	52
Social anxiety	25	39
Social-skills deficit	59	50
Substance use/abuse		
Alcohol	42	23
Other substances	14	7

[a]Percentage of sample
[b]Note. From "Relapse Prevention of Sexual Aggression" by W. D. Pithers, K. Kashima, G. F. Cumming, L. S. Beal, and M. Buell. In *Human Sexual Aggression: Current Perspectives* (p. 246), Eds. R. Prentky and V. Quinsey, 1988, New York: New York Academy of Sciences. Copyright 1988 by New York Academy of Sciences. Reprinted by permission.

Other precursors occurred in similar proportions among the rapists and pedophiles. Variables noted in relatively high proportions in both samples included: cognitive distortions (72% of rapists; 65% of pedophiles), low self-esteem (56% vs. 61%), and emotional inhibition or overcontrol (58% vs. 51%). Psychosexual evaluation data revealed that the majority of both groups exhibited a disordered sexual arousal pattern (69% vs. 57%). The discrepancy between self-reported deviant preferences and objectively measured deviant preferences

TABLE 5.2. Early Precursors to Sexual Aggression[b]

Precursor	Rapists[a]	Pedophiles[a]
Divorce (more than 5 years before act)	14	15
Exposure to violent death of human or infrahuman	22	2
Familial chaos	86	49
Maternal absence/neglect	41	29
Parental marital discord	59	45
Paternal absence/neglect	59	54
Physically abused as child	45	7
Prior arrest for nonsexual offense	44	15
Sexual anxiety	39	58
Sexual dysfunction	11	11
Sexual victimization		
Prior to age 12	5	56
Between ages 12 and 18	11	6
Use of female prostitutes	30	8

[a]Percentage of sample
[b]Note. From "Relapse Prevention of Sexual Aggression" by W. D. Pithers, K. Kashima, G. F. Cumming, L. S. Beal, and M. Buell. In *Human Sexual Aggression: Current Perspectives* (p. 245), Eds. R. Prentky and V. Quinsey, 1988, New York: New York Academy of Sciences. Copyright 1988 by New York Academy of Sciences. Reprinted by permission.

(via the penile plethysmograph) was greater for rapists (17% by self-report; 69% by objective measurement) than for pedophiles (51% vs. 57%).

Table 5.2 reveals that among early precursors to sexual offenses, a greater proportion of rapists than pedophiles had witnessed the violent death of a human (e.g., hunting accidents) or an animal (e.g., pig slaughtering) during childhood (22% of rapists; 2% of pedophiles), experienced chaotic family lives (e.g., spousal abuse, extramarital affairs viewed by the subject; 86% vs. 49%), and been subjected to physical abuse as a child (45% vs. 7%). More pedophiles (56%) than rapists (5%) revealed sexual victimization prior to age 12. In contrast, a slightly greater proportion of rapists (11%) than pedophiles (6%) were sexually victimized during adolescence.

These data demonstrate that precursors to sexual offenses are identifiable through analysis of criminal and clinical records. The nature of these precursors suggests that truly impulsive, unplanned sexual offenses are exceptionally rare. Identification of offense precursors enables many of the client's high-risk situations to be outlined. On the basis of this outline, a tentative treatment plan may be delineated.

Reliability of Risk-Factor Identification
from Record Reviews

In order for relapse prevention to have practical utility, professionals must agree on the factors that should be considered offense precursors for a sexual aggressor. Since, in the Vermont Treatment Program for Sexual Aggressors (VTPSA), relapse prevention is implemented by both mental health and correctional professionals, all parties involved in the treatment effort must be able to specify the same precursors for an individual offender.

To assess the extent of agreement in risk-factor identification among professional groups, two psychologists and two probation and parole officers reviewed case records of ten convicted pedophiles (Pithers, Buell, Kashima, Cumming, & Beal, 1987). The level of agreement in identification of immediate precursors reached 85% among the psychologists and 75% among the officers. For early precursors, the psychologists agreed on 76% of their ratings, while the officers' ratings coincided 57% of the time. Comparing level of agreement across professions, the clinicians and officers agreed on 76% of the immediate precursors and 66% of the early precursors.

Thus levels of agreement on immediate and early offense precursors, both within and across two professional groups, were relatively high. It must be emphasized that these ratings were not performed on predetermined, dichotomous variables where the chance probability of rater agreement is 0.5. Since ratings were based solely on information gleaned from reading case files, with no structure provided to guide reporting of risk factors, the probability of chance agreement between raters was closer to zero than to 0.5. Therefore, the percentage of agreement in risk factors identified within and between the two professional groups is impressive. Given this high level of agreement, offense precursors (i.e., risk factors) appear to represent meaningful concepts among psychologists and probation officers acquainted with the relapse prevention model.

Efficacy of Training in Identifying Risk Factors
from Records

In order for relapse prevention to be adopted widely, it must be demonstrated that training enables professionals to discern offense precursors from clinical records. To assess transfer of skills to professionals inexperienced with relapse prevention, social workers participating in a 6-hour training session completed a pretest and posttest that required them to identify risk factors contained in a fictional narrative about an adolescent offender (Pithers, Buell, Kashima, Cumming, & Beal, 1987).

The training session, conducted by the VTPSA staff, covered the central concepts of relapse prevention, interviewing strategies, introducing relapse prevention to clients, working within the treatment model, dealing with lapses in a therapeutic manner, assessing the potential of imminent relapse, and suggestions to enhance relationships with other mental health professionals. Didactic presentations, videotaped interviews, illustrative slides, and case vignettes were employed as training media.

Upon reviewing the narrative, four expert raters reached consensus that 21 risk factors were present. Prior to the workshop, participants correctly identified 38% of the risk factors contained in the disposition summary. On conclusion of the training, an average of 68% of the offense precursors were correctly reported, a statistically significant increase. The percentage of erroneously identified risk factors (6%) did not change. Additional supervised experience after the workshop was expected to further hone participants' skills. Therefore, brief training in the relapse prevention model effectively increased perception of precursive risk factors.

IDENTIFICATION OF RISK FACTORS
THROUGH CLINICAL INTERVIEWS

Evaluation Sequence

* If an interview is to be conducted as part of a complete psychosexual evaluation, it should be the last component of the evaluation. The offender may disclose information during other procedures that the examiner may want to pursue in the interview. If the offender is aware that he has responded to deviant sexual stimuli in a plethysmographic assessment, his responses to questions about sexual fantasies may be more revealing than if the interview had been completed prior to the physiological evaluation. In this fashion, information derived from other assessment procedures may be used to motivate the offender to make greater disclosures during the interview.

Dealing with Denial of Responsibility
during Clinical Interviews

Salter (1988) has observed that denial is not an all-or-none phenomenon, but rather a continuum. One can deny responsibility for an entire offense, acknowledge portions of the offense but disclaim others, refute the frequency with which the abuse purportedly took place, minimize the severity of harm to the victim, attempt to displace responsibility onto the victim, or attribute the act to a drug-altered consciousness.

Regardless of the form that denial takes, treatment for a propensity toward sexual aggression cannot take place until the offender at least acknowledges that the abuse occurred. An individual cannot be helped to deal with a problem until he admits one exists. Therefore, gaining the offender's admission is necessary if an adequate clinical interview is to proceed. We have developed the following methods to assist in gaining the offender's admission during an interview:

1. *Attempt to create a "yes" response set.* Establishing even minor agreements with the offender at an early stage of the interview can foster agreement on more difficult issues later in the session. In this fashion, opposition normally encountered in discussing the offender's abuse history can be minimized.

2. *Demythologize stereotypes about sex offenders.* Society endorses many myths about sexual offenders. The client, as a member of society, also subscribes to these beliefs. Therefore, offenders may be reluctant to admit responsibility, since they believe they will be acknowledging far more than the sexual offense. We dispel these fears with statements such as the following:

"You may have heard, and you may well believe, what society believes about men who have sexually abused children (or raped). You may think that the only people who do things like that are morally bankrupt, emotionally depraved individuals who foam at the mouth as they continually fantasize about sexual abuse and constantly search for the next person they can kidnap and violate.

"I want to let you know that sex offenders usually aren't at all like society's stereotypes of them. I've evaluated hundreds of men who have committed sexual offenses. Some have been outstanding teachers, successful bankers, governors' aides, drug abusers, attorneys, psychologists, and members of the clergy. Most of the men I've met aren't monsters. They're men, who for the most part have led decent lives, but who have a major problem when it comes to their sexual behaviors. The men who commit sexual abuse are men just like you. Some of them choose to make the problem worse by not admitting it exists. Others recognize they need help in order to stop."

3. *Mix confrontations with supportive comments.* "You may have a lot of people who trust you and who think they are your friends. However, they're not really your friends because you have never really allowed anyone to know just who you are. You only permitted them to see the trustworthy side of you. In this way, you created an illusion of friendship that you used to gain sexual access to your victims.

"Throughout most of your life, loss of these 'friendships' never really mattered since you got what you wanted out of it. However, now that your secret is out and all the people who once considered themselves your friends have left you and are wondering if you were trying to set them up, too, you realize, perhaps for the first time, how really alone you are in the world. It can't be easy for you to go through times like this alone. I can imagine that now you wish there was someone you could really trust."

4. *Emphasize relief of acknowledging his secrets.* "It must be difficult for you to go through life being unable to talk with anyone about the secrets you've had to keep all alone. It can't be easy for you to keep your secret 24 hours a day, especially now that you're feeling all alone.

"At the same time, I realize that it could feel risky for you to talk about what you've been doing. Getting started is the hard part. Once you've started it will get easier. In fact, you'll find that it feels good to get all this off your chest. A lot of men have told me that they felt relaxed for the first time in years after talking about what they'd done."

5. *Discuss the strength demonstrated by disclosure.* Many offenders feel inadequate. By describing ability to admit responsibility as a manifestation of personal strength, offenders can be motivated to do so.

"You may think that, if you admit everything you've done to victims over the years, you'll be telling everyone how weak willed you are. But just the opposite is the case. Everyone knows that you've made some mistakes. By taking responsibility for what you've done, you can show yourself and everyone else that you are strong enough to admit your mistakes. Not everyone has that kind of strength. I think you do."

6. *Stress the importance of not making a second mistake.* "You made a mistake that may have lasted no more than a few seconds in time on several occasions. All of us make mistakes. I imagine you'd agree that the worst thing you could do is make the situation worse by making a second mistake by not acknowledging the first one. You have a chance to start changing your life today. Don't blow it."

7. *Make use of strong religious beliefs.* "You mentioned that you are a devout Roman Catholic. I'm aware that your religion is one of the most ancient and that many rituals exist, particularly when it comes to being forgiven for one's sins. All people sin and, fortunately, the church has procedures for absolution. Tell me, in order to be forgiven for your sins, what is the first thing you need to do? So, although you will not be forgiven for your criminal acts by participating in treatment, what do you need to do in order to start clearing your life of this problem?"

8. *Ask "successive approximation" questions.* Offenders may deny that a specific abusive act occurred yet acknowledge that they approximated the act. By leading the offender through successively closer approximations to the act, he may reach the point of admitting it took place. One may also discover that the offender maintains idiosyncratic definitions of abuse. For example, some offenders may deny performing intercourse since they did not ejaculate inside the victim. They examiner may ask:

"You mentioned that you masturbated by rubbing your penis against the back of the victim's thighs. How often did you find yourself sliding your penis up between the victim's buttocks? . . . So you might rub yourself there a bit. How often did you just touch your penis against the victim's anus? . . . I imagine, once there, you probably nudged your penis up against the victim's anus . . . Whenever you nudged it, did it happen to go in just a little?"

9. *Confront contradictions.* The interviewer should confront inconsistencies in the offender's responses and request explanations. Confrontation may reach various levels, from the indirect approach ("There's just one thing I don't understand. Do you remember when you said. . . .") to more direct assertions ("Your story makes no sense. First you said . . . but then you said . . . Just what's the truth here?").

10. *Repeat questions periodically.* Simply repeating questions at various points during the interview often leads offenders to disclose more accurate information about the abuse. Asking several times "How old was Jimmy when you began touching him?" or "How many times did you say you touched Jimmy?" often elicits a younger age for the victim and a greater frequency of abuse than given in the prior response.

Using Information from Record Reviews in Clinical Interviews

Information acquired from the record review may enable specific strategies to be employed during the clinical interview. In one instance, an adolescent male who had abused his younger sister was referred to one of us (W. D. P.) for evaluation. Case files revealed that the diminutive adolescent, who preferred to be called Sly rather than by his given name, Willard, was denying responsibility for the abuse. Sly, whose school records indicated he was frequently picked on for being "puny," apparently had adopted the nickname of his idol, Sylvester Stallone. Based on this background information, the examiner adopted a tough demeanor during the interview, confronting the adolescent with the notion that "it takes a real man" to admit having sexually abused someone. Sly soon acknowledged his responsibility and then revealed his own sexual victimization.

Obviously, case reviews do not always provide such useful information. However, points to be followed up during the interview may be suggested by the record review. For instance, in another case, records revealed that a first-time convicted rapist had (1) committed several breaking-and-entering offenses, (2) moved frequently without apparent reason, (3) been divorced several times, and (4) received a premature, but honorable, discharge from the military service. By following up these issues in the interview, the "first-time" rapist was discovered to have (1) broken into residences at night intending to rape and, whenever the house was unoccupied, taken only feminine undergarments;

(2) changed jobs upon sensing that police suspected him as a rapist or that a victim might be able to identify him, (3) battered his spouses and forced them to submit to sexual acts they regarded as degrading, and (4) attempted to rape several women while in the service but been discharged in lieu of civil or military prosecution. Thus, the first-time-convicted rapist was found to be a compulsive sex offender. Had the record review not been conducted, the offender may have been considered less dangerous than he actually was. Such exploration of informational gaps can yield critical clinical details.

In order to create a relatively comfortable environment that may maximize initial disclosures, we recommend that the interview begin by examining non-threatening topics. Care must be exercised in deciding how to begin the interview. Safe topics are not the same for everyone. While one offender may be totally at ease discussing his educational background, another may view his academic performance as the worst embarrassment of his life. Generally, safe topics can be discerned during the case record review.

During the interview, both process and content issues should be examined. Does the offender openly discuss most issues but become suddenly reticent when his sexual or criminal behaviors are questioned? When summarizing his sexual offense, does the offender become more animated, developing the glazed appearance of complete absorption in an exciting event that he is reliving, or evidence disgust? How socially adept does the individual appear? To what extent does the offender accept responsibility for his sexually aggressive acts (e.g., denies the abuse took place, displaces responsibility onto the victim, accepts factual responsibility for the offense but denies any harm to the victim, minimizes extent of harm, acknowledges physical and emotional trauma)? To what degree does the offender's story correspond to the victim's report of the abuse? Does this person seem always to have been walking on the edge of criminality? How does the offender's affect compare to the topic he is discussing? Are there any periods of time that the offender is reluctant to discuss? How does this individual respond to confrontation, support, or expression of incredulity about aspects of his responses? Each of these observations may yield information important to risk assessment and treatment.

CONCLUSION

Record reviews and clinical interviews are essential elements of a comprehensive assessment. Record reviews enable generation of hypotheses that can be investigated during a clinical interview. Confronting offenders with information from other assessment procedures (e.g., penile plethysmography) is an effective method of countering denial of responsibility. Both procedures can be employed to identify high-risk situations that have precipitated sexual abuse and to gain information about the client's treatment needs.

REFERENCES

Pithers, W. D., Buell, M. M., Kashima, K., Cumming, G., & Beal, L. (1987, May). *Precursors to relapse of sexual offenders.* Paper presented at a meeting of the Association for the Behavioral Treatment of Sexual Abusers, Newport, OR.

Pithers, W. D., Cumming, G. F., Beal, L. S., Young, W., & Turner, R. (1989). Relapse prevention: A method for enhancing behavioral self-management and external supervision of the sexual aggressor. In B. Schwartz (Ed.), *A practioner's guide to treatment of the incarcerated male sex offender* (pp. 121–135). Washington, DC: National Institute of Corrections.

Pithers, W. D., Kashima, K., Cumming, G. F., Beal, L. S., & Buell, M. (1987, January). *Sexual aggression: An addictive process?* Paper presented at the New York Academy of Sciences, New York, NY.

Pithers, W. D., Kashima, K., Cumming, G. F., Beal, L. S., & Buell, M. (1988). Relapse prevention of sexual aggression. In R. Prentky & V. Quinsey (Eds.), *Human sexual aggression: Current perspectives* (pp. 244–260). New York: New York Academy of Sciences.

Salter, A. (1988). *Assessment and treatment of child sexual offenders: A practical guide.* Beverly Hills, CA: Sage.

6

Use of Autobiographies in the Assessment and Treatment of Sex Offenders

J. DAVID LONG
ALICIA WUESTHOFF
WILLIAM D. PITHERS

A thorough evaluation should assess an offender's present and past sexual, criminal, psychological, interpersonal, developmental, and cognitive functioning. This information is often obtained through various sorts of structured interviews, record reviews, formal psychological tests, and physiological measures of sexual arousal.

In assessing sex offenders we also find it useful to include an assignment requiring offenders to write an autobiographical essay. A tool requiring clients to reflect on themselves and their behaviors, an autobiography offers a foundation for the identification and evaluation of significant life events (Groth, 1983). In contrast to many other assessment devices, writing an autobiography requires the client to assume a responsible role in examining his own behaviors and sets the stage for treatment that relies on the client to become his own agent of control (Marlatt, 1985a).

The material generated in an autobiography depends entirely on the client's phenomenological world. A client's view of his strengths, difficulties, life experiences, goals, and values improves our understanding of what he views as important and assists in identification of problem areas in need of therapeutic attention.

In order to expeditiously obtain relevant clinical information, most assessment techniques focus on identification of deviant characteristics. In contrast, the absence of a strong deviance focus in this task promotes an understanding of the broader life context of sexual offenses, including the more positive aspects of a person's experience. This provides clients an opportunity to reveal information about themselves under less anxiety-provoking conditions, resulting in increased disclosure of relevant clinical data from resistant clients.

Autobiographical tasks are used to address a variety of assessment and treatment concerns. One sex offender treatment program finds that an autobiography task orients offenders to the group treatment process by familiarizing them with each other and by making them aware that their histories are not unique (Knopp, 1984). Marlatt (1985b) conceptualizes the autobiography task as the best means of obtaining information about self-image factors that can contribute to the increased likelihood of recurrence of an undesirable behavior.

We have found that, in the initial phases of treatment, clients are often quite confused about the process of group therapy. The autobiography task presents a structured introduction to group therapy and organizes the initial treatment activity of both clients and therapists. It also demonstrates to clients that therapy will not consist of their passive participation in something akin to a "class" but rather will require their active involvement.

PROCEDURE

The autobiographical assignment[1] is adaptable for use during various phases of assessment and treatment. It can be assigned prior to treatment and used in conjunction with other assessment devices to direct therapy. Used in this manner, reviewing the essay with the client often elicits additional information, further clarification, and a reconsideration of purposefully distorted or missing information.

We have found it most useful to assign this task shortly after the inception of group treatment. At this point, a client's curiosity is often piqued, and there may exist a strong desire on his part to answer the question "Why did I commit this reprehensible act?" The autobiography task may be viewed as a safe means of beginning to explore this question. Since some clients may not be so ready to disclose information early in treatment, they should be instructed to continually revise their autobiography throughout the therapeutic process.

Clients are informed that the objectives of the autobiography task include their (1) learning more about themselves and others; (2) becoming better able to reflect on their own lives, identifying both positive and negative aspects of their experiences; (3) becoming more aware of their strengths and coping skills; and (4) identifying both long-standing and more immediate factors that contributed to their deviant behavior. They are asked to consider beliefs, emotional states, experiences, and behaviors that increased the likelihood of their offending.

Questions are posed about the client's upbringing and functioning over the years. Clients are also asked to discuss significant events in their lives and their

[1]The autobiography task discussed in this chapter is available from J. David Long, Rutland Mental Health Services, 78 South Main Street, Rutland VT 05701.

feelings, roles, behaviors, and interactions with others surrounding these events. Descriptions of their goals and values are also requested. The content of the questions is designed to give clients an opportunity to emphasize those experiences that they view as important.

Initially, we did not specifically ask clients to discuss their offenses in the autobiography task, since we assigned another structured task to elicit descriptions of the immediate antecedents and consequences of offending behaviors. However, clients often chose to discuss their offenses and the subsequent criminal proceedings, and we now include questions about these. In retrospect, it does not seem at all surprising that offenders were somewhat preoccupied with their arrests and convictions, given the immediacy of those experiences.

Autobiography writing may be delivered as a single assignment or broken up into several discrete tasks. Responding to a few questions at a time can prove less overwhelming for clients, particularly if their writing skills are limited. The essay written as a whole, though, enables clients to better consider the relationships and sequences among the events about which they write.

Once returned, assignments are reviewed by therapists, who formulate additional questions. Each client then recites his autobiography in group. Group members are encouraged to ask questions, provide feedback, and identify beliefs, values, emotional states, and circumstances that have played significant roles in their own lives or have contributed to their own sexual offenses. This discussion further educates group members about the relapse prevention model by providing numerous concrete examples of apparently irrelevant decisions and risk factors.

As they become identified, risk factors are listed on newsprint and displayed on walls of the group-therapy room in subsequent sessions. These lists function as visual aids to assist clients in committing their risk factors to memory. They are referred to and amended throughout the course of treatment.

It is not uncommon for clients to be unresponsive to some questions included in the task. Discussion in the group session assists clarification as to whether their unresponsiveness is due to a lack of understanding, insufficient information, avoidance, guilt, or denial. The disclosures and confronting questions of other group members are quite helpful in this regard.

Clients are often asked to do additional work on areas of their essays that they have not completed to the satisfaction of other group members and group leaders. This process is aided by modeling those individuals who have done the task well and by the "permission" given to uncomfortable clients by those who can frankly discuss their deviant thoughts and behaviors.

Inability to write need not preclude the completion of this assignment. Clients who cannot write are encouraged to ask for help from other group members, family, or friends. Their requests for assistance frequently facilitate communication at home about issues that have never been discussed. They may also use a tape recorder to dictate their autobiographies. In addition, we make referrals to adult basic education for evaluation and tutoring of those clients who have skill deficits in reading or writing.

IDENTIFICATION OF RISK FACTORS

The autobiographical essay, as well as subsequent presentation and discussion of the essay in group treatment, provides a wealth of information about the beliefs, attitudes, feeling states, and behaviors that play a role in offending and increase the probability of reoffense. One rather frequent finding has been the presence of negative emotional states preceding offenses (Pithers, Marques, Gibat, & Marlatt, 1983). Men who have committed sex offenses often describe antecedent feelings of loneliness, worthlessness, depression, anger, or resentment, as well as discomfort with expressing those emotions.

The initial focus of offenders is often on those risk factors that are the most concrete, external, and proximal to abuse. These are generally circumstances over which they have the least control and, therefore, feel the least responsible. Offenders also have an easier time accepting responsibility for the sexually abusive act itself than for all the planning and setting up of situations that preceded it.

For instance, being alone with a child is readily recognized as a high-risk situation by many child molesters. Their initial conception of a relevant coping strategy often consists of avoiding situations in which they are alone with children. Although avoidance strategies are supported as short-term interventions, pedophiles frequently observe that children are everywhere and that such situations cannot always be circumvented.

Clients are encouraged to develop a more thorough understanding of risk factors by attending less to situational variables and more to those over which they can gain control. They are instructed to examine the way in which their behaviors, beliefs, and attitudes have led to sexual abuse of children. For example, substance use may be discovered to have played a direct role in the relapse process (impairing judgment and disinhibiting behavior) as well as indirectly contributing to offending by magnifying such negative emotional states as depression.

Autobiographies also reveal the false beliefs and distortions that offenders so often evidence (Carnes, 1983). These cognitions can rationalize or justify sexually abusive behavior in a number of ways. Some beliefs create psychological distance (such as when clients think that coercive sexual activity that does not involve violent physical force is not harmful or painful). Others might represent a minimizing of the degree of forethought ("I didn't think about it; it just happened") or an overestimation of the extent to which an addictive behavior is under control ("This will be the last time").

"Apparently irrelevant decisions" (AIDs) (Pithers et al., 1983) often come to light in the autobiographical essay. These are steps taken by offenders that result in their setting up high-risk situations with seemingly little awareness of the implications for relapse. There is a nondeviant motive (the route to work with the favorite coffee stop . . .) that conceals a deviant one (. . . also happens to go past a playground). Because these decisions will often be repeated many times in an offender's lifetime, the autobiography is particularly useful for bringing to light the patterns involved and their relationship to deviant behaviors.

EARLY ANTECEDENTS

In addition to its utility in assessing specific high-risk attitudes, beliefs, and behaviors, a client-generated autobiography can prove useful in identifying more pervasive, long-standing personality characteristics. These early antecedents appear to predispose toward, or reflect, problems in life generally rather than precipitate sexually abusive behaviors in particular. They may be the result of conditions encountered during early developmental periods (e.g., familial alcoholism, physical abuse) or adulthood (e.g., divorce, physical impairment).

For example, an individual's sense of self-esteem is often reflected in both his responses to the autobiographical questions and in his attitude toward the task itself. We have found that individuals who hold themselves in low esteem, as many child molesters do (Panton, 1978; Pithers, Kashima, Cumming, Beal, & Beull, 1988), have particular difficulty completing this task. However, disdain for oneself is seldom fully generalized. Use of broad content in autobiographical questions, rather than a narrow focus on solely criminal and sexual behaviors, fosters assessment of the variations in an individual's self-esteem across a variety of situations or roles. The client describes not only how he feels about himself generally but also how he regards himself as an employee, a father, a husband, or a friend.

Descriptions of social experiences often shed light on clients' attitudes about interpersonal relationships and about their self-efficacy. Sex offenders in general, and child molesters in particular, are noted for their social-skills deficiencies and inordinate fear of negative evaluations by others (Overholser & Beck, 1986). In assessing the offender's perceptions, we ask a number of questions. Does he tend toward insular activities? Does he value spending time with others? Does anyone hold importance in his life? Has the influence of others been experienced primarily in negative or positive terms? Are there differences in the way he describes interactions with children, same-sex adults, and opposite-sex adults?

The autobiography also reveals features of personality style. To what extent are clients preoccupied with meeting their own needs at the expense of others? How much are they able to disclose about themselves? To what extent is the writer able to reveal successes and failures, and what is the relative emphasis? Do clients see themselves as having the power to influence significant moments of their lives, or do they view themselves as the victims of events beyond their control?

It is important to include questions relating to the individual's own history of sexual and physical victimization because of the frequency of these experiences among sex offenders (Groth & Burgess, 1979; Pithers et al., 1988) and because of the profound impact these experiences may have on a person's view of himself (Becker, Skinner, & Abel, 1983; Groth, Hobson, & Gary, 1982). The autobiography gives access not only to the events as the offender–victim experienced them but also to the way in which he has understood himself in light of those experiences.

The relative emphasis that a writer places on various aspects of his life can also yield valuable insights into his phenomenology. Some offenders are preoccupied with recent events, such as their offenses, arrest, and conviction, and with conveying their version of these events. Descriptions of these events enable clinicians to determine if a client's apparent remorse reflects an increased awareness of the victim's trauma or his own humiliation at the public revelation of his offense. Other clients are more concerned with understanding or conveying their childhood experiences or their difficulties in adult relationships. Career criminals may organize significant life events around offenses for which they were incarcerated at the time. Fixated pedophiles may describe interactions with children more enthusiastically than those with adults.

TREATMENT ASPECTS

While the autobiography task is typically employed primarily for assessment purposes, our procedure requires clients to read and discuss their autobiographies in the treatment group. The utility of the autobiography task as a structured group activity has been noted by others (Adkins, Taber, & Russo, 1985; Silver, 1976). We concur with their observation that having group members present autobiographies orally within group sessions can have beneficial treatment effects. As they have noted, this procedure enhances development of what Yalom (1975) labeled the "curative factors" in group therapy. For example, clients become aware that they are not alone in their unacceptable impulses or aberrant behaviors. As a result, they are more likely to accept ownership of, and learn to deal with, these problems.

Because writing an autobiography requires self-reflection, the task also represents an opportunity to enhance self-monitoring skills, which are crucial to relapse prevention treatment procedures (MacDonald & Pithers, Chapter 7, this volume; Marlatt, 1985c). Looking at their experiences from a historical perspective, clients learn to appreciate that their offenses have antecedents and consequences. After writing and rewriting their responses following the advice, feedback, and confrontation of other group members, clients generally improve their self-monitoring skills. Inability to perform satisfactorily on this sort of task may be predictive of a poor outcome in relapse prevention treatment.

Group discussion of the autobiography provides an opportunity for clients to integrate their offending behavior into the context of a whole life. This is not to say that clients are permitted to avoid discussion of the specific problems that brought them into treatment. Rather, we believe it is also important for offenders to become more aware of, and make better use of, those aspects of their functioning that are positive and adaptive.

Like all group activities, oral presentation of an autobiography is an opportunity for a group member to increase his awareness of his interpersonal functioning and social skills. This group process has both an assessment role, as members become more aware of how they and others function in a group, and a treatment role, as individuals are encouraged, by other group members and leaders, to improve their facility for discussing their own lives and relating their views and experiences to those of other group members.

The response of group members to the autobiographical information presented by other members is often quite revealing. Some clients appear preoccupied with the lives of others and less willing to discuss their own. This may appear to be a demonstration of compassion; however, in many cases, it represents avoidance of personal issues or issues related to their offenses. Others seem, for the most part, to take no interest in the experiences of their fellow group members. These individuals often stress the differences between themselves and other group members. Such posturing may manifest a desire to remain isolated from the group or represent a belief that other group members are more disordered.

Special note is taken of the way in which offenders respond to descriptions of the abuse of other group members. We make a point of encouraging all members to express their thoughts and feelings at these times, and we carefully observe the degree to which other offenders are able to empathize with the experience of the presenter. If the capacity for empathy appears diminished, offenders are made aware of that fact and of the relationship between their lack of empathy and their likelihood of victimizing.

Our use of the autobiography task as a homework assignment and group activity in the early phases of treatment, rather than during a pretreatment evaluation, challenges the offender to begin immediately to make use of the products of his own reflections, as well as the observations of other group members and therapists. In a concrete and personally meaningful way, the client is made aware of many of the issues he will need to address during the rest of his treatment. He may have already begun to put into practice appropriate coping strategies based on the feedback he receives. He has now become informed as to the process and expectations of treatment, and is thus more prepared for the task that remains.

REFERENCES

Adkins, B. J., Taber, J. I., & Russo, A. M. (1985). The spoken autobiography: A powerful tool in group psychotherapy. *Social Work, 30,* 435–439.

Becker, J. V., Skinner, L. J., & Abel, G. G. (1983). Sequelae of sexual assault: The survivor's perspective. In J. G. Greer & I. R. Stuart (Eds.), *The sexual aggressor: Current perspectives on treatment* (pp. 240–266). New York: Van Nostrand Reinhold.

Carnes, P. J. (1983). *Out of the shadows: Understanding sexual addiction.* Minneapolis: CompCare Publications.

Groth, A. N. (1983). Treatment of the sexual offender in a correctional institution. In J. G. Greer & I. R. Stuart (Eds.), *The sexual aggressor: Current perspectives on treatment* (pp. 160–176). New York: Van Nostrand Reinhold.

Groth, A. N., & Burgess, A. W. (1979). Sexual trauma in the life histories of rapists and child molesters. *Victimology, 4,* 10–16.

Groth, A. N., Hobson, W., & Gary, T. (1982). The child molester: Clinical observations. *Journal of Social Work and Human Sexuality, 1,* 129–144.

Knopp, F. H. (1984). *Retraining adult sex offenders: Methods and models.* Syracuse, NY: Safer Society Press.

Marlatt, G. A. (1985a). Relapse prevention: Theoretical rationale and overview of the model. In G. A. Marlatt & J. R. Gordon (Eds.), *Relapse prevention* (pp. 3–70). New York: Guilford.

Marlatt, G. A. (1985b). Cognitive assessment and intervention procedures for relapse prevention. In G. A. Marlatt & J. R. Gordon (Eds.), *Relapse prevention* (pp. 201–279). New York: Guilford.

Marlatt, G. A. (1985c). Situational determinants of relapse and skill-training interventions. In G. A. Marlatt & J. R. Gordon (Eds.), *Relapse prevention* (pp. 71–127). New York: Guilford.

Overholser, J. C., & Beck, S. (1986). Multimethod assessment of rapists, child molesters, and three control groups on behavioral and psychological measures. *Journal of Consulting and Clinical Psychology, 54,* 682–687.

Panton, J. H. (1978). Personality differences appearing between rapists of adults, rapists of children, and non-violent sexual molesters of children. *Research Communications in Psychology, Psychiatry and Behavior, 3,* 385–393.

Pithers, W. D., Kashima, K. M., Cumming, G. F., Beal, L. S., & Buell, M. M. (1988). Relapse prevention of sexual aggression. In R. A. Prentley & V. L. Quinsey (Eds.), *Human sexual aggression: Current perspectives* (pp. 244–260). New York: Annals of the New York Academy of Sciences.

Pithers, W. D., Marques, J. K., Gibat, C. C., & Marlatt, G. A. (1983). Relapse prevention with sexual aggressives: A self-control model of treatment and maintenance of change. In J. G. Greer & I. R. Stuart (Eds.), *The sexual aggressor: Current perspectives on treatment* (pp. 214–239). New York: Van Nostrand Reinhold.

Silver, S. N. (1976). Outpatient treatment for sexual offenders. *Social Work, 21,* 134–140.

Yalom, I. D. (1975). *The theory and practice of group psychotherapy* (2nd ed.). New York: Basic Books.

7

Self-Monitoring to Identify
High-Risk Situations

RITA K. MacDONALD
WILLIAM D. PITHERS

Identification of high-risk situations is an essential component of relapse prevention. Information about offense precursors can be obtained through several assessment strategies: (1) review of case records, which reveal information about offense characteristics and historical antecedents, (2) thorough interviews, which elicit information about the offender's cognitive and emotional state before, during, and after his offenses, and (3) penile plethysmography, which yields information about the extent to which the offense may have been motivated by excessive sexual interest in children or a fusion of sexuality and violence. These procedures build an excellent foundation for thorough assessment but yield information that is static in time, reflecting the way things *were* at some moment in time. Although skilled evaluators can make inferences about an offender's risk factors based on this information, assessment is incomplete at this point. Comprehensive assessment of risk must include an understanding of the offender's current, ongoing, internal processes.

Knowing that a rapist was angry at the time of his offense does not provide sufficient information to direct treatment. It is essential to know the types of frustrations that provoke his anger and what he does to cope with that emotion. Does he even recognize that he is angry? What self-statements does he employ, and how do they modify his experience? Does being angry enable him to feel powerful, or does it frighten him? Each of many possible answers to such questions holds different implications.

By training an offender to monitor his negative emotional states, deviant fantasies, and thoughts about offending, one can ascertain elements of an offender's day-to-day reality that promote relapse. Self-monitoring provides a very powerful means of access to an offender's cognitive and emotional processes. While many assessment procedures yield highly abstract information that may have little meaning to an offender, information obtained by self-

96

monitoring is concrete. Since self-monitoring records are created by the client, they contain only information that he regards as meaningful.

Any meaningful form of assessment is, in itself, therapeutic, and self-monitoring capitalizes on this interrelationship. Learning to observe cognitive, affective, and behavioral patterns across situations can enhance an offender's self-management abilities.

PREPARATION FOR SELF-MONITORING

Self-monitoring is a very simple strategy. Some clients learn the strategies in a single session. Others require repeated instructions or direct assistance. Careful preparation enhances a client's ability to benefit from the process. A client's motivation to learn the procedure can be heightened by telling him that the process will teach him a powerful system with which to understand himself.

SELF-MONITORING PROCEDURES

Journals of daily events are used to develop hypotheses about circumstances leading to problematic behaviors. Thus a client may discover that the comfort he experiences by isolating himself from others is, in reality, a precursor to his deviant fantasies and offenses. Once offense precursors have been identified through journals of daily events, clients can begin to monitor the occurrence of these specific risk factors.

Many types of self-monitoring devices exist, ranging from mechanical counters to elaborate behavioral diaries. When choosing among these systems, the therapist should consider ease of use, simplicity, and compatibility with the behavior being monitored. Easily used systems lead to more frequent and consistent observations, particularly among cognitively impaired clients. The monitoring procedure must be compatible with the behavior of interest in order for data to be clinically useful. In assessing precursors to sexual aggression, emotional, cognitive, and behavioral *processes* are monitored. For this reason, narrative records are recommended.

Narrative Self-Monitoring

A highly structured format is recommended initially to teach the client to detect the moods, fantasies, planning, and behaviors that predispose toward sexual abuse. Clients are instructed to carry a pocket-sized notebook at all times. Inside the front cover is a list of cues that help the client recognize experiences that should be recorded. Also listed are several questions that help clients identify situational and personal variables that precede occurrence of risk factors.

Research has demonstrated that negative affective states, deviant sexual fantasies, and planning represent three major precursors to sexual abuse (Pithers, Kashima, Cumming, Beal, & Buell, 1987, 1988). These internal events are the focus of self-monitoring.

Whenever a precursive emotion, fantasy, thought, or behavior is experienced, a brief notation is made in the pocket-sized notebook. This entry need not be greatly detailed, but it should include sufficient cues to facilitate recall of that information later. These notations can be accomplished quickly without attracting attention.

At the end of each day, more detailed accounts of these events are written in a daily journal. Included should be the date, time, antecedent events and mood, a description of the event (e.g., content, duration, affect), and mood after the event. (Clients who cannot write may record the information on audiotapes). One event may involve the interaction of several precursors. For example, an offender may become angry at a female, use self-statements to heighten the emotion, and attempt to cope with his affect by masturbating to a rape fantasy. Each element should be appropriately and separately labeled in the margin as either emotion, fantasy, thought, or behavior. This process enhances the client's differentiation of his internal states.

Clients are instructed to set aside a regularly scheduled half hour to complete this process. Clients are asked to spend a few minutes during that half hour thinking about their entries to make sure they have included all the important information. They are also requested to speculate about the relationship of these elements, encouraging self-evaluation. A half-hour time limit is recommended, however, so that the task does not become so cumbersome that it is neglected.

The incidental method of recording information may not be appropriate in some cases. Some clients initially overlook many occurrences of significant events, since they either are unaccustomed to watching for them or are passively resisting. For those clients, a more structured approach is helpful initially. Such clients are asked to make entries at several specified times each day and to record any significant experiences that have occurred. This is a more intrusive system of information gathering and thus is less likely to be maintained for long periods, but once the habit of self-monitoring is established, scheduled writing can be replaced with incidental recording.

SELF-MONITORING OF
NEGATIVE AFFECTIVE STATES

Dealing with Resistance to Monitoring of Emotion

Sexual aggressors often experience a great deal of fear when asked to attend to unpleasant emotions. At the beginning of therapy this is seldom expressed as fear but more often as an angry resistance, a blustering insistence that they do not have those feelings, or a more passive stance of confusion or inability to remember emotions. It is helpful for the therapist to see beyond that anger or passivity and to keep in mind the fear that motivates these defenses. Unless that fear is dealt with, the client's self-monitoring is likely to be superficial and incomplete.

The reasons for that fear are easily understood after even a cursory review of an offender's history. Many offenders come from extremely chaotic, dysfunctional families in which the expression of emotion was distorted and often used coercively. Offenders with this background view emotions with fear, for they have experienced them as weapons of manipulation. Negative emotional states may be constant for them, leaving them unable to discriminate any change in their emotional state. For other offenders, "normal" may have been defined as having everything, including emotions, tightly under control. For these individuals, any emotion is frightening, for they have equated affect with chaos and loss of control. In families in which the goal has been rigid control, the experience of emotion represents failure. Offenders from these sorts of families have not experienced emotions as tools for intimacy, trust, communication, or problem solving.

Many offenders experience the world as divided into two groups—victims and aggressors. They perceive emotional statements as attacks and conceptualize the process of communication as a battle to be won. Disclosing emotion becomes a traitorous act that provides top-secret information to an enemy, and the experience of emotion becomes aversive because of its association with combat and failure.

An additional reason for offenders' fears of emotion is that, despite occasional protestation, they understand very clearly the connection between negative emotion and sexual aggression. Often when angry, lonely, or worried, they have fantasized about sexual aggression to gain momentary escape from these emotions. This connection may seem automatic to them. Offenders may fear that allowing themselves to actually experience emotions could result in a loss of self-control.

Dealing with these fears is very important if the offender is to be enlisted as an active partner in his assessment. Offenders are encouraged to consider their ability to cope with fear as a sign of therapeutic progress and personal strength. Maintaining a stance of active collaboration assists clients in overcoming fears, while extreme confrontation is usually not effective. Journeys into unexplored areas seem less frightening when clinicians are viewed as traveling companions rather than as mule drivers.

Analysis of any affective state can be broken down into three components—emotion, physical sensation, and cognition. Special problems encountered in self-monitoring of these three components of emotion are presented below.

Negative Affective States: Emotional Component

Therapists can begin to prepare clients for the self-monitoring of negative affect by explaining that they are going to talk briefly about the idea of uncomfortable emotions.

> We're going to talk about the ways in which people feel bad sometimes. That's important in understanding why people sexually abuse others. We know that nobody does those things because he feels good; there's always some bad feeling happening. We're going to start to learn what that was like for you.

If clients show resistance to this initial effort, a therapist acting as an active collaborator can utilize that information by reframing it as compliance and moving on to the next step.

> I'm glad that you're able to show me so clearly that you're hesitant to do this. That tells me that you can express your emotions pretty clearly and that you already understand a lot of what we'll be talking about. I'm not surprised that you're cautious. A lot of people are uncertain about how to do this. Let's put "uncertainty" on the list.

> I understand what you mean when you say you don't remember what you felt and that you were confused. Bad feelings are hard sometimes, and they're so upsetting that we often feel mixed up and confused. Those are bad feelings right there. Let's put them on the list. And how does it feel to not remember? We can put that down too.

The therapist should list whatever negative emotions the client can think of and then help the client augment the list. Any negative emotions he has discussed in his interview should be added. Examples of various situations can be pulled from his history, or made up, and the offender can be asked "How would someone feel in this case?" If he is unable to answer, the presentation of forced choice may be helpful initially.

> Just about all feelings come under four headings: mad, sad, glad, and scared. Which one do you think someone would feel in this situation?

Clients should be complimented on any effort to augment their lists. The goal during the assessment phase is not to have a list that is perfectly logical or exhaustive but to initiate a process within the offender. At this point, the work consists of instilling a desire for self-exploration. The therapist's job is to begin to teach a new attitude toward emotions.

> I'm glad you could add to your list. Emotions give us a way of connecting with people around us and of feeling alive. Imagine someone who could only feel two emotions. He would be like a robot most of the time.

If the therapist can instill a desire for self-awareness, the client will be much more involved and effective when self-monitoring begins.

Negative Affective States: Physical Component

Some clients may approach the experience of emotion by recognizing physical sensations. If this is the client's strongest mode of experience, it is helpful to begin there.

As with the emotional component of affect, it is good to begin with the client's current level of understanding and then to expand on that. After giving an example involving stress and shoulder tension (an experience known to most individuals), the therapist can choose an emotion that the client has already identified and ask where the client usually feels that in his body. Therapist and client can then go through various body parts, systems, and muscle groups to help identify other negative emotions. This exercise may help a client to identify emotions he had not previously been aware of or to identify additional cues to familiar emotions. The therapist can ask questions such as:

> What sorts of feelings could you have in your forehead? What might cause those? Is there anything you could do with your teeth to indicate the emotion? How about your neck? Your chest? Your breathing? Shoulders? Fists? Stomach?

Some clients may be very unaware of physical sensations. For some of these, just initiating the discussion will cause increased awareness. Others may require guided muscle relaxation so that they can begin to discriminate between tension and relaxation.

Negative Affective States: Cognitive Component

This is the most complex part of preparing clients to self-monitor negative affect, especially for those clients who have trouble distinguishing between thought and emotion and who relate what they think when asked what they feel. Understanding this aspect of emotionality can greatly augment an individual's self-awareness.

The cognitive component of emotion can be described as self-statements that reveal emotions. For example, an offender may think that he is handling a conflict without becoming angry. However, he finds himself thinking "Why did he have to bring that up in front of all these people?" The irritated, almost querulous, tone of that question indicates that the offender is feeling something about what the other individual did. Other examples include thinking "I really need . . ." instead of "I really want . . . ," indicating a sense of desperation or, perhaps, entitlement; or describing oneself as "hurt" instead of "sad," indicating that some expectation or assumption was not met and that there is an element of anger involved over having been injured or slighted.

Other cognitive clues to emotion can be derived from an examination of word choice. Clients who revert to calling adult females "girls" after they have learned the correct word are obviously experiencing something related to women. Similarly, clients who begin to speak to other individuals as "them" or "those caseworkers" are expressing some emotion by that depersonalization.

A simple way for a therapist to teach this sort of self-monitoring is to comment on those choices in word, tone, and self-statements whenever there is evidence of their occurrence. As clients sharpen their skills in this area, they become aware of subtle nuances of emotion they had not previously experienced.

SELF-MONITORING OF FANTASY

When self-monitoring of fantasy is discussed, it is from the standpoint that deviant fantasies are occurring or will occur. The therapist's stance is:

> You'll have these, of course, because you have not learned yet to handle some of the difficult emotions you experience, and these fantasies have been a way to make difficult situations feel better.

The expectation that fantasies are occurring or will occur reinforces the initial work done to prevent the abstinence violition effect (Marlatt & Gordon, 1985, Pithers, Marques, Gibat, & Marlatt, 1983). This stance encourages offenders to take an objective view of fantasy, and to view it as a reaction to certain feelings, and to begin to dissociate themselves from the fantasy material.

As in the preparation for other components of self-monitoring, clients are asked their current understanding about the concept to be monitored. Clients often deny having sexual fantasies. That response can be incorporated into teaching statements:

> I'm glad you recognize that you don't have any sexual fantasies that are long, drawn-out, movie-like scenarios. Many people think that's what fantasies are. However, people usually experience fantasies as brief flashes or images or ideas, things that come and go very quickly.

An important element in preparation to monitor sexual fantasies is to dispel the myth that only long, movie-like scenarios count as fantasies. If a client waits to report fantasy material until it is that extensive, he has already experienced a lapse. Self-monitoring of fantasy is designed to detect the very early occurrence of change in fantasy material, and therefore the preparation focuses on encouraging clients to report fantasy elements.

You see the little girl by the swing-set and notice the sun shining on her red hair. You see how shiny it is and think about how warm it must be from the sun. It looks soft. That's a fantasy. You notice something specific, begin to think about it, and find your thoughts drifting. You begin imagining something about what you're seeing. That's a fantasy.

You see a woman walking toward you. You notice the movement of her breasts and wonder, just for a second, what she would look like without her blouse. That's a fantasy, even though it only lasted for a few seconds.

SELF-MONITORING OF OFFENSE PLANNING

The concept of teaching clients to monitor and report small elements rather than whole scenarios applies to the self-monitoring of offense planning also. It is important to teach clients to report these elements as soon as they occur. If they wait until the plan has achieved the status of a step-by-step scenario, they are much closer to relapse than if they had reported their initial thoughts.

Preparation starts with eliciting a client's description of the process of planning his offense. Again, even a negative response can be utilized to ally with an offender and elicit his participation.

I understand that when you say you didn't plan your offense you mean that you didn't have a step-by-step plan worked out. I'm glad you understand that. Most plans are not like that. Plans often consist of quick little ideas that come and go. They may not seem connected in any conscious way. I'm sure you'll remember some of the little bits and pieces you experienced as we discuss this.

Clients are then given information about what sorts of information the therapist is looking for.

A good example of what I mean is a rapist who is arguing with a woman. He just happens to notice that they're all alone and that there is no one else in the building. That's an element of a plan. I'm sure you can see that the addition of just a few more pieces would make that a full-fledged rape scenario. Each of those pieces is an element of a plan.

You see the little boy in the parking lot. He's by himself. You find yourself scanning the parking lot, looking for adults. That's part of a plan.

The maintenance of an objective stance is essential in self-monitoring elements of planning. Any sense of alarm can lead clients to experience the abstinence violation effect. Clients may learn that brief flashes of this sort occur when certain emotional states are experienced and that the goal is to deal with them effectively by talking about them when they occur.

CONCLUSION

Self-monitoring is a powerful assessment tool that can provide vital information about an offender's emotional and cognitive processes on an ongoing basis. There is no magic in the actual procedure. However, encouraging clients to become active investigators of their own processes, as well as teaching them the importance of noting and reporting as many small elements of negative affect, deviant fantasy, and elements of offense planning as possible, can have great benefits. Only the offender himself can know his own emotional and cognitive experience. It is essential that treatment personnel gain access to as much of that information as possible.

Information obtained through effective self-monitoring is essential to understanding an offender's daily reality. This information enables the offender and his therapist to develop a comprehensive view of the operation of risk factors in his daily life. That understanding is essential to the development of effective relapse prevention strategies for sexual aggressors.

REFERENCES

Marlatt, G. A., & Gordon, J. R. (Eds.). (1985). *Relapse prevention.* New York: Guilford.

Pithers, W. D., Kashima, K., Cumming, G. F., Beal, L. S., & Buell, M. (1987, January). *Sexual aggression: An addictive process?* Paper presented at the New York Academy of Sciences, New York, NY.

Pithers, W. D., Kashima, K., Cumming, G. F., Beal, L. S., & Buell, M. (1988). Relapse prevention of sexual aggression. In R. Prentky & V. Quinsey (Eds.), *Human sexual aggression: Current perspectives* (pp. 244–260). New York: New York Academy of Sciences.

Pithers, W. D., Marques, J. K., Gibat, C. C., & Marlatt, G. A. (1983). Relapse prevention with sexual aggressives: A self-control model of treatment and maintenance of change. In J. G. Greer & I. R. Stuart (Eds.), *The sexual aggressor: Current perspectives on treatment* (pp. 214–239). New York: Van Nostrand Reinhold.

8

Direct Monitoring by
Penile Plethysmography

D. RICHARD LAWS

To this point we have considered various ways to assess high risk for sex offenders through clinical interviews, analysis of clinical and criminal records,
autobiography, and self-monitoring. Despite their obvious utility, most of these
sources of information are open to influence by the client, who may use them to
diminish and minimize his involvement in deviant sexual activity.

Pithers and Laws (1989) recently described the problem:

> [T]he sexual aggressor has not entered therapy on his own accord in an effort to
> diminish feelings of distress. More typically, sexual offenders reluctantly seek
> therapy after their abuse of others has been discovered by authority figures or
> significant others. Often, the offender views his disorder as problematic solely
> because it led to his arrest, conviction, and imprisonment. For such individuals,
> leaving prison and treatment as soon as possible, rather than achieving attitud-
> inal and behavioral change, represent the goals of therapy. Due to these
> characteristics, the sexual aggressor's self-report may be a particularly suspect
> measure of change.
>
> Since many sexual aggressors prefer not to accurately describe their deviant
> sexual interests, therapists must have access to an evaluative procedure that
> objectively and reliably measures an individual's sexual arousal pattern (p. 83).

SEXUAL AROUSAL MEASUREMENT

That evaluative procedure is called penile plethysmography, or phallometry, a
technology used to measure the erectile response in males (Rosen & Keefe,
1978). Technically, plethysmography is defined as the use of an instrument for
"determining and registering variations in the size of an organ or limb"
(*Webster's Unabridged Dictionary*, 1971, p. 1740). In the procedure, the client

attaches an electronic sensor, called a penile transducer (Bancroft, Jones, & Pullan, 1966; Barlow, Becker, Leitenberg, & Agras, 1970; Laws, 1977), around the shaft of his penis. The sensor detects changes in the size of the organ from a state of complete flaccidity to one of complete engorgement. Erotic stimuli, usually in the form of slides or audiotaped descriptions of deviant and nondeviant sexual behavior, are presented to the client while his erection response is measured. Clients respond more to some stimuli than others, and these measured differential amplitudes of response give an indication of his sexual interests and preferences (Laws & Osborn, 1983). The technology is primarily used in two ways: (1) to assess deviant and nondeviant interests prior to and following treatment and (2) to periodically index progress in treatment (i.e., successful treatment should produce a decline in deviant sexual arousal).

Many researchers and clinicians believe that the erectile response is a highly powerful measure for purposes of assessment and treatment. This is particularly so when it is used in conjunction with other data, such as card sorts (Laws, 1986) and psychometric devices intended for use with sexual deviants (Langevin, 1983; Nichols & Molinder, 1984), as well as self-reports of urges, sexual fantasies, frequency of masturbation, and content of masturbatory fantasies. Recent evaluative research has shown that penile plethysmography possesses psychometric properties that equal or exceed those shown for traditional measurement techniques (Murphy & Barbaree, 1988).

It is my belief that penile plethysmography is an essential component of an effective sex offender treatment program. In this chapter pre- and posttreatment assessment results are reported, but the primary focus is on the utility of plethysmography as a treatment progress indicator. Sometimes, even when used in conjunction with clinical and self-report measures that show changes in the desired direction, plethysmographic measures will reveal that one of the core elements of a deviant sexual orientation—deviant sexual fantasy and arousal— is not being affected by the treatment program. In the absence of this measure, then, spurious conclusions regarding the effectiveness of treatment might be made. This chapter is a report of such a case.

CASE STUDY

The Client

The client was a 30-year-old white male, divorced, unemployed, and disabled. He referred himself for treatment due to depression and suicidal ideation. The depression, purportedly related to deviant sexual fantasies about teenage boys, had become so severe that he had attempted to shoot himself. He succeeded only in wounding himself, causing no neurological impairment. These suicidal gestures had been evident for the preceding 10 years. As a child, he had been physically and emotionally abused by his parents. During his teens he engaged in infrequent homosexual encounters with peers. He successfully completed 2 years of college but was unable to maintain a job as an auto mechanic. At the time he presented for treatment he reported an inability to sleep, poor appetite although he was overweight, and thoughts of suicide. He ruminated constantly about sex with teenage boys. He showed some insight into his problems and possessed good intellectual ability and good verbal skills. At the time he was first seen, existing diagnoses were major depression, recurrent; and pedophilia (fantasy).

The Treatment Program

The treatment regime that the client experienced is reported in more detail later by Jenkins-Hall, Osborn, Anderson, Anderson, and Shockley-Smith (Chapter 23, this volume). He first experienced 20 weeks of rational–emotive therapy (RET; Walen, DiGiuseppe, & Wessler, 1980; Wessler & Wessler, 1980) to deal with illogical, irrational thinking, deviant sexual cognitions, assertion training, and social skills. He concurrently experienced behavior therapy (BT) to reduce deviant sexual arousal, which continued throughout the treatment program. In these procedures he was twice exposed to olfactory aversion and once to masturbatory satiation (Laws & Osborn, 1983). He next experienced 20 weeks of relapse prevention (RP) training (Marlatt, 1985; Pithers, Marques, Gibat, & Marlatt, 1983) to provide him with an individualized program for managing his behavior in high-risk situations (HRSs). Following the formal RP training, he was placed in individual follow-up (IFU) based on RP principles.

Throughout this process the client's sexual arousal was measured. He underwent a comprehensive psychophysiological and self-report assessment at (1) the pretreatment baseline; the entire psychophysiological and portions of the self-report were then repeated at (2) the end of 20 weeks of RET; (3) the end of 20 weeks of RP; and (4) after 6 weeks of individual follow-up. Independent of these major assessments, his sexual arousal to deviant and nondeviant audio-taped stimuli was assessed every 2 weeks.

Figure 8.1 shows the three phases of treatment experienced by the client. The data are erectile response scores obtained biweekly by penile plethysmography. The ordinate shows the measurement scale as relative deviant arousal (that is, the percentage that deviant arousal represented relative to all arousal produced to *both* deviant and nondeviant stimuli (RDA = D / [D + ND]). The abscissa shows the weeks for each phase of treatment. Only the biweekly measurement data are reported as RDA. All other assessment data described below are reported as a percentage of full erection.

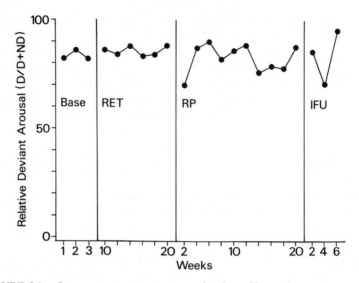

FIGURE 8.1. Progress in treatment expressed in biweekly penile erection scores. Data are shown as relative deviant arousal (i.e., the percentage that deviant arousal represents of the total of deviant and nondeviant arousal produced: RDA = D /[D + ND].

Baseline Assessment

There are two parts to the psychophysiological assessment, a slide procedure and an audiotaped procedure.

The client was presented with 12 categories of slides of male and female children and adults of various age levels. He observed each slide for 2 minutes while his sexual response was measured.

He was also presented with twelve 3-minute audiotaped descriptions of violent and nonviolent sexual and nonsexual activities with male and female children, as well as with two 3-minute descriptions of consenting activities with adults.

It was here that the first indication of the client's actual sexual interests emerged. In the slide procedure he did not respond to depictions of teenage boys; rather he showed high response (66% to 68%) to very young boys, aged from infancy to about 7 years. Response to adult stimuli was insignificant. In his responses to the audiotapes he showed high to very high arousal (54% to 91%) to descriptions of fondling, consenting sex, psychologically coercive sex, rape, and sadism with boys, and high to very high arousal (51% to 77%) to descriptions of fondling, consenting, coercive, and sadistic sex with girls. These measurements strongly suggested that this was not a client who merely "ruminated" about consenting sex with teenage boys. Response was moderate (39%) to adult male stimuli and insignificant to adult females.

Rational–Emotive Therapy

RET was conducted as group therapy for 1.5 hours per week for 20 weeks. All sessions were guided by treatment manuals that explicitly stated what was to be covered in each session. Clients were expected to attend and actively participate, and missed sessions were made up in tutorials. Homework was provided in every session, and this formed the basis of part of the following week's work. In addition, clients kept a daily self-report of urges, fantasies, masturbations, and deviant sexual contacts. At the end of each session, the client and therapist completed goal-attainment scales on which they indicated the client's progress in treatment.

Throughout RET the client's participation was reported to range from "insignificant" to "minimal" to "fairly active," although he was usually reported as being "attentive." The therapist frequently noted that he did not seem to grasp the basic principles of RET, but here and there his homework seemed to improve. When the group therapy activity became more concrete—for example, assertion training—he seemed to do better. Toward the end of RET he expressed fear of relationships with adult women. Importantly, he refused to destroy a collection of pornographic pictures, and his daily self-reports indicated a high level of deviant fantasizing and masturbation.

Behavior Therapy

The client was first exposed to olfactory aversion treatment (Laws, Meyer, & Holmen, 1978; Laws & Osborn, 1983). In this treatment the client was to pair the inhalation of the fumes of spirits of ammonia with the spontaneous production of deviant sexual fantasy. He was to do one session in the clinic under supervision and two at home, recording his fantasies on a portable deck. Figure 8.1 shows that the client's relative deviant arousal at baseline averaged above 80%. There was essentially no response to nondeviant stimuli throughout treatment.

Behavior therapy did not begin until the eighth week of RET, thus only six data points (10th–20th weeks) are shown in Figure 8.1. It is quite clear that the treatment had no effect on his arousal, averaging about the same to somewhat higher than baseline (very high arousal). His homework sessions were considered to be satisfactory. In behavior therapy the client was quite honest about his deviant interests, the fantasies focusing on anal intercourse with young boys. As treatment proceeded, he began to describe the victims as noncompliant.

After 6 weeks of olfactory aversion treatment, it was clear that no effect was being produced, and he was switched to masturbatory satiation (Laws & Osborn, 1983; Marshall, 1979). In this treatment he was to masturbate to ejaculation using a nondeviant fantasy, then, when he was refractory to further stimulation, he was to switch to a deviant fantasy, thus pairing inability to become aroused with favored fantasy themes. He agreed to participate but expressed concern about fantasizing about adult partners.

Although the change initially appeared to have an effect, the client was poorly motivated to complete homework sessions and was switched back to olfactory aversion at the beginning of the RP segment.

Assessment 1

Following the completion of RET, the client was reassessed on the psychophysiological measures. Very little change was evident. His response to slides of very young males remained quite high (58% to 79%) and at moderate levels (13% to 38%) to females in the same age groups. Response to adults was insignificant. Responses to audiotaped descriptions of both violent and nonviolent activities with males and females ranged from high to very high (52% to 87%). Response to adult males was high (64%), and no response to adult females was observed. Given that no results were shown for behavior therapy and that therapist goal-attainment scores showed little progress in RET, these results are not surprising.

Relapse Prevention

In the initial RP (George & Marlatt, 1986; Marlatt & Gordon, 1985) group sessions, the client remained as resistant as he had been during RET and continued to report deviant fantasies and masturbations. The clinical notes show that he vacillated, shifting back and forth from stating that he wanted to change his behavior and could control his fantasies and masturbations, to stating that he was not motivated or willing to do anything. In treatment he minimized his deviant behavior and its inappropriateness.

Although the clinical notes do not reflect why it happened, the client then began to participate in RP treatment, showing greater interest in its more concrete way of dealing with behavior management. He stated that his perspective on his deviant behavior had changed and that he felt more motivated. Although initially his participation was minimal and he failed to complete homework assignments, by midphase he was actively participating, using RP concepts correctly, and doing the homework. His self-reports began to show less fantasizing and masturbatory activity. Therapist goal-attainment scores for the period showed substantial progress.

Behavior Therapy

Olfactory aversion was resumed at the onset of RP. In these sessions the client often remarked that the ammonia fumes were not affecting him adversely, and the dose was doubled. He was reported to be cooperative in laboratory sessions, and his homework sessions were satisfactory. His sexual arousal ranged from moderate to quite high during laboratory treatment sessions. In these sessions as well as on homework tapes, his fantasies began to be quite violent, describing forced fellatio and anal rape with both boys and girls. Figure 8.1 (weeks 12–18 of RP) shows some decrease in relative deviant sexual arousal but not what is usually observed in successful olfactory aversion treatment. Note that in the final 2 weeks of treatment, deviant arousal increased once more. Behavior therapy was discontinued at this point. A number of behavior-therapy homework tapes remained to be reviewed at this point, and their evaluation showed that his fantasies had become even more violent than previously reported.

Assessment 2

Although deviant sexual arousal decreased from the levels observed in Assessment 1, they remained high. Response to slides of very young males averaged 50% to 60%, and response to young females was insignificant. Response to adults was also insignificant. Response to audiotapes of violent and nonviolent activities with males ranged from 50% to 72% and to females, from 29% to 50%. Despite the progress measured in RP and some change in behavior therapy, the measured responses to males did not represent substantial changes from the previous assessment. Response to adults was insignificant.

Individual RP Follow-Up

The client remained in treatment for an additional 6 weeks. Although the self-reports indicated continued reduced deviant activity, he reported encountering numerous HRSs. He described adequate coping skills in response to these situations, primarily escape, avoidance, and self-talk. However, his therapist reported that his motivation seemed to be decreasing and that he was expressing inability to believe that he could control his fantasies and urges. Figure 8.1 shows that his relative deviant arousal during these individual sessions averaged between 70% and 80%, essentially what it had been at the end of RP.

Assessment 3

A final assessment was conducted during the follow-up period. Response to male slides ranged from 51% to 62%, and insubstantial change across treatment; moderate response (40%) to one female category was evident. There was no response to adults. Response to audiotapes of activities with males showed high response to fondling (58%) and rape (63%) and moderate response to psychological coercion (45%). These represented changes but remained alarmingly high. Response to audiotaped descriptions of sex with females showed moderate response to psychological coercion (48%). There was no response to adults.

Disposition of the Case

The client was not a resident of Tampa and coming to treatment represented something of a hardship for him. Recognizing that the client continued to pose a danger to the community, the staff attempted to obtain a commitment from him to continue treatment on a biweekly basis. He refused, but he did agree to attend monthly sessions to evaluate his sexual arousal. At termination it was agreed that (1) he would receive services for his sexual deviance at a mental health center or with a private practitioner in his area of residence, (2) the treatment staff would provide consultation as needed, (3) he would receive services for his depression, (4) he would attend monthly measurement sessions in Tampa, and (5) he could apply for readmission to treatment if he felt it necessary. Under these conditions, all of them totally out of the treatment staff's control, after 18 months of intensive treatment, the client was terminated.

SUMMARY AND CONCLUSIONS

This case of a not very unusual sex offender was reported at some length to indicate the degree to which the treatment staff attempted to monitor and document his behavior as well as provide him mechanisms to control it. Despite this effort, as well as the changes observed in the client, this could not be counted a successful treatment case.

The case is in many ways illustrative of the problems facing all workers in this field. A recent nationwide survey (Knopp, Rosenberg, & Stevenson, 1986) identified 297 adult sex offender treatment programs in the United States. Many of these programs, whether based in insitutions, community clinics, or private practice, do not have the resources to train staff in sex offender treatment, to hire clinical, research, or technical staff, or to obtain expensive hardware and software that would improve their service capability. These programs would accept a client such as this since he was self-referred and admitted to deviant interests, even though he had no known history. They would treat him to the limit of their ability and hope for the best. If he was not exposed to any explicit demands or contingencies to be self-revealing, if he participated minimally, if he slightly modified his denial, minimization, and rationalization, he might escape effective treatment yet be counted a "successful" case.

Consider, however, what *did* happen to him; he walked into a program that *did* have highly trained staff and all the necessary resources. He experienced a very comprehensive intake interview specifically focused on sexual deviance. He completed numerous self-report inventories and psychological instruments. He completed daily self-reports on urges, fantasies, and masturbations for 18 months. He completed four psychophysiological assessments. He participated in two highly systematic group therapies and two behavior therapies. And finally, he had his sexual arousal measured every other week for the entire period. Considering his low motivation and continuous resistance, what is remarkable is that he stuck it out. You may ask why the staff stuck with him. There are two answers. First, he intermittently provided sufficient reason to hope that he could be a successful case. Second, and most important, when it became apparent how potentially dangerous he actually was, it became an ethical imperative to hold on to him as long as possible. When the treatment was complete, there was no further justification for retaining him against his wishes.

Consider also what would have happened had penile plethysmography and behavior therapy not been central elements of this treatment program. In my judgment, the penile measures told the whole story throughout treatment, and it was the direct monitoring by plethysmography that sealed this case as a failure. At the completion of the pretreatment baseline assessment, this man's responses to the slides clearly indicated that he was lying about the target of his deviant interests. His responses to the audiotapes indicated strong attraction to violent sexual activities, presumably with young male children. His fluctuating moderate to high levels of sexual arousal in laboratory behavior therapy sessions, and the content of his fantasies, which progressively deteriorated to more and more violent activities, confirmed these initial observations. The total lack of change in the biweekly erectile measures and the lack of substantial change in the pre- and postassessment measures between phases clearly showed that the treatment package had not been effective. These simple measures told more about this man's secret life than anyone had ever known.

Had the penile measures been absent, as they are in 73% of the sex offender programs in the United States (Knopp et al., 1986), this would have been judged just one more marginal case. The therapist's notes, the goal-attainment scores, the self-reports, and the various other items of the assessment battery—the usual details of a standard clinical program—would suggest that the case was not a total failure, that the client received some benefit from treatment, but that, given his motivation, he probably needed continued supervision. The penile measures speak more loudly, and they tell us that he probably needs a great deal of watching.

REFERENCES

Bancroft, J., Jones, H. G., & Pullan, B. R. (1966). A simple transducer for measuring penile erections, with comments on its use in the treatment of sexual disorders. *Behaviour Research and Therapy, 4,* 239–241.

Barlow, D. H., Becker, J., Leitenberg, H., & Agras, S. (1970). A mechanical strain gauge for recording penile circumference change. *Journal of Applied Behavior Analysis, 3,* 73–76.

George, W. H., & Marlatt, G. A. (1986). *Relapse prevention with sex offenders: A treatment manual*. Unpublished manuscript, Florida Mental Health Institute, Tampa.

Knopp, F. H., Rosenberg, J., & Stevenson, W. (1986). *Report on nationwide survey of juvenile and adult sex-offender treatment programs and providers, 1986*. Syracuse, NY: Safer Society Press.

Langevin, R. (1983). *Sexual strands: Understanding and treating sexual anomalies in men*. Hillsdale, NJ: Erlbaum.

Laws, D. R. (1977). A comparison of the measurement characteristics of two circumferential penile transducers. *Archives of Sexual Behavior, 6*, 45–51.

Laws, D. R. (1986). [Sexual deviance card sort: Assessment scores]. Unpublished raw data.

Laws, D. R., Meyer, J., & Holmen, M. L. (1978). Reduction of sadistic sexual arousal by olfactory aversion. *Behaviour Research and Therapy, 16*, 281–285.

Laws, D. R., & Osborn, C. A. (1983). How to build and operate a behavioral laboratory to evaluate and treat sexual deviance. In J. G. Greer & I. R. Stuart (Eds.), *The sexual aggressor* (pp. 293–335). New York: Van Nostrand Reinhold.

Marlatt, G. A. (1985). Relapse prevention: Theoretical rationale and overview of the model. In G. A. Marlatt & J. R. Gordon (Eds.), *Relapse prevention: Maintenance strategies in the treatment of addictive behaviors* (pp. 3–70). New York: Guilford.

Marlatt, G. A., & Gordon, J. R. (Eds.). (1985). *Relapse prevention: Maintenance strategies in the treatment of addictive behaviors*. New York: Guilford.

Marshall, W. L. (1979). Satiation therapy: A procedure for reducing deviant sexual arousal. *Journal of Applied Behavior Analysis, 12*, 10–22.

Murphy, W. D., & Barbaree, H. E. (1988, September). *Assessment of sex offenders by measurement of erectile responses: Psychometric properties and decision making*. Paper presented at the meeting of the Association for Behavioral Treatment of Sexual Abusers, Atlanta, GA.

Nichols, H. R., & Molinder, I. (1984). *Multiphasic Sex Inventory*. (Available from Nichols & Molinder, 437 Bowes Drive, Tacoma, WA 98466)

Pithers, W. D., & Laws, D. R. (1989). The penile plethysmograph: Uses and abuses in assessment and treatment of sexual aggressors. In B. Schwartz (Ed.), *A practitioner's guide to treatment of the incarcerated male sex offender* (pp. 83–91). Washington, DC: National Institute of Corrections.

Pithers, W. D., Marques, J. K., Gibat, C. C., & Marlatt, G. A. (1983). Relpase prevention with sexual aggressives: A self-control model of treatment and maintenance of change. In J. G. Greer & I. R. Stuart (Eds.), *The sexual aggressor* (pp. 214–239). New York: Van Nostrand Reinhold.

Rosen, R. C., & Keefe, F. J. (1978). The measurement of penile tumescence. *Psychophysiology, 15*, 366–376.

Walen, S. R., DiGiuseppe, R., & Wessler, R. L. (1980). *A practitioner's guide to rational-emotive therapy*. New York: Oxford University Press.

Webster's new international unabridged dictionary of the English language. (1971). New York: Merriam.

Wessler, R. A., & Wessler, R. L. (1980). *The principles and practice of rational–emotive therapy*. San Francisco: Jossey-Bass.

9

Assessment of Sexual Arousal by Means of Physiological and Self-Report Measures

DAVID M. DAY
MICHAEL H. MINER
V. HENLIE STURGEON
JOSEPH MURPHY

This chapter is directed at the issue of how to characterize sex offenders in quantifiable ways so that hypotheses about them can be tested. The Sex Offender Treatment and Evaluation Project (SOTEP; Marques, Day, Nelson, & Miner, Chapter 22, this volume) employs a multimodal approach to the treatment of sex offenders. One component of the program is the use of a sexual behavior laboratory for the assessment and treatment of offenders with deviant sexual arousal patterns. In our standard laboratory assessment, the number of stimuli to which subjects respond is quite large. When our concern is with testing hypotheses about changes in behavior as a result of treatment in the laboratory, the number of subjects required in order to apply the appropriate statistical procedures is prohibitive. Therefore, some method is necessary to make possible the reduction of the amount of data available for analysis without losing the information the data contain.

There have been other efforts to develop procedures for summarizing sexual behavior laboratory data. For example, Abel, Barlow, Blanchard, and Guild (1977) developed the Rape Index, which was designed to characterize the arousal patterns of rapists; Avery-Clark and Laws (1984) developed the Dangerous Child Abuser Index, a similar indicator for pedophiles. It should be noted, however, that both of these indices tap only one attribute, arousal to depictions of violent acts. What is needed are methods of data reduction that capture the complete range of available stimulus characteristics, such as age and sex of victim, as well as violence.

A second issue that must be addressed in the utilization of data produced in sexual behavior laboratories concerns their validity as accurate representations of individuals' actual sexual preferences. Validation studies of such data have relied on three primary data sources: (1) self-reports of arousal made by subjects to the stimuli presented during physiological assessment, (2) self-reports of past sexual behavior and interest made by means of paper-and-pencil tests in nonlaboratory situations, and (3) group comparisons made among persons known to have engaged in sexually deviant behaviors in the past.

Examples of the first approach, concurrent self-estimates of arousal, are the most commonly reported and typically produce correlations of moderate magnitude (Farkas, 1978; Geer, 1976; Hall, Binik, & Di Tomasso, 1985). The second approach, self-report scales, is exemplified by Freund, Chan, and Coulthard (1979). These investigators, concerned with the accuracy of physiological assessments in the identification of deviant arousal, developed two self-report scales to capture pedophilic tendencies. Using a sample of males known to exhibit such behaviors, these authors found that subjects scoring high on either scale ("admitters") were more accurately assessed by physiological measures than were those scoring low ("nonadmitters").

Validation of physiological assessments using known groups is exemplified by Avery-Clark and Laws (1984), who had independent raters evaluate accounts of their subjects' offenses with respect to amount of violence used. These authors found that pedophiles whose offenses were rated as violent showed higher responses to audiotaped scenarios involving nonconsenting and aggressive sex with children than to audiotaped scenarios involving consenting sex. Those whose offenses were rated nonviolent manifested the opposite pattern.

This chapter presents one approach to the goal of reducing the amount of data produced in sexual behavior laboratories: aggregating individual measures into composites. In addition, the validity of these composites is assessed, using the second and third validation methods. That is, the relationship between physiological assessments and self-reports of prior sexual deviance is evaluated; and then each of these assessment procedures is validated, using subjects grouped according to the nature of their sex-offense histories.

METHOD

Subjects for this study were 66 persons assessed in the sexual behavior laboratory at intake to the program. An examination of the offense histories of these persons revealed that 50 had been found guilty of child molesting and 16, of rape. All of the rapists' victims were female, as were 28 of the child molesters' victims. Sixteen of the molesters had male victims, and 6 had both male and female victims.

In an attempt to replicate Avery-Clark and Laws's (1984) findings that physiological assessments can distinguish violent from nonviolent offenders, we used the arrest and probation reports prepared at the time of sentencing for each of these subjects to identify those who had injured or verbally abused their victim(s) or used a weapon in the commission of their offenses. In accord with these criteria, 32% of the subjects were classified as having used violence in their offenses and 68% were not.

Physiological Assessments

Penile circumference was assessed for each subject by means of a mercury-in-rubber strain gauge and a plethysmograph. The stimulus materials consisted of sets of slides portraying nude male and female children and adults of various ages (Laws & Osborn, 1983), a series of audiotapes presenting scenes of sexual encounters with male and female children that varied in terms of the amount of coerciveness involved in the encounter (Avery-Clark & Laws, 1984), videotaped presentations of sexual encounters between males and females that varied in terms of the coercion involved in the encounter (Abel, Blanchard, Becker, & Djenderedjian, 1978), and a set of audiotapes that roughly paralleled the videotapes in content (Abel, Blanchard, Barlow, & Mavissakalian, 1975).

Altogether 96 stimuli were presented, 72 with deviant and 24 with nondeviant content, and measures of subjects' arousal in response to them were combined into rational composites in terms of common stimulus content. The final determinations of the items included in composites were made so that the maximum reliabilities were obtained for each, as measured by coefficient *alpha* (Lord & Novick, 1968).

The mean arousal to the stimuli composed of audiotaped narratives and video depictions of rape and aggression toward women was computed for use as a measure of rape arousal. This composite was named Rape and had a reliability that was quite high (*alpha* = 0.89), indicating that arousal to any one of these stimuli was predictive of arousal to the others.

The procedure used in the development of the Rape composite was applied to the development of a set of child molester arousal scores. The first of these was computed as the mean arousal to slides showing nude boys of three age groups and audiotaped narratives portraying sex with consenting male child victims. This composite was named Male Child Consenting, and its reliability was 0.95. The second, named Male Child Nonconsenting, was computed as the mean arousal to audiotaped narratives concerned with coerced sex with male children, and it had a reliability of 0.87. Parallel stimuli concerning female children were composited to produce Female Child Consenting, which measured arousal to slides of female children of various ages and narratives portraying sex with consenting female children, and Female Child Nonconsenting, which measured arousal to narratives portraying sex with nonconsenting female children. The reliabilities for these composites were 0.86 and 0.91, respectively.

The nondeviant stimuli produced two composites. The first used responses to audiotaped narratives concerned with consenting sex with adult males to form a measure, Homosexual Arousal, which had a reliability of 0.82. The second used slides displaying adult females and video depictions and audiotaped narratives of sex with consenting adult females to produce Heterosexual Arousal, which had a reliability of 0.85.

Self-Report Behaviors

Self-reports of sexual behaviors were obtained by means of a standardized assessment instrument, the Multiphasic Sex Inventory (MSI; Nichols & Molinder, 1984). The MSI is a 300-item inventory consisting of statements about sexual activities, problems, and experiences. Respondents evaluate each statement and indicate its relevance to themselves as either true or false. Responses are composited as the numbers of items checked true or false, depending on the scoring direction of the item for a given scale.

There are 25 scales in the MSI (Nichols & Molinder, 1984), but only 9 were selected for analysis. In this section, the selected scales will be presented, along with descriptions of item content and reliabilities.

Child molesting was assessed by means of three scales: Child Molest, Male Preference, and Female Preference. Examination of the item content of the Child Molest Scale as described by Nichols and Molinder (1984) revealed considerable overlap between it and the two gender-preference scales. Additionally, the initial reliabilities of all three scales for these subjects were not high enough to be acceptable. In order to guarantee that all scales were reliable and consisted of unique sets of items, alterations were made so that the Child Molest Scale was composed of six items selected from the original scale. These items requested subjects to report various deviant behaviors with children, and the scale reliability was 0.90. The two gender-preference scales were composed of two items each and had reliabilities of 0.72 for Female Preference and 0.86 for Male Preference.

Self-reports of rape behaviors were obtained by using items from two MSI scales: Rape and Sadism. Items were deleted or assigned to one or another scale in order to maximize reliability and eliminate item overlap, as was done with the three child molest scales above. The reliabilities of these modified scales were 0.75 for Rape and 0.72 for Sadism.

To assess subjects' hetero- or homosexual orientation, a Sexual Orientation Scale was constructed from the MSI item pool. The reliability for this scale was 0.74. Nichols and Molinder's (1984) Voyeurism Scale was also included in order to make possible the statistical control of subjects' preferences for or aversions to pornographic displays. Its reliability was 0.70. Finally, two measures of response set, Sexual Obsessions and Social Sexual Desirability, were included to assess subject tendencies to "fake bad" or "fake good." The Sexual Obsessions Scale had a reliability of 0.85 and Social Sexual Desirability, a reliability of 0.88.

Statistical Analyses

Two sets of multivariate analyses were used in this study. The first was canonical correlation analysis, a procedure that permitted investigation of the relationships between the two sets of variables. This procedure first derived weights for linear composites of each set of variables and then computed a correlation between them (Levine, 1977; see Morrison, 1976, for a mathematical treatment of the topic). Estimates of the redundancy of measures were computed in order to describe the proportion of variance each set accounted for in the other. Also, descriptions of the nature of the relationships found between the sets of variables were based on an examination of the correlations between them and the composites.

The second procedure was linear discriminant analysis (Klecka, 1980; Morrison, 1976), which permitted the differentiation of two or more groups of subjects with respect to a set of variables (e.g., physiological and self-report measures were compared in terms of their relative adequacy in discriminating groups). As was the case in canonical correlation analysis, this statistical procedure produced sets of weights that allowed the combination of predictor variables to yield composite scores. In the case of linear discriminant analysis, the composite permitted classification of subjects. The classification entailed computation of the weighted composite and application of a decision rule that assignment to one group or another be made on the basis of whether it was above or below a given cutoff. Separate analyses were performed based on subjects' commitment offenses, the sex of victims, and the violence involved in offenses. Cohen's *kappa* (1960) was used to evaluate the overall agreement in classification for each function.

RESULTS AND DISCUSSION

The results of the canonical correlation analysis revealed that the physiological and self-report measures were strongly associated, sufficiently so to exceed accepted levels of statistical significance. The redundancy of the two sets of variables, on the other hand, indicated that they shared only 25% common variance. Examination of the specific linkages among the self-report and physiological measures suggests that this association arises from a complex dimension that is anchored at one end by homosexual, noncoercive sexual preference and at the other, by heterosexual, coercive sexual preference. Apparently, for subjects in this sample of sex offenders, gender preference and preference for coerced sexual activity were related, not independent, phenomena.

The results of the linear discriminant analyses for the physiological assessment data produced significant results for only two of the three analyses performed. The first of these was for the discrimination of groups of offenders formed on the basis of the sex of victim: male, female, and both sexes. Because rapists had had only female victims, this analysis was made for child molesters only. While two functions could be derived in the analysis of the three groups, only the first was statistically significant. Examination of the correlations between this discriminant function and each physiological measure of arousal revealed that those who showed arousal to themes including male sex partners were more likely to have molested male victims, while those who showed arousal to rape themes were more likely to have molested female victims. This function could not adequately discriminate those who had molested both male and female victims from the other two groups.

The second function of physiological measures, derived for the discrimination of groups in terms of the violence used in the offense, revealed that arousal to all of the themes involving male sex partners, as well as those involving consenting female children, was associated with nonviolent offending behavior. Arousal to rape themes was associated with offenses of a more violent nature.

The linear discriminant analyses for the self-report measures revealed all three to have statistically significant results. Examination of the associations between the discriminant function derived for offense groups—rapists and child molesters—and the individual self-report variables showed the child molest scales (Child Molest, Male Preference, and Female Preference) to be associated with child molesting and the Rape Scale, and to some extent Voyeurism, to be associated with rape. Examination of the function discriminating sex of victim for the child molesters revealed that those with high scores on Sexual Orientation, Male Preference, and Sexual Obsessions tended to have had male victims, while those with high scores on Female Preference, and to a lesser extent on Rape and Sadism, tended to have had female victims. As was the case for the physiological measures, the self-report measures could not adequately discriminate bisexual from heterosexual and homosexual molesters. Finally, those with high scores on Child Molest, Female Preference, Male Preference, and Sexual Orientation were less likely to have included violent elements in their offenses, while those with high scores on Rape, and to a lesser extent on Sadism and Voyeurism, were more likely to have included such elements.

Each of the six functions developed in the linear discriminant analyses were used to classify subjects, and the derived classifications were cross-tabulated with actual group membership. This permitted a comparison of the relative accuracy of each set of measures in making three separate discriminations.

Overall, the self-report measures performed better than the physiological measures in discriminating groups for this sample of subjects. For the self-report measures, 95% of the sample were classified correctly with respect to offense using the linear discriminant function (*kappa* = 0.85); 86% of the child molesters were classified correctly with respect to the sex of victim (*kappa* = 0.74); and 85% of the sample were classified correctly with respect to violence included in the offense (*kappa* = 0.64) It should be noted that these *kappa* values were all quite large and statistically significant.

For the physiological measures, only 74% of the sample were correctly classified with respect to their offenses (*kappa* = 0.04); 82% of the child molesters were correctly classified with respect to sex of victim (*kappa* = 0.65); and 74% of the sample were correctly classified with respect to violence (*kappa* = 0.31). Only the second and third of these *kappa* values were statistically significant.

It is interesting that for each of the discriminant analyses, the self-report measures performed better than did the physiological measures. This finding is consistent with that reported by Freund et al. (1979): Those who admit their offenses are more accurately assessed by physiological measures than those who do not. However, it is often the expressed opinion of investigators concerned with sex offenders that physiological assessment is necessary because these persons cannot be taken at their word. Of course, the subjects for the present study might have been more forthright about their deviant sexual histories and their preferences for activities of a nonconventional nature because they had been convicted and sentenced for their offenses and admission of responsibility was required when they volunteered for treatment.

The attempted replication of Avery-Clark and Laws (1984) produced some noteworthy results for the physiological measures. It was expected that scenarios presenting consenting victims would anchor one end of the predictor dimension, while those concerned with rape and nonconsenting victims would anchor the other. While some of this pattern emerged, the two nonconsenting pedophile scenarios (Male Child Nonconsenting and Female Child Nonconsenting) did not correlate as predicted. Instead, arousal to scenarios containing presentations of nonconsenting sex with female children was unrelated and arousal to scenarios containing nonconsenting male children was positively associated with nonviolent offenses. This finding indicates that molesters of male children are not as likely as other offenders to harm or verbally abuse their victims, even though such actions might be arousing to them. Thus the present study would have to be described as inconclusive in its attempt to replicate Avery-Clark and Laws's study (1984).

CONCLUSIONS

The results of this study indicate that the MSI scales used as self-report measures were superior to the physiological measures of arousal derived from our standard sexual behavior laboratory assessments in discriminating between groups classified on the basis of the characteristics of past criminal behavior. The two sets of measures were related to one another by a single common dimension, one which confounded heterosexual with coerced sexual preference. Indeed, arousal to stimuli depicting coerced sexual acts with boys was not reflective of violent elements in the actual criminal behaviors of this sample.

In interpreting these results, it must be remembered that the discriminant analyses reported here bear on the validity of the physiological and self-report data in a postdictive, rather than predictive, sense. The assessments that produced the data for these analyses were made after the commission of the offenses. Therefore, the arousal exhibited in the assessments may have been reflective of, and not necessarily a contributing factor to, offending.

Physiological arousal is one element making certain situations, those involving children or aggressive behavior, a high risk for sex offenders. As such, measures of it may be viewed as tapping some aspects of the potential to offend. The self-report measures, on the other hand, measure the degree to which subjects have acted on this potential in the past.

For much of the current research literature concerned with sexual behavior laboratory data, either hypotheses are tested using separate, univariate statistical analyses of responses to sets of individual stimuli, or profiles are constructed showing comparative levels of arousal and interpreted using rationally derived criteria. These research strategies impose limitations both on the nature of the research questions that can be answered and on the generalizability of results. The present study employed composites of measures of arousal and used two types of multivariate procedures, canonical correlation analysis and linear discriminant analysis, in an effort to elucidate the relationships between measures produced in the physiological assessment of sex offenders. In general, the results supported the conclusion that composites formed from responses to scenarios presented in the sexual behavior laboratory can be made and analyzed without significant loss of information.

REFERENCES

Abel, G. G., Barlow, D. H., Blanchard, E. B., & Guild, D. (1977). The components of rapists' sexual arousal. *Archives of General Psychiatry, 34,* 895–903.

Abel, G. G., Blanchard, E. B., Barlow, D. H., & Mavissakalian, M. (1975). Identifying specific erotic cues in sexual deviation by audiotaped descriptions. *Journal of Applied Behavior Analysis, 8,* 247–260.

Abel, G. G., Blanchard, E. B., Becker, J. V., & Djenderedjian, A. (1978). Differentiating sexual aggressives with penile measures. *Criminal Justice and Behavior, 5,* 315-332.

Avery-Clark, C. A., & Laws, D. R. (1984). Differential erection response patterns of sexual child abusers to stimuli describing activities with children. *Behavior Therapy, 15,* 71-83.

Cohen, J. (1960). A coefficient of agreement for nominal scales. *Education and Psychological Measurement, 20,* 37-46.

Farkas, G. M. (1978). Comments on Levin et al. and Rosen and Kopel: Internal and external validity issues. *Journal of Consulting and Clinical Psychology, 46,* 1515-1516.

Freund, K., Chan, S., & Coulthard, R. (1979). Phallometric diagnosis with "nonadmitters." *Behaviour Research and Therapy, 17,* 451-457.

Geer, J. H. (1976). Genital measures: Comments on their role in understanding human sexuality. *Journal of Sex and Marital Therapy, 2,* 164-172.

Hall, K. S., Binik, Y., & Di Tomasso, E. (1985). Concordance between physiological and subjective measures of sexual arousal. *Behaviour Research and Therapy, 23,* 297-303.

Klecka, W. R. (1980). *Discriminant analysis.* Beverly Hills, CA: Sage.

Laws, D. R., & Osborn, C. A. (1983). How to build and operate a behavioral laboratory to evaluate and treat sexual deviance. In J. G. Greer & I. R. Stuart (Eds.), *The sexual aggressor* (pp. 293-335). New York: Van Nostrand Reinhold.

Levine, M. S. (1977). *Canonical analysis and factor comparison.* Beverly Hills, CA: Sage.

Lord, F. M., & Novick, M. R. (1968). *Statistical theories of mental test scores.* Reading, MA: Addison-Wesley.

Morrison, D. F. (1976). *Multivariate statistical methods.* New York: McGraw-Hill.

Nichols, H. R., & Molinder, I. (1984). *The Multiphasic Sex Inventory manual.* (Available from Nichols and Molinder, 437 Bowes Drive, Tacoma, WA 98466)

B · COPING SKILLS

10

Assessment of Coping Skills: Development of a Situational Competency Test

MICHAEL H. MINER
DAVID M. DAY
MARY K. NAFPAKTITIS

In the preceding chapters on assessment, high-risk situations were addressed. Such situations have been defined as ones containing internal or environmental elements that threaten a person's sense of control and, thus, increase the risk that he will indulge in an illegal sexual behavior (Nelson, Miner, Marques, Russell, & Achterkirchen, 1988). By defining the concept in terms of perceived control, we include noncompetency as an integral part of our definition of a high-risk situation. That is, a situation is defined to be high risk to the extent that it exceeds the individual's ability to cope adequately with the elements present. It is for this reason that coping skills are at the core of relapse prevention (RP). Relapse is most likely to occur in situations that present an offender with problems that he cannot inadequately address due to a lack of coping skills (Litman, Eiser, Rawson, & Oppenheim, 1979; Nelson et al., 1988; Pithers, Marques, Gibat, & Marlatt, 1983; Shiffman, Read, Maltese, Rapkin, & Jarvik, 1985).

This chapter addresses the development and uses of a procedure for assessing the coping skills of individuals convicted of sex offenses: the Situational Competency Test. Such a test is based on a concept of competence first presented by Goldfried and D'Zurilla (1969). Their behavioral–analytic model defines competence operationally in terms of an individual's interactions with his/her environment; that is, by the occurrence of adaptive behaviors in a specific situation or class of situations (Hops, 1983; Scheidt & Schaie, 1978). Using this definition, an assessment procedure designed to evaluate competence must involve the presentation of a variety of specific situations germane to the inappropriate behavior in question and allow the person being assessed to display his/her mode of response to those situations. The development of such a test involves situation sampling, the selection of situational attributes, and, finally the construction of the measurement instrument itself (Goldfried & D'Zurilla, 1969; Scheidt & Schaie, 1978).

PREVIOUS SITUATIONAL COMPETENCY TESTS

The first Situational Competency Test (SCT) was developed by Chaney, O'Leary, and Marlatt (1978) to evaluate a skills-training intervention for alcoholics. Chaney et al. used a number of sources to generate situations that were likely to be problematic to an inpatient population of excessive drinkers. These sources included (1) descriptions of relapse situations collected by Marlatt (1978) from follow-up interviews, (2) suggestions of treatment personnel at two alcohol treatment facilities, (3) interviews with alcoholics at an alcohol treatment program, and (4) modifications of situations from several inventories designed to assess assertive behavior (Chaney et al., 1978). This procedure resulted in 80 items that were presented to 40 patients who were instructed to rank them with regard to the difficulty each would present if encountered in the natural environment. The 32 most difficult situations were selected and classified by two independent raters into four categories: (1) frustration and anger, (2) interpersonal temptation, (3) negative emotional states, and (4) intrapersonal temptation (see Chaney et al., 1978, for a description of these categories and the items included in each). From these items an SCT was developed that consisted of 16 tape-recorded descriptions of high-risk situations.

Chaney and Roszell (1985) subsequently modified the SCT to address the coping skills of opiate addicts. This revision involved having a group of clinicians from several drug treatment programs review the original SCT situations and suggest changes in wording to reflect the demographic and substance-use differences between alcoholics and opiate addicts. New situations were added to the original item pool from interviews conducted with opiate addicts in a methadone maintenance program who had a relapse episode following at least 1 month of abstinence (Chaney, Roszell, & Cummings, 1982). Based on this information, the original SCT was expanded from 16 to 20 items to reflect situations that could be characterized by six categories: (1) intrapersonal negative emotional states, (2) intrapersonal negative physical–physiological states, (3) intrapersonal testing control or giving in to temptation, (4) enhancement of intra- or interpersonal positive emotional states, (5) interpersonal conflict, and (6) social pressure (see Chaney & Roszell, 1985, p. 275, for a listing of the situations).

Coping-skills assessment procedures similar to those used by Chaney and his colleagues (Chaney et al., 1978; Chaney & Roszell, 1985) have been developed for use in smoking cessation programs (Davis & Glaros, 1986), interventions aimed at the academic performance of college freshmen (Goldfried & D'Zurilla, 1969), and problem identification in adolescent populations (Hunter & Kelley, 1986). In each of these applications, the SCT has provided information useful for identifying coping-skills deficits and for assessing the impact of interventions based on skills training. Therefore, it was deemed essential to produce a similar test for sex offenders.

DEVELOPMENT OF THE SEX OFFENDER SITUATIONAL COMPETENCY TEST (SOSCT)

The development of an assessment tool for evaluating coping skills in incarcerated male sex offenders was undertaken using the behavioral–analytic method (Goldfried & D'Zurilla, 1969). This method involved four steps: (1) situational sampling, (2) selection of situational attributes, (3) the development of a pool of test items, and (4) the construction of the assessment instrument itself (see Day, Miner, Nafpaktitis, & Murphy, 1987, for an in-depth treatment of the information presented in this section).

Situational Sampling

In the situational-sampling phase of test development, male sex offenders were interviewed individually by staff from the Sex Offender Treatment and Evaluation Project (SOTEP) at Atascadero State Hospital. Forty-one subjects participated; 34 were men who had volunteered for treatment in the SOTEP (see Marques, Day, Nelson, & Miner (Chapter 22, this volume, for a complete description of this population) and 7 were men committed to the state hospital as mentally disordered sex offenders (MDSOs) prior to 1981, when that commitment was abolished by the California State Legislature. The population represented by these 7 subjects may be atypical of the mainstream of sex offenders, since they had been in treatment for a long period of time and had been deemed inappropriate for transfer to a less secure environment. The MDSOs who remained in the hospital would have been perceived by the staff to be a dangerous, but treatable, class of offenders. The offenses committed by the 41 subjects included rape, molestation of a female child (heterosexual molester), molestation of a male child (homosexual molester), and molestation of children of both sexes (bisexual molester).

Using a structured interview procedure, subjects were asked to present a chronology, beginning immediately after their commitment offense and proceeding backward in time through a period of 24 to 48 hours before the offense. The intention was to identify a wide range of high-risk situations for sex offenders. Because of requirements imposed by California's Child and Elderly Abuse Reporting Acts, and the need to guarantee subject confidentiality, subjects were discouraged from discussing sex offenses for which they had not been charged. Interviews lasted 30 to 90 minutes, were tape recorded, and were later transcribed.

Transcripts were content analyzed using a standardized rating form in order to determine the salient characteristics of the offender's lifestyle at the time of the offense, the offense itself, the offender, and his victim or victims. This analysis was used to develop concise statements of the situations described by the 41 men. These statements were then used in the next phase of test development, the selection of situational attributes.

It should be noted that the situations derived from this procedure were not necessarily relapse situations. Other investigators developing Situational Competency Tests have started with persons who originally had made a commitment to give up their indulgent behavior (Marlatt, 1978; Shiffman, 1982, 1984). Our sample may have included some individuals who had made such commitments, but it may also have included individuals who had never committed themselves to abstain from illegal sexual behavior; for example, first-time offenders. One must, therefore, be careful in the interpretation of the results of this sampling. The situations sampled may be more representative of situations in which persons are likely to commit sex crimes than of situations that are likely to lead to the relapse of sex offenders. For example, it may be that the characteristics of the abstinence violation effect (Marlatt, 1985a; Russell, Sturgeon, Miner, & Nelson, Chapter 4, this volume) are such that our sampling provided only a subset of the situations in which treated sex offenders are likely to relapse.

Selection of Situational Attributes

Following the classification system used by Chaney and Roszell (1985), we sorted situations derived from the interviews of our subjects into six categories. After the initial classification was completed, the results for each narrative were discussed, differences resolved, and a final classification agreed on. The overall agreement between raters was high and exceeded accepted levels of statistical significance (*kappa* = 0.522, $p < .0001$) (Day et al., 1987).

The results of the situational analysis indicated that high-risk situations for sex offenders can be reliably described using the same classification scheme that had previously been used to develop situational competency tests for other indulgent behaviors. However, it also appears that the characteristics of sex offenders differ with respect to the age and gender of their victims. Bisexual child molesters, heterosexual child molesters, homosexual child molesters, and rapists reported offense situations that were categorized very differently from one another. Also, an initial assessment of offenders' lifestyles indicated differences across offender types. At the time of their offenses, rapists were more likely to have been involved in criminal lifestyles, most frequently subsisting as drug dealers. Bisexual and homosexual child molesters were more likely to have been involved in ongoing relationships with their victims, to have had multiple victims, and, in the case of the first group, to have been preference offenders (see Howells, 1981, for a definition of preference vs. situational offenders). Homosexual child molesters did not appear to have been users of alcohol and drugs to the extent that the other three offender types were. Heterosexual child molesters were more likely to have been leading criminal lifestyles than were other child molesters, and they were more likely than rapists to have had familiar relationships with their victims. Child molesters as a group tended to have had positive feelings toward their victims, to have perceived the victims as being willing participants, and to have victimized children living in their immediate households.

These findings suggested that different assessment tools should be developed to evaluate coping skills in the four offender types. It was clear that the types of situations that would prove to be high risk, as well as the types of behaviors that could be viewed as appropriate coping strategies, would differ with both the age and gender of the victim.

Development of Item Pool

Using the information obtained from the exploration of situational attributes, items were prepared to represent each of the six situational categories described in Chaney and Roszell (1985), with different forms of the assessment tool created for the different types of sex offenders. Some of the items were specific to rape and some to child molesting. Of the latter, some of the items were specific to female victims, others were specific to male victims, and still others, were mute on the subject of victim gender. Finally, some items were generic, not addressing specific offenses at all. This strategy produced an item pool that reflected coping challenges at each stage of a cognitive–behavioral chain of reoffense (Nelson et al., 1988), while at the same time reflecting the wide range of possible high-risk situations discovered during the situational-sampling and attributes-selection phases of this procedure. A total of 98 tentative test items were developed.

Item difficulties for the 98 situations were determined using a card-sorting task. Each of the 98 situations was printed on a 3 × 5 card, and these cards were sorted into ten piles that corresponded to the degree of difficulty each situation would present to an ex-offender attempting to abstain from illegal sexual behavior. The resultant composite estimates of item difficulty showed high agreement between four independent raters (Day et al., 1987). Items with low interrater agreement were then eliminated from the item pool. This resulted in a 59-item pool.

Final Test Composition

Four alternate forms of the SOSCT were constructed, one each for rape and homosexual, heterosexual, and bisexual child molesting. They were equated in terms of overall item difficulty and were composed of 14 items each. In constructing the four versions of the SOSCT, it was decided that each, in addition to being balanced with respect to item difficulty, should contain a set of core, generic items so that comparisons could be made across types of offenders. Items were also selected in such a way that there was representation from all six situational categories. Each version included situations of varying levels of difficulty presented in random order. The mean difficulty scores of each of the four tests were determined to be sufficiently close to one another to conclude that they were of comparable difficulty (Day et al., 1987).

ADMINISTRATION AND SCORING OF THE SOSCT

In order to standardize administration of the situations that make up the SOSCT, audiotaped versions of the test were developed.[1] Each situation is described by a female voice with a 15-second interval between situations. Each description ends with the question "What would you do?"; this is followed by a click to signal the end of the situation.

The first step in administering the SOSCT is to carefully determine which version of the test to use. In choosing the version, we consider not only the patient's instant offense but also any historical information we have that may indicate involvement in illegal sex acts other than the one responsible for his arrest. This procedure is fairly straightforward for men convicted of rape. In distinguishing between the homosexual, heterosexual, and bisexual child molester versions, we consider whether there is any indication in the patient's background that he might have been involved with children of both genders. If that seems to be the case, we use the bisexual child molester version.

Individual test administration takes 30 to 45 minutes per subject. The entire assessment session is videotaped for future evaluation. Situations are

[1]Copies of the taped Sex Offender Situational Competency Test and the instruction manual are available from David M. Day, Evaluation Director, Sex Offender Treatment and Evaluation Project, California Department of Mental Health, 1600 9th Street, Sacramento, CA 95814.

played, one at a time, until all 14 have been presented. The subject responds to each situation by describing what action he would take, what he would be thinking, and/or what he would say if confronting each one in real life. The test administrator does not ask any questions during the SOSCT. However, once all the situations have been presented, the tester will often probe items that the subject failed to answer or where the nature of the response was ambiguous.

Scoring the Responses

The purpose of developing the SOSCT was twofold: to assess patient competence and coping-skills deficits and to evaluate the acquisition of coping skills taught as part of our treatment model. With these two goals in mind, we developed a scoring system that both describes the characteristics of the coping response within each situation and assesses the effectiveness of that response in addressing the high-risk elements of that situation.

Effective coping involves a process that can only be evaluated within a specific context. The subject must assess the situation to determine the high-risk elements, formulate a plan to address each of these elements, and, finally, implement that plan (Lazarus & Folkman, 1984). Errors in any of these activities lead to inadequate coping and thus leave the subject vulnerable to stress. While our scoring procedure does not directly address the formulation of the problem or plan of action, it infers the completeness of these activities from the report of the coping strategy presented by the subject.

The rating scale consists of yes/no judgments as to whether the response addressed the situation as presented and whether the subject attempted to resist the temptations within the situation. The response is then rated on a number of dimensions designed to describe the response in terms of factors salient to our treatment program and relapse prevention in general.[2]

A number of studies have determined that coping responses that include both cognitive and behavioral strategies are more effective than either alone (Litman et al., 1979; Shiffman, 1982, 1984). Relapse prevention also advocates intervention in high-risk situations on both the cognitive and behavioral levels (Marlatt, 1985b). Therefore, the presence of cognitive factors in the subject's response is important, and it is noted as present or absent. The presence or absence of assertiveness in the subject's response is also rated, since this characteristic would have a bearing on the effectiveness of the response. Integral to our intervention are the identification of possible escape and avoidance strategies for high-risk situations (Nelson, 1987) and a strong dependence on relapse prevention terminology. Therefore, our assessment of a subject's response to an

[2]Copies of the scoring manual are available from Michael H. Miner, Sex Offender Treatment and Evaluation Project, Atascadero State Hospital, Box 7001, Atascadero, CA 93423-7001.

item on the SOSCT includes a rating of his use of these strategies and whether or not the response explicitly contains RP concepts. Responses are also characterized with respect to how specifically the coping strategy is described, its complexity, the number of alternative actions included in the response, and whether the use of alcohol or drugs is included. All of these factors influence the competence of the subject within a possible relapse situation.

Effectiveness of the response is rated on a 5-point Likert Scale in accordance with the criteria described by Goldfried and D'Zurilla (1969): (1) the degree to which the response alters the high-risk situation such that it no longer is problematic and (2) the extent to which it produces a maximum of other positive consequences and a minimum of negative ones. In addition to effectiveness, two scores derived from Chaney et al. (1978) are also used in the SOSCT. The first is response latency, defined as the elapsed time from the end of the situation description to the onset of the subject's coping response, excluding dysfluencies and hedging. The second is duration, the total length of the subject's response, also exclusive of dysfluencies and other verbal fillers.

DISCUSSION

We have, in this chapter, described the development of an instrument for assessing coping skills in sex offenders. This task has involved determining the situations in which men are likely to commit sex crimes, describing the salient characteristics of these, and, finally, using this information to develop a measurement tool.

The SOSCT is in its infancy in terms of instrument development. At the present time, it appears to have face validity and to be consistent with other instruments, such as the Situational Competency Test (Chaney et al., 1978) and the Problem-Solving Test (Davis & Glaros, 1986). Developing a representative set of high-risk situations for sex offenders proved to be more complex than appears to have been the case for such indulgent behaviors as alcohol abuse, drug abuse, and smoking. The characteristics of the situations and the strategies that could be considered indications of competence necessitated the development of alternate forms of the test for rapists, homosexual child molesters, heterosexual child molesters, and bisexual child molesters.

The Sex Offender Situational Competency Test is an analogue task that attempts to assess how an individual would behave in real-life situations. As such, it is limited, since behaviors observed in analogue situations may not be indicative of how a person would behave in the real world (Hops, 1983). However, while assessment procedures such as the SOSCT may not access naturalistic performance, they are reasonable measures of response capability (Kern, Miller, & Eggers, 1983) and as such are useful for both clinical and evaluation purposes. The SOSCT has the potential to be a useful tool for identifying the coping-skills deficits of men who have committed child molestation and rape and for evaluating the impact of a relapse prevention program such as ours, in so far as performance on it is indicative of the repertoire of behaviors available to the subject.

REFERENCES

Chaney, E. F., O'Leary, M. R., & Marlatt, G. A. (1978). Skill training with alcoholics. *Journal of Consulting and Clinical Psychology, 46,* 1092–1104.

Chaney, E. F., & Roszell, D. K. (1985). Coping in opiate addicts maintained on methadone. In S. Shiffman & T. A. Willis (Eds.), *Coping and substance abuse* (pp. 267–293). New York: Academic.

Chaney, E. F., Roszell, D. K., & Cummings, C. (1982). Relapse in opiate addicts: A behavioral analysis. *Addictive Behaviors, 7,* 291–297.

Davis, J. R., & Glaros, A. G. (1986). Relapse prevention and smoking cessation. *Addictive Behaviors, 11,* 105–114.

Day, D. M., Miner, M. H., Nafpaktitis, M. K., & Murphy, J. F. (1987). Final report: Development of a situational competency test for sex offenders. (Available from David M. Day, California Department of Mental Health, 1600 Ninth Street, Sacramento, CA 95814)

Goldfried, M. R., & D'Zurilla, T. J. (1969). A behavior–analytic model for assessing competence. In C. D. Spielberger (Ed.), *Current topics in clinical and community psychology* (Vol. 1; pp. 151–196). New York: Academic.

Hops, H. (1983). Children's social competence and skills: Current research practices and future directions. *Behavior Therapy, 14,* 3–18.

Howells, K. (1981). Adult sexual interest in children: Considerations relevant to theories of aetiology. In M. Cook & K. Howells (Eds.), *Adult sexual interest in children* (pp. 55–94). Toronto: Academic.

Hunter, N., & Kelley, C. K. (1986). Examination of the validity of the adolescent problems inventory among incarcerated juvenile delinquents. *Journal of Consulting and Clinical Psychology, 54,* 301–302.

Kern, J. M., Miller, C., & Eggers, J. (1983). Enhancing the validity of role play tests: A comparison of three role play methodologies. *Behavior Therapy, 14,* 482–492.

Lazarus, R. S., & Folkman, S. (1984). *Stress, appraisal and coping.* New York: Springer.

Litman, G. K., Eiser, J. R., Rawson, N. S., & Oppenheim, A. N. (1979). Differences in relapse precipitants and coping behavior between alcohol abusers and survivors. *Behaviour Research and Therapy, 17,* 89–94.

Marlatt, G. A. (1978). Craving for alcohol, loss of control and relapse: A cognitive behavioral analysis. In P. G. Nathan, G. A. Marlatt, & T. Loberg (Eds.), *Alcoholism: New directions in behavioral research and treatment* (pp. 271–314). New York: Plenum.

Marlatt, G. A. (1985a). Relapse prevention: Theoretical rationale and overview of the model. In G. A. Marlatt & J. R. Gordon (Eds.), *Relapse prevention: Maintenance strategies in the treatment of addictive behaviors* (pp. 3–70). New York: Guilford.

Marlatt, G. A. (1985b). Cognitive assessment and intervention procedures for relapse prevention. In G. A. Marlatt & J. R. Gordon (Eds.), *Relapse prevention: Maintenance strategies in the treatment of addictive behaviors* (pp. 201–279). New York: Guilford.

Nelson, C. (1987). *Core relapse prevention group manual.* Unpublished instruction manual.

Nelson, C., Miner, M., Marques, J., Russell, K., & Achterkirchen, J. (1988). Relapse prevention: A cognitive–behavioral model for treatment of the rapist and child molester. *Journal of Social Work and Human Sexuality, 7,* 125–143.

Pithers, W. D., Marques, J. K., Gibat, C. C., & Marlatt, G. A. (1983). Relapse prevention with sexual aggressives: A self-control model of treatment and maintenance of change. In J. G. Greer & I. R. Stuart (Eds.), *The sexual aggressor: Current perspectives on treatment* (pp. 214–239). New York: Van Nostrand Reinhold.

Scheidt, R. J., & Schaie, K. W. (1978). A taxonomy of situations for an elderly population: Generating situational criteria. *Journal of Gerontology, 33,* 848–857.

Shiffman, S. (1982). Relapse following smoking cessation: A situational analysis. *Journal of Consulting and Clinical Psychology, 50,* 71–86.

Shiffman, S. (1984). Coping with temptations to smoke. *Journal of Consulting and Clinical Psychology, 52,* 261–267.

Shiffman, S., Read, L., Maltese, J., Rapkin, D., & Jarvik, M. E. (1985). Preventing relapse in ex-smokers: A self-management approach. In G. A. Marlatt & J. R. Gordon (Eds.), *Relapse prevention: Maintenance strategies in the treatment of addictive behaviors* (pp. 472–520). New York: Guilford.

11

Self-Efficacy Ratings

RODERICK L. HALL

DEFINITION OF SELF-EFFICACY

Self-efficacy refers to one's belief that he/she has the ability to perform a task successfully or adequately in a given situation. A person who has quit smoking may believe, for example, that he can avoid smoking when in the company of others who are smoking or when experiencing an emotional crisis. A person who has a fear of snakes may believe that he can approach and touch a live snake. Similarly, a person who has abused children sexually may believe that he can resist the temptation to fantasize about molesting a child when feeling depressed or believe that he can avoid molesting when alone with a child while engaging in deviant fantasy. As reflected in the above examples, one's perceived personal efficacy may vary across situations. That is, the ex-smoker may believe that he can successfully cope (avoid a lapse) when in the company of others who are smoking—but not if he is also drinking. There is, however, evidence (Tipton & Worthington, 1984) that people also have generalized self-efficacy, which facilitates competent performance across a broad range of situations.

The self-efficacy construct was introduced by Bandura (1977) to explain behavior changes that occur across different modes of treatment. Bandura asserts that all treatment interventions, no matter what form they take, create and/or enhance expectations of personal efficacy and that efficacy expectations are the primary causal factors in behavior change. The client with a phobia about snakes is able to change his fear and avoidance of snakes through expectations that he can successfully cope with an encounter with a snake. The client who has quit smoking remains abstinent mainly through expectations that he can successfully cope with situations that, without a successful coping response, would lead to resumption of smoking. The client who has molested children abstains through expectations that he can succesfully cope with high-risk situations, such as feeling lonely and depressed.

How does self-efficacy facilitate behavior change? According to Bandura (1977), the client who has a high level of self-efficacy in a given situation will attempt to cope, while one having a relatively low level will not make the attempt. A person's perceptions about his own potential effectiveness will determine whether he tries to cope in the first place, that is, whether he initiates behaviors that may lead to a desirable outcome. Furthermore, efficacy expectations also determine how much effort the client will expend and how long he will sustain effort in the face of obstacles and aversive experiences. Thus self-efficacy mediates one's motivation and ability to cope with a given stressful situation.

Bandura (1977) points out that efficacy expectations are not the only determinants of behavior:

> Expectation alone will not produce desired performance if the component capabilities are lacking. Moreover, there are many things that people can do with certainty of success that they do not perform because they have no incentives to do so. Given appropriate skills and adequate incentives, however, efficacy expectations are a major determinant of people's choice of activities, how much effort they expend, and of how long they will sustain effort in dealing with stressful situations. (p. 194)

Bandura also distinguishes efficacy expectations (beliefs that one can successfully execute behavior required to produce a desirable outcome) from outcome expectations (beliefs that a given behavior will lead to a given outcome). A client may believe that a particular sequence of behaviors will lead to a desirable outcome but may not initiate these if he has serious doubts about whether he can perform them. Thus, according to Bandura, efficacy expectations interact with, but are independent of, outcome expectations.

Bandura (1977) posits four sources of efficacy expectations: (1) performance accomplishments, (2) vicarious experience, (3) verbal persuasion, and (4) emotional arousal. These are briefly described here because of their treatment implications. Performance accomplishments are based on personal mastery experiences and are the most influential of the four. In general, repeated successes increase self-efficacy, while repeated failures decrease it. Vicarious experience involves seeing others perform required tasks or behaviors with positive outcomes (reinforcements). The modeling of required behaviors may be live (actually done by another person) or symbolic, that is, imagined by the client (covert modeling). Verbal persuasion involves the use of suggestion (by others or self) to convice clients that they can cope successfully with situations that have overwhelmed them in the past. Verbal persuasion is quite limited in its ability to produce enduring personal efficacy and can undermine self-efficacy if used with clients who do not have requisite skills. It might better be used to raise outcome expectancies (when clients have the ability to perform) than to enhance self-efficacy. Emotional arousal is generally associated with stressful and taxing situations. Such arousal generally lowers coping ability (via cognitive distortions) and debilitates performance, especially when it is high. In turn, reduced coping ability and inadequate performance reduce one's expectation for success. Therefore, one is more likely to expect success when one is not confronted with high, aversive arousal.

While it goes beyond the scope of this chapter to evaluate the conceptual accuracy of Bandura's use of the self-efficacy construct, the reader should be aware that Kirsh (1985) has raised several questions in that regard. Kirsh claims, for example, that Bandura uses the term *outcome expectancy* in two different ways, each implying a different relation to self-efficacy. Kirsh also suggests that Bandura's self-efficacy concept is functionally equivalent to Rotter's (1954) expectancy of success concept. Finally, contrary to Bandura's self-efficacy theory, Kirsh suggests that self-efficacy is affected by the reinforcement value of the coping response and the perceived difficulty of the task.

THE ROLE OF SELF-EFFICACY IN
THE PREVENTION OF RELAPSE

Relapse prevention relies heavily on the client's ability to learn and to initiate appropriate coping behaviors at the earliest possible point in the relapse process. The extent to which the client is able to cope successfully with situations that threaten his control over undesirable behavior (high-risk situations) will ultimately determine whether he will engage in a lapse or full-blown relapse. As noted previously, the probability that one will initiate a coping response in a given situation, the degree of effort he will expend in the situation, and how long he will expend effort in the face of adversity will mainly depend on his belief that he can successfully cope with the situation (Bandura, 1977).

According to Marlatt (1985a, 1985b), self-efficacy is highest at the point of abstinence. Each movement closer to relapse will theoretically be accompanied by decreases in self-efficacy. At the point of lapse (initial indulgence in the target behavior), self-efficacy is low. The client often believes that he has already failed and that his future chances of success are equally slim. He may feel excessively guilty and ashamed about the lapse (abstinence violation effect), which may further reduce self-efficacy. The client must have enough self-efficacy remaining to use cognitive restructuring and other coping skills to deal effectively with these aversive feelings. If he is able to cope successfully, he experiences increased self-efficacy and returns to abstinence. If, on the other hand, the client is unable to cope successfully, the lapse is likely to escalate into a full-blown relapse. Thus self-efficacy plays a pivotal role in the relapse prevention model by determining whether the client will avert the escalation of a lapse into a relapse by performing an appropriate coping response.

SELF-EFFICACY AND TREATMENT OUTCOME

There are no studies that have examined the relationship between self-efficacy and the treatment of abusive sexual behavior. However, a fair number of research studies have demonstrated that self-efficacy is predictive of treatment outcome with respect to phobias (Bandura, Adams, & Beyer, 1977; Barrios, Somervill, Henke, & Merritt, 1981; Biran & Wilson, 1981) and obesity (Mitchell & Stuart, 1984). Several studies have also examined the relation between self-efficacy and treatment of smoking behavior. In a study by Yates and Thain (1985), subjects who had voluntarily quit smoking 1 year earlier were administered a 14-item self-efficacy questionnaire, asking them how certain they were of being able to resist smoking in different circumstances (e.g., when feeling impatient, when worried). Data were also collected on 10 additional variables (e.g., age, income, years smoked, age started smoking, and percentage of family who smoked). Smokers who scored higher on the questionnaire were less likely to relapse after a 1-year period than those who scored low. A discriminant function analysis showed that the efficacy scores were as effective in classifying the subjects as abstainers or relapsers as were all 11 variables or the best combination of them.

To determine if the predictor equation obtained in the above retrospective study would be equally effective in a prospective study, Yates and Thain obtained measures on the same 11 variables in a group of subjects who had recently quit smoking and whose eventual status was not known. Using the predictor equation obtained from the retrospective study, the self-efficacy scores accurately predicted the status of all 15 relapsers and 7 abstainers in a 4-month follow-up period. The predictive power of the efficacy scores was maintained at 8-months follow-up.

In a similar study, Coelho (1984) administered a 31-item self-efficacy questionnaire to adult smokers enrolled in treatment that had a social learning focus. Ratings of self-efficacy were obtained at four points: pretreatment, treatment cessation, and 1 and 3 months posttreatment. Abstinent subjects had significantly higher efficacy scores at all assessments except pretreatment, and their level remained relatively constant from treatment cessation to 3 months posttreatment. In contrast, the efficacy scores of smokers decreased significantly over the same period. Furthermore, the pretreatment efficacy scores of the smokers were not significantly different from their 3 month posttreatment scores.

Similar findings have been reported by DiClemente (1981) and by Condiotte and Lichtenstein (1981). These results, along with the findings of Yates and Thain (1985) and Coelho (1984), suggest that self-efficacy ratings may be effective in identifying persons at risk for relapse, at least with certain addictive behaviors. They may also prove helpful in pinpointing situations that are most risky for the client as well as revealing the client's expected reaction to a lapse. Similar studies must be conducted with sex offenders before these promising findings can be generalized to that group.

Finally, it might be prudent to briefly review a study by Shiffman (1984) that failed to support the relationship between self-efficacy and relapse predicted by Marlatt (1985a; 1985b). Shiffman obtained efficacy ratings and various coping and effects-of-smoking measures on ex-smokers who called a relapse prevention hotline. Contrary to Marlatt's prediction that persons who successfully cope with a crisis (avert a lapse) would experience increases in self-efficacy, all subjects in this study experienced significant decreases in self-efficacy regardless of whether they had averted a lapse. Apparently, some people experience feelings of failure and decreased personal efficacy even if they have coped successfully with a high-risk situation. Shiffman also found that subjects who had lapsed had higher levels of self-efficacy than did subjects who had been able to cope successfully with the crisis and thereby avert a lapse. This latter finding, which is just the opposite of the predicted positive relationship between self-efficacy and abstinence, suggests that in some situations actual probability of success may be low despite high self-efficacy.

SELF-EFFICACY IN SEX OFFENDERS

Sex offenders, particularly sexual abusers of children, have been described as personally and socially inadequate (Finklhor, 1984; Laws, 1985; Marshall & McKnight, 1975). Psychoanalytic formulations of pedophilia describe the pedophile as sexually inadequate and fearful of contact with women (Karpman, 1959). Others view the inadequacy of the sex offender as a skills deficit (Laws, 1985; Vetter & Silverman, 1986). Laws (1985) states:

> Sex offenders may never have learned appropriate social behaviors and so possess a skills deficit. It is more likely that they have learned inappropriate behavior in criterion situations which have been reinforced a sufficient number of times that, even if they possess the appropriate skills, the inappropriate performances have a higher probability of occurrence. (p. 33)

Pedophiles often report that they feel inadequate in adult social situations. They fear rejection from adults and avoid situations in which rejection might be forthcoming. They feel most comfortable around children and come to value their interactions with children more highly. By avoiding adult situations, they miss the opportunity to gain experiences in interpreting the nonverbal and other social cues needed to form and maintain successful adult relationships. Laws (1985) states further:

Sex offenders often experience repeated failures in successfully initiating, performing, and sustaining reciprocal adult social and sexual relationships and are
therefore likely to experience and report an expectation of self-inefficacy in
those situations. Their "efficacy expectation" is often that they lack the skills to
succeed and their "outcome expectation" is that they will fail if they try, which
can lead to the faulty deduction that they are therefore condemned to remain
sexual deviants. (p. 33)

With respect to feelings of sufficient self-efficacy to abstain from further
deviant sexual fantasy or behavior in high-risk situations, rapists and pedophiles
are likely to differ, with the former having generally higher self-efficacy levels.
This may be the case for two reasons. First, the frequency of deviant sexual
behavior (including fantasies and urges) will typically be much greater in the
pedophile than in the rapist, so much so that the pedophile may experience his
deviant fantasies and behaviors as having a quality of compulsiveness. Considering the relative compulsion that the pedophile experiences in his deviant
sexual behavior, it is reasonable to expect that he will be less confident about his
ability to resist deviant urges.

Second, pedophiles are more likely than rapists to feel personally inadequate, especially in adult social situations. Pedophiles are also more likely to
attribute difficulties, including lapses into deviant fantasy, to personal deficits.
This personal attribution and self-blame, with associated feelings of guilt (abstinence violation effect), tend to reduce the pedophile's sense of self-efficacy. In
contrast, because the rapist is more likely to attribute difficulties to external
versus internal factors, he is thereby able to maintain high self-efficacy despite
occasional or even repeated lapses.

It is also possible that rapists may have higher generalized self-efficacy than
pedophiles. Limited support for this speculation is provided in a study by Hall
(1986) that examined rapists' and child molesters' expectations of success on a
novel learning task. In that study, subjects were asked to indicate their chances
of getting at least 80% of the learning-task items correct. Subjects rated their
chances for success on a scale that ranged from 0 (no chance at all) to 100
(completely certain). Rapists tended to give relatively high success estimates,
some as high as 100, even though the subjects had no information about the
nature of the learning task prior to making their estimates.

Finally, if Marlatt (1985b) is correct in asserting that an "abstinence
violation effect" (AVE) occurs when one experiences a lapse in the face of strong
commitment to abstinence, then the sexually abusive client may experience a
less intense AVE, and hence fewer decrements in self-efficacy, than do other
self-indulgent clients (e.g., overeaters and smokers). The reasoning here is that
the sexually abusive client may be less committed to abstinence, owing to his
generally involuntary status in treatment, his relative lack of immediate incen-

tives to avoid a lapse, and the relative lack of personal discomfort he experiences directly from engaging in the prohibited behavior.

Considering the sexually abusive client's hypothesized lowered commitment to abstinence, it may not be particularly upsetting to him when he violates weak convictions. The end result is likely to be unrealistically high self-efficacy and increased risk of relapse, which, as Shiffman (1984) suggests, may stem from the highly confident person's tendency to put himself in situations that might best be avoided. Shiffman (1984) states further:

> The data relating self-efficacy to performance are strongest in cases, such as phobias, when the subject is capable of performing, but avoids doing so. In these instances, high self-efficacy promotes efforts to master the task. In some cases, however, attempts offer no guarantee of success. As Bandura points out, "expectations alone will not produce desired performance if the component skills are lacking." As a result, "acting on misjudgments of personal efficacy can produce adverse consequences." Self-efficacy may be related to outcome only when it is backed up by relevant competence. In the absence of competence, high self-efficacy may lead to unsuccessful attempts to deal with dangerous situations. (p. 307)

ASSESSMENT OF SELF-EFFICACY
IN SEX OFFENDERS

The assessment of self-efficacy is important for several reasons. First, it may help to identify clients who are at high risk for relapse so that appropriate preventive interventions can be employed. Second, efficacy ratings can help to reveal the most risky of the client's high-risk situations that might warrant special attention in therapy. Third, efficacy ratings may be used to anticipate the client's reaction to an initial lapse into deviant sexual fantasy. This information can be used to prepare the client for the inevitable lapse in order to avoid escalation of the lapse to a relapse. Fourth, efficacy ratings provide self-evaluations of coping capacity, which can highlight areas in which additional skills training is needed.

Techniques to assess self-efficacy in sex offenders are relatively new and unvalidated. The few scales that are available borrow heavily from those used in alcohol and smoking cessation research. Most rating scales are comprised of a list of specific high-risk situations and an accompanying 5- or 7-point Likert Scale. Clients are typically asked to rate the degree of temptation they would likely experience and their degree of confidence in their ability to cope successfully (avoid a lapse) in each situation.

Laws (1985), for example, uses a number of scales adapted from self-efficacy scales for substance abuse to assess the frequency with which clients engage in high-risk behaviors (e.g., being in an uncomfortable social situation, drinking alcohol or using drugs, feeling bored with nothing to do, and experiencing strong frustration), the degree of temptation associated with the high-risk behavior, and the degree of confidence in resisting that temptation. All three of the above scales contain essentially the same 12 high-risk behaviors, and all are rated using a 7-point Likert Scale. Three additional scales assess coping responses across three situations: feeling depressed, having an argument with someone close, and finding oneself in the company of children. Nine coping responses are provided for each of the three situations, and the client uses a 5-point scale (ranging from "not at all likely" to "extremely likely") to indicate how likely he would be to make each response.

The several self-efficacy scales described above are comprehensive, but they nevertheless have several shortcomings. None of them assess the frequency of the sex offender's unacceptable sexual fantasy (lapse) or, more importantly, assess the degree to which the sex offender would be tempted to fantasize about unacceptable sexual behavior. The scales also fail to assess the client's confidence that he could resist the temptation to fantasize about unacceptable sexual behaviors in high-risk situations. Instead, the scales focus on the client's temptation to molest (relapse) and his ability to resist that temptation. The addition of scales that assess the use of the ability to control deviant fantasy would greatly improve the utility of the existing scales.

CONCLUSION

Although there is a growing body of research suggesting that self-efficacy ratings may be useful in the treatment of addictive behaviors such as obesity (Mitchell & Stuart, 1984) and smoking (Yates & Thain, 1985), no known studies have examined the relationship between self-efficacy and treatment of abusive sexual behavior. The paucity of research in this area compels one to use caution in applying the generally positive findings obtained in studies of obesity and smoking.

The lack of sufficient research in the area of self-efficacy and treatment of sexually abusive behavior is reason enough to continue to assess self-efficacy routinely as part of any treatment effort. Such practice will facilitate much-needed research regarding the utility of the self-efficacy construct in predicting relapse among sex offenders.

Furthermore, the paucity of research notwithstanding, self-efficacy ratings are likely to be useful in (1) identifying clients who are at high risk for relapse, (2) revealing the most risky of the client's high-risk situations that might warrant special attention in therapy, (3) anticipating the client's reaction to an initial lapse into deviant sexual fantasy, and (4) evaluating the client's use of effective coping responses.

In using self-efficacy ratings as described above, the therapist should consider that more than a few sex offenders may tend to report unrealistically high self-efficacy, for the reasons already stated. Caution is especially advised against the use of self-efficacy ratings to predict low probability or decreased probability of relapse. As stated previously, the available research data do not justify such uses. Furthermore, Shiffman's (1984) finding that self-efficacy is inversely related to abstinence in ex-smokers may be especially relevant to sex offenders, given their general use of denial and their relatively lowered abstinence conviction. The actual probability for relapse for many sex offenders will be high, despite their ability to maintain high self-efficacy about their ability to cope successfully with high-risk situations.

REFERENCES

Bandura, A. (1977). Self-efficacy: Toward a unifying theory of behavioral change. *Psychological Review, 84*, 191–215.

Bandura, A., Adams, N. E., & Beyer, J. (1977). Cognitive processes mediating behavioral change. *Journal of Personality and Social Psychology, 35*, 125–139.

Barrios, F. X., Somervill, J. W., Henke, K. J., & Merritt, B. R. (1981). Comparison of modelling and cognitive rehearsal in reduction of snake avoidance. *Psychological Reports, 49*, 635–642.

Biran, M., & Wilson, G. T. (1981). Treatment of phobic disorders using cognitive and exposure methods: A self-efficacy analysis. *Journal of Consulting and Clinical Psychology, 49*, 886–889.

Coelho, R. J. (1984). Self-efficacy and cessation of smoking. *Psychological Reports, 54*, 309–310.

Condiotte, M. M., & Lichtenstein, E. (1981). Self-efficacy and relapse in smoking cessation programs. *Journal of Consulting and Clinical Psychology, 49*, 648–658.

DiClemente, C. C. (1981). Self-efficacy and smoking cessation maintenance. *Cognitive Therapy and Research, 5*, 175–187.

Finkelhor, D. (1984). *Child sexual abuse: New theory and research.* New York: Free Press.

Hall, R. L. (1986). *The relationship between psychopathy and avoidance learning as mediated by success expectancy.* Unpublished doctoral dissertation, University of South Florida, Tampa.

Karpman, B. (1959). *The sexual offender and his offenses.* New York: Julian.

Kirsh, I. (1985). Self-efficacy and expectancy: Old wine with new labels. *Journal of Personality and Social Psychology, 49*, 824–830.

Laws, D. R. (1985). *Prevention of relapse in sex offenders.* (Grant No. 1R01 MH42035). Rockville, MD: National Institute of Mental Health.

Marlatt, G. A. (1985a). Cognitive factors in the relapse process. In G. A. Marlatt & J. R. Gordon (Eds.), *Relapse prevention: Maintenance strategies in the treatment of addictive behaviors* (pp. 128–200). New York: Guilford.

Marlatt, G. A. (1985b). Relapse prevention: Theoretical rationale and overview of the model. In G. A. Marlatt & J. R. Gordon (Eds.), *Relapse prevention: Maintenance strategies in the treatment of addictive behaviors* (pp. 3–70). New York: Guilford.

Marshall, W. L., & McKnight, R. D. (1975). An integrated treatment program for sexual offenders. *Canadian Psychiatric Association Journal, 20,* 133–138.

Mitchell, C., & Stuart, R. B. (1984). Effect of self-efficacy on dropout from obesity treatment. *Journal of Consulting and Clinical Psychology, 52,* 1100–1101.

Rotter, J. B. (1954). *Social learning and clinical psychology.* Englewood Cliffs, New Jersey: Prentice-Hall.

Shiffman, S. (1984). Cognitive antecedents and sequelae of smoking relapse crises. *Journal of Applied Social Psychology, 14,* 296–309.

Tipton, R. M., & Worthington, E. L. (1984). The measurement of generalized self-efficacy: A study of construct validity. *Journal of Personality Assessment, 48,* 545–548.

Vetter, H. J., & Silverman, I. J. (1986). *Criminology and crime: An introduction.* New York: Harper & Row.

Yates, A. J., & Thain, J. (1985). Self-efficacy as a predictor of relapse following voluntary cessation of smoking. *Addictive Behaviors, 10,* 291–298.

12

Relapse Fantasies

GENELL G. SANDBERG

G. ALAN MARLATT

One important assessment procedure in evaluating the client's coping skills is the relapse fantasy. Relapse fantasies can be a useful self-report indicator of a client's strengths and weaknesses in coping capacity. To develop relapse fantasies, the client is asked to fantasize a set of circumstances that might lead to a possible future relapse. These guided fantasies are used to elicit information concerning specific characteristics and details of that relapse that a client must be prepared to handle to prevent reoffending in the future. Being less structured, relapse fantasies often elicit idiosyncratic factors that might otherwise be missed in more structured assessment measures, such as the Situational Competency Test and ratings of self-efficacy.

To introduce the rationale for this assessment procedure, the therapist could state the following:

> You and I both hope relapse never happens in your case, and we're going to work hard so you will be able to prevent yourself from reoffending. However, it would be very helpful to our work toward that goal if, for just the next few minutes, you pretend you're no longer in treatment and you're having difficulty controlling your urge to rape (molest a child). I would like you to sit back comfortably in your chair and close your eyes. Relax and breathe slowly and deeply. Pretend it is sometime in the future. You are having difficulty keeping your mind off raping (molesting a child). Imagine a situation that would make it very difficult to resist your growing urge to rape (molest) again. Allow yourself to actually see yourself in that situation. When you can imagine the scene vividly, just allow yourself to start describing your feelings and the situation as clearly as you can.

It may be necessary for the therapist to give additional nonspecific prompts, such as "How else would you feel?" or "Tell me more about that," to develop the most detailed situation possible. The fantasies can be audiotaped for later transcription and review, or the therapist can note specific high-risk situations that increase the risk of reoffense, paying special attention to the absence of adaptive coping responses and the use of maladaptive coping behaviors. This procedure can reveal important clinical material for developing a treatment plan individually tailored to a client's particular coping-skill deficits.

We recommend that a thorough assessment involve having the client provide at least two relapse fantasies during the assessment procedure. The exercise can also be repeated midway through treatment to obtain more in-depth information about potential high-risk situations and coping responses.

An example of a relapse fantasy given by a rapist who is verbal, articulate, and has no difficulty with imagery follows:

> I go home after a hard day at work, and my wife gets on my case about not taking out the garbage that morning like I promised and forgetting to pick up our daughter's medication from the pharmacy. She tells me I'm irresponsible, a lazy good-for-nothing, and that I only care about myself. We get in a big argument, there's lots of yelling, and I decide to go for a drive to get away from her and cool off. When I go into the garage to back out the car I see my hunting knife on the workbench, and I pick it up and throw it on the seat beside me. I drive around for a while and then go to a café where I often have lunch with the guys, and I order a sandwich and a beer. After all the hassle I've gone through during the day, I end up with this smart-ass waitress who has waited on me before. She tells me to go to hell when I try to start up a conversation with her. I watch her waiting on other customers and being polite and nice to them, but not to me, as I'm eating my food. I have one more beer and then leave the restaurant and drive around some more. I really start thinking about that waitress and what a bitch she is. I get madder and madder and finally park the car outside the café and wait for her to get off her shift. When she comes out I watch her drive away, and I follow her to her apartment. I park down the block and walk up behind her car, making sure she doesn't see me. As she's getting out of her car and fumbling with her keys, I come up behind her, put my arm around her neck, and with my other hand hold the knife in front of her face. All she can do is plead, "Don't hurt me, don't hurt me." I tell her to shut up and that she should have been nice to me when she had the chance! I drag her off onto a side street behind some bushes and rape her. I am really mad during all of this and keep thinking about how she snubbed me in the restaurant and how she is so scared of me now. I like it that she is frightened. It makes me feel real powerful and in control.

By reviewing this fantasy with the client, a number of potentially high-risk factors can be ascertained, such as marital conflict and feelings of powerlessness, self-pity, shame, rejection, and anger. Further, this fantasy suggests that the client's aggressive style probably involves weapons and drinking. In reviewing this fantasy, the therapist attempts to focus on the client's cognitions, emotions, behaviors, and repertoire of coping responses that emerge as significant factors. Further, this information would be combined with other assessment data in the development of a highly individualized relapse prevention plan. Because even minimal stress may precipitate a relapse for a rapist who lacks adaptive coping skills, assessment of fantasies (in combination with other assessment data) is a crucial part of the overall evaluation of a client's strengths and weaknesses.

The following case example illustrates a relapse fantasy described by a pedophile:

> I'm living in an apartment complex where there are a lot of single mothers with kids. The children are always running around outside my window, playing games and having a lot of fun together. I work at a camera store and don't have any close friends; consequently, I spend most of my leisure time alone. One Saturday morning after finishing my household chores, I'm sitting in my living room watching a boring television program when Timmy, one of the boys in the complex who is about 9 years old, knocks on my door. He asks if I have seen the ball he and his friends were playing with yesterday. I tell him no, I haven't seen it, and I invite him in for some chocolate-chip cookies. While Timmy eats two cookies, he sees my collection of nature photographs on the wall. When I tell him that photography is my hobby, he gets very excited and says he's always wanted to have his own camera and learn to take and develop pictures by himself. I take out my Polaroid camera and show him how to work it. As I am explaining the procedure to him. I stand behind him, leaning up against his body with my arms extended over his shoulders. I allow Timmy to take a picture of me, and I take several of him, giving him one to take home. I also invite him to go on a picture-taking excursion to the park the next day if his mother will give her permission.
>
> When Timmy leaves, I prop his picture on the mantel above the fireplace and lay down to take a nap. I find my mind wanders to him, and I begin to fantasize about undressing him and fondling him, and I masturbate to this fantasy.
>
> The next day we go to the park and take pictures for several hours. As we sit in the car before leaving the park, looking at the pictures we took, I feel really turned on. I edge close to Timmy and put my arm around him. While he's looking at the pictures and laughing I place my other hand on his thigh and slide it gradually over to rest on his genitals. Timmy doesn't say anything, and he continues to look at the pictures. I feel highly sexually aroused now, but I decide not to try anything further until the next time we're together. In a few moments I slide over behind the wheel and casually mention that I have an old camera lying around I don't want. I ask Timmy if he would like to have it and try it out next weekend. He excitedly says yes, and we agree to come to the park again next Saturday. As we drive home, I replay the molestation over in my mind and still feel sexually excited, and also a little anxious about whether Timmy realizes what happened and whether he will tell anyone. To stop feeling anxious, I just think about how much fun it will be to plan next week's outing with Timmy and what I'll try with him next.

In reviewing this relapse fantasy, several high-risk factors that highlight coping-skill deficits emerge, including proximity to potential child victims, loneliness, lack of interpersonal relationships with adults, and engaging in sexual fantasy involving children. Again, the task of the therapist is to identify the absence of adaptive coping responses and the use of maladaptive coping behaviors. Self-report data obtained in the fantasy are then combined with information from the Situational Competency Test, self-efficacy ratings, and the client autobiography to provide a cumulative picture of the client's repertoire of coping behaviors.

When using assessment information to determine specific target areas for skill training, it is important to ascertain the extent to which a deficiency in responding to a specific high-risk situation represents a deficit in past learning experience or a current block in performance (of an already learned response) because of the inhibiting effects of anxiety, fear of evaluation, or other emotional reactions. For clients whose coping responses are blocked by fear or anxiety, the therapist may attempt to disinhibit the behavior by using an appropriate anxiety-reduction procedure, such as systematic desensitization. However, for most clients who demonstrate coping deficits, a systematic and structured skills-training approach is in order. In the example given above, if the pedophile's relapse fantasy is illustrative of his general response capacity, then his degree of loneliness and lack of interpersonal relationships with adults suggest a need for social-skills and/or dating-skills training. In the rapist case example, specific skill training for anger management and assertiveness is called for. The relapse prevention approach combines specific skill training with instruction in general problem-solving ability. Adopting a problem-solving orientation to stressful situations permits the client greater flexibility and adaptation to new problem situations.

For a client who lacks good imagery skills, his description of past sexual episodes can also provide useful assessment data. Asking the client to recall thoughts, feelings, or behaviors that occurred prior to the relapse may facilitate the recall of valuable information. What were the situational or intrapersonal determinants, and how did the client react to the relapse? Assessment of both a client's attitudes toward past relapses and that client's ability to control his own behavior will assist the therapist in developing an intervention program. Negative attributions about the client's own capacity to change, feeling devoid of any self-control abilities, and fearing the prospect of yet another failure are all attitudes to focus on in the treatment plan. On the other hand, clients may overestimate their capacity to change and may harbor unrealistic ideas about their ability to bring about desired changes based on distorted notions about past relapses (or lack of them).

A final cautionary note relates to the timing of relapse fantasies in the assessment process. Because these fantasies require the client to generate a scenario that leads to offending behavior, this procedure may evoke a great deal of guilt and other negative reactions. For this reason, clients may be highly resistant to giving relapse fantasies early in treatment. If it is determined that a guided relapse fantasy would evoke intense guilt feelings or dangerous urges, this procedure should be delayed or, in some instances, omitted entirely. Alternatively, for the client who is resistant to this technique primarily because of a dislike for feeling guilty, the therapist may frame the exercise as an opportunity for the client to begin to confront his guilt.

III

SOLUTIONS: TREATMENT

This section also considers solutions to problems facing sex offenders. Here we emphasize solutions through treatment, first through specific skills training and then through more global interventions.

SPECIFIC SKILLS TRAINING

The decision matrix is also a procedure borrowed from original RP, and Jenkins-Hall describes its adaptation to sex offenders. The matrix is a very simple method that permits the client a quick look at the positive and negative aspects, both short and long term, of sexual offending. Especially interesting in this chapter is the authors' discussion of decision-making processes in criminal and sexual offenders.

The cognitive–behavioral chain, as described by Nelson and Jackson, is essentially a sorting out of the typical thoughts and behaviors used by an individual in planning and implementing a sex offense. The procedure allows the client to identify relevant cognitions and behaviors that have previously served as antecedents to sex offenses. He may thus identify specific high-risk elements that can serve as cues to implement coping responses. In this way, they say, the offender can anticipate where events can lead and so take responsibility for the outcome.

Following from this analysis, Steenman, Nelson, and Viesti describe the development of coping strategies for high-risk situations. The goal is to intervene in the sequence of events leading to offending at the earliest sign of risk, substituting adaptive thoughts and behaviors for the previous maladaptive ones. This is a difficult task, since generalized high risks and their consequences cannot be fully anticipated in every possible situation. Therefore, the procedure teaches the importance of imagination, flexibility, and speed in implementing coping behaviors.

Carey and McGrath suggest a variety of methods that might be used to cope with urges and craving. In so doing they depart from the more typical and familiar RP strategies. They suggest the use of such diverse techniques as covert sensitization, masturbatory satiation, thought stopping, biological interventions, and changing contingencies in the offender's environment, as well as more familiar RP strategies, such as self-statements and relapse contracts. This type of flexibility, as Marlatt has long advocated, should be a hallmark of RP.

Related to the assessment procedure of relapse fantasies is relapse rehearsal. Hall recommends that this procedure be used only with clients who have made substantial gains in treatment, since it deliberately reinstitutes some of the conditions that promote a lapse. Additionally, since it involves deliberate deviant fantasy, it can produce the "abstinence violation effect" (AVE). As in his previous discussion of self-efficacy (see Chapter 11, this volume), Hall is skeptical of the use of this procedure with rapists, who may not experience the AVE.

Cognitive restructuring is a standard procedure in cognitive–behavior therapy, and Jenkins-Hall describes its use in RP. Her discussion weaves together the joint use of rational–emotive therapy (RET) and RP. She gives an extremely detailed analysis of typical irrational, self-defeating thinking in sex offenders from the RET perspective, than shows how a technique learned in one treatment may be easily applied in another. This is yet another example of the adaptability of the RP framework.

GLOBAL INTERVENTIONS

Major lifestyle interventions with sex offenders represent one of the most difficult of the RP goals. Thompson notes that such relevant research as exists comes mainly from treatment of addictive disorders. Drawing on that research, he suggests meditation, aerobic exercise, alteration of food and sleeping habits, and development of hobbies and adaptive social activities as possibilities that might be useful with sex offenders. He also correctly cautions that suggestion and encouragement are unlikely to be effective and that reinforcement-based contingency contracting may be necessary.

The PIG is a lifestyle problem, and feeding it can be a full-time occupation for some people. Marlatt suggests ways to handle it. He notes, as Thompson does, that lifestyle balancing can reduce the PIG's influ-

ence. Its influence is so pervasive that more specific techniques, such as coping responses for urging and craving as well as the use of aversive conditioning and masturbatory satiation, may be required to reduce it.

Finally, Hilderbran and Pithers treat a subject that is a very difficult task for many therapists, the promotion of offender empathy for their victims. They note that while RP teaches specific skills for training people how not to reoffend, it does not necessarily teach them anything about the consequences of their offenses against others. The technique they report uses books, reports, videos, and role-plays, all designed to engage the offender empathically with his victims. "How does it feel to have this done to you?" they ask the offender. Not surprisingly, the authors say that clients often find this the most difficult part of their treatment.

A · SPECIFIC SKILLS TRAINING

13

The Decision Matrix

KATURAH D. JENKINS-HALL

DEFINITION OF CONCEPT

Human beings are constantly processing information and making decisions regarding courses of action. In fact, most human behaviors can be analyzed in terms of the conscious or unconscious decisions made to get from point A to point B. Likewise, decision making is an important component in the chain of events leading to relapse (Marlatt, 1985). The concept of decision making is one that is relevant to all aspects of the process from abstinence to relapse. One chooses to engage in situations that invoke negative emotional states, to involve oneself in high-risk situations, and ultimately to engage in lapse and relapse behavior.

The perception of choice regarding engaging in the precursors of relapse affords the individual a sense of control over the behavior from which he/she is choosing to abstain. For example, the overweight man who believes that obesity is hereditary and that he will always be fat, regardless of his diet, feels very little control and is therefore likely to eat more. Similarly, a child molester who was sexually victimized as a child and who believes that these past conditions dictate his future inappropriate sexual behaviors perceives himself as having little control and is therefore more likely to engage in future molestations. The belief that, despite past conditions, one has choices about the future is a powerful therapy tool in that it provides the client with a sense of hope, self-efficacy, and self-control. It is imperative, then, that clients learn to make good choices regarding the course of their behaviors.

Because humans have a limited capacity for processing information in complex choice situations and in considering all alternatives, including the trade-offs implied by making one choice over another, decision aids are needed (Hogarth, 1980). Both in business and in psychological settings, efforts are made to train others in the making of sound decisions.

The idea that clients can be trained in using decision aids and decision-making techniques is not new. Many cognitive therapies teach decision-making strategies as part of problem-solving techniques (Meichenbaum, 1977; Nezu & D'Zurilla, 1981). These strategies usually include a system for defining the problem, generating alternative solutions, weighing the solutions in terms of their relative value, and making the decision. Nezu and D'Zurilla (1981) found that training in a decision-making strategy significantly increased the decision-making effectiveness of those trained compared to a control group of untrained subjects.

The concept of "utility," the subjective value of a given alternative (Tedeschi & Lindskold, 1976), is usually heavily relied on in the majority of decision-making strategies. In fact, most strategies for decision making are based on the utility rule: a method of problem solving that maximizes positive consequences and minimizes negative consequences, both long and short term, both social and personal (Nezu & D'Zurilla, 1979). This rule is based on a major assumption of social psychology—that humans are basically hedonistic and that, given the opportunity, they will seek to maximize utilities in decision making (Tedeschi & Lindskold, 1976). "Whenever [a] person must make decisions among alternative actions, it may be assumed he will act to maximize the utility available to him under the circumstances" (Tedeschi & Lindskold, 1976, p. 20).

The decision matrix is a tool used in relapse prevention that is based on the utility rule. It is designed to get the client to consider both short- and long-term consequences of abstinence versus relapse. As stated by Marlatt (1985), it is:

a 2 × 2 × 2 matrix with the following factors: the decision to resume the old behavior or to maintain abstinence, the immediate versus delayed effects of either decision, and, within each of the former categories, the positive and negative consequences involved. (p. 58)

This chapter examines the use of the decision matrix in working with sex offenders and the special problems inherent in working with this population using such an approach. Because sexual offending is a criminal behavior, the chapter provides a brief overview of criminal decision making, followed by an examination of problems in decision making specific to sex offenders. Finally, the use of the decision matrix as a therapeutic tool in increasing motivation to refrain from sexually deviant behavior is addressed.

CRIMINAL DECISION MAKING

It is a commonly held view that people who chronically engage in criminal activity use different decision-making strategies than those who do not. Most decisions made by the criminal are made on the basis of his perception of the immediate positive consequences of his actions (Hare, 1970). Although the criminal may be aware on an intellectual level that he might get caught and

punished for the antisocial behavior, he usually has no emotional insight into these negative consequences. Therefore, he mainly concerns himself with what is tangible and what he feels in the present (Hare, 1970).

Yochelson and Samenow (1976), in their description of criminal thinking, state: "In most of the criminal's decision-making there is no weighing of pros and cons, no careful evaluation of course of action" (p. 402). The criminal has not learned that there are a number of alternative courses of actions. In fact, he does not need to consider alternatives because he trusts his own initial assumptions over all others. He therefore bases his decision on unvalidated assumptions and his immediate desires (Yochelson & Samenow, 1976). This, of course, presents problems for the criminal who makes major life decisions based on his drive for immediate gratification and the likelihood that he will benefit in the short run.

Hare (1970) posits that this "inability to delay gratification" is perhaps related to the criminal's low expectancies of positive long-term consequences. In other words, the criminal lacks the foresight to perceive long-term positive consequences as having an equal or greater positive valence than short-term positive consequences.

In addition to not evaluating alternative courses of action and not being able to appreciate the value of long-term positive consequences, the criminal is also unable to evaluate adequately the negative consequences of his behaviors on others. As stated by Yochelson & Samenow (1976): "There is no realistic long-term planning, no consideration of injury to others, and no putting himself in the place of others" (p. 403). Numerous writers have emphasized the criminal's apparent lack of empathy (e.g., Cleckley, 1964; Hare, 1970; Schalling, 1978; Yochelson & Samenow, 1976). It is important to note that without empathy, the offender is unable to appraise the severity of short- and long-term negative consequence to his victim(s).

THE DECISION-MAKING PROCESS
OF SEXUAL OFFENDERS

Sexual offenders have the same flaws in their decision making as other criminals. They have problems foreseeing long-term consequences (positive or negative), they do not generate or weigh alternative solutions, and they are unaware of the impact of their behaviors on their victims.

The problem of not being aware of long-term consequences has been described (e.g., George & Marlatt, 1986; Marlatt, 1985; Pithers, Marques, Gibat, & Marlatt, 1983) as a problem of immediate gratification.

> After a client has been abstinent for some period of time, a shift in attitudes and beliefs about the effects of the foregone . . . activity often occurs. Positive

> outcome expectancies for the immediate effects become an especially potent motivating force to resume [the deviant behavior] when the client is faced with a high risk situation ... the temptation to [indulge] in the formally taboo activity is a powerful influence to contend with. (Marlatt, 1985, p. 57)

Sexual gratification is a primary reinforcer, and because sexually deviant behavior is pleasurable, it is easy for the offender to forget the long-term consequences of the deviant behavior and to indulge in the positive feelings of the here-and-now. The decision matrix is a useful tool for addressing the problems of immediate gratification.

With respect to not being able to generate alternative solutions when confronted with a critical decision point (e.g., a high-risk situation), the sexual offender will often describe how he felt compelled to act or how he had no other choice or alternative. For example, a pedophile in outpatient treatment was dating a woman with two sons the age of his desired victims. He had managed to avoid being alone with the boys until, one day, he agreed to go to the movie with the family. The mother of the boys was driving and remembered that she needed to dash into the drugstore before the movie. She asked the client if he would please wait in the car and supervise the boys. At the time, the client could see no other choices but to wait with the boys and, predictably, found himself experiencing deviant urges. In session, the client was assisted in generating alternatives, such as observing the boys from outside the car, supervising the boys in the store while their mother shopped, and offering to go into the store for the mother.

Regarding the issue of empathy, when asked to consider the effects of his behavior on his victims, the sexual offender will minimize, rationalize, deny, and distort reality. For example, the pedophile fails to see any harm done unless he has physically assaulted or penetrated his young victim. It is also very difficult for the pedophile to acknowledge ill effects on a child with whom he has felt some personal connection.

On the other hand, many rapists believe that their victims somehow deserved the treatment they received. They project blame onto the victim with such statements as "I never would have hit her if she hadn't screamed" or "She shouldn't have been dressed like that if she didn't want any action." Some rapists have been so bold as to ask the women they have brutally raped for dates afterwards, denying the victims' extreme disdain.

Both rapists and pedophiles generally are unaware of the rippling effect of victimization. That is, even if they acknowledge the impact of their behavior on given victims, they are ignorant of the impact on the victims' parents, siblings, mates, and friends. Because impact of behavior on the victim is an area so easily dismissed by most offenders, many clinicians using the decision matrix require that factors regarding the impact of the sexual assault be included.

THE USE OF THE DECISION MATRIX IN THERAPY

The decision matrix is a simple therapeutic aid for handling very complex chunks of information regarding the consequences of offending. It may be used as a tool to reinforce the client's motivation to be deviance-free as well as a tool for teaching the client a general decision-making strategy. The therapist introduces the decision matrix after the client understands the problems of immediate gratification (his tendency to focus on the short-term positive effects). The matrix is introduced as a systematic way of examining both short- and long-term consequences, positive and negative. It is generally helpful to begin by using another addictive behavior (e.g., smoking) as an example of how to complete the matrix. This provides the client with the opportunity to learn to use the matrix in a nonthreatening way. For example, an offender will respond more readily to questions related to the short- and long-term consequences of smoking than he will to ones related to sexual offending. Most will recognize and readily admit to the immediate relief and tension reduction associated with taking the first cigarette after a period of abstinence. However, when asked the same question about the sexual offense, because he is concerned about social desirability, the offender will not as easily volunteer that the deviant sexual behavior was pleasurable. Similarly, while the offender will likely recognize the immediate consequences of not taking the initial cigarette (e.g., increased anxiety, irritability), he may not be as insightful about his own negative reactions when he chooses not to offend.

After the matrix is completed with the nonthreatening example, the therapist then assists the client in making entries related to the decision to offend or not to offend (to perform or to refrain). "All effects that the client regards as important should be listed in the matrix, whether or not the therapist agrees" (Pithers et al., 1983, p. 236). However, the therapist should be active in assisting the client in defining long- versus short-term consequences, whether a particular consequence is positive or negative, and the effect of the offense on the victim.

Figure 13.1 is a decision matrix completed by a pedophile in outpatient treatment at the Center for Prevention of Child Molestation (see Jenkins-Hall, Osborn, Anderson, Anderson, & Shockley-Smith, Chapter 23, this volume). As can be seen in the figure, the client had the most difficulty in thinking of positive long-term consequences resulting from the decision to offend and negative long-term consequences resulting from the decision not to offend. This is very typical and expected. Clients mull over what they should enter in these cells and are relieved when they discover that there are very few entries that would be appropriate. When the matrix is complete, they gain the insight that there is little to be gained in the long run by offending and little to lose by not offending.

	Short-term Consequences		Long-term Consequences	
	Positive	Negative	Positive	Negative
To Offend	1. It feels good 2. It's exciting 3. I feel in control over victim	1. Depression/Guilt/ Fear 2. Worried about getting caught 3. Negative response of victim 4. Loss of control of myself 5. Anxiety over keeping the secret	1. Pleasure 2. Exciting/Risky lifestyle 3. No rejection from adults	1. Loss of freedom 2. Loss of family support 3. Loss of job if incarcerated 4. Loss of self-esteem 5. Negative effect on victims 6. Shame
Not To Offend	1. Feelings of power over sexuality 2. Self-respect 3. No victim 4. Approval from others	1. Sexual frustration 2. Some increase in urges	1. Deviant-free lifestyle 2. Increased adult relationships 3. Freedom from legal system 4. Self-respect 5. Respect of friends & family 6. Feelings of self-control 7. No victims	1. No sexual pleasure from kids (adults only) 2. Some anxiety over new lifestyle (will go away in time)

FIGURE 13.1.   Decision matrix.

In preparation for use of the decision matrix, the therapist may wish to use two exercises described by George and Marlatt (1986) in the earlier stages of therapy: the problem list and benefits of changing. The instructions for the problem list exercise are as follows: "List all the problems and negative consequences you have experienced in your life as a result of your deviant sexual practices. Include various life areas: emotional, family, health, legal, economics, [and] vocational" (p. 19). The completion of the list, if done in the initial sessions of relapse prevention, can be used as a means for catharsis. The client is more than eager to share with the group how miserable his life has become (usually as a result of being "unfairly" apprehended). Many clients begin treatment a short time after they have been released from incarceration or soon after the offense has been discovered. Many have recently lost jobs, gone through divorce, or given up visitation rights.

After some time in therapy, when the client is engaging in lifestyle modifications, the following exercise, referred to as "benefits of changing" (George & Marlatt, 1986), may be useful:

> We hope that by now you are experiencing a few improvements in your daily lifestyle as a result of giving up your involvement with the deviant sexual activities. We have been encouraging you to engage in pleasurable activities and to learn how to manage stress. Take a few moments to reflect on the benefits you are experiencing. . . . Touch on various aspects of your life in which you have noticed benefits, . . . social relations, family relations, personal growth, economic, legal, occupational, etc. (p. 64)

After completing the matrix, the client (in a group setting) has the benefit of hearing the entries of other offenders and should be instructed to add to the matrix as appropriate. After the matrix is completed, an examination and count of the number of entries in each cell will guide the client to the most adaptive decision. That is, the decision with the greatest number of positive outcomes and lowest number of negative outcomes should be undertaken. (In working with a number of sex offenders using the decision matrix, I have found that the decision not to offend has always won out.) Other clinicians (e.g., Pithers et al., 1983) have suggested that the client assign numerical ratings to each entry, indicating their relative importance. This extra step may be well worth it to higher-functioning clients who understand the concept of weighing. The results of a simple count and the adding of weights should be the same—the decision not to offend. Clients are instructed to carry the decision matrix with them and to examine the long-term consequences whenever their motivation is waning.

THE USE OF THE MATRIX
AS A GENERAL STRATEGY

Many clients are taken with this simple but effective method of decision making and voluntarily will use the matrix for other decisions of daily living. Matrices have been used as aids in deciding whether or not to stay in a given relationship, remain on a given job, move to certain areas, and even remain in therapy. The decision matrix is reported by clients to be one of the most valuable tools offered in relapse prevention treatment.

REFERENCES

Cleckley, H. (1964). *The mask of sanity.* St. Louis: Mosby.
George, W. H., & Marlatt, G. A. (1986). *Relapse prevention with sexual offenders:* A *treatment manual.* Unpublished manuscript, Florida Mental Health Institute, Tampa.

Hare, R. D. (1970). *Psychopathy: Theory and research.* New York: Wiley.

Hogarth, R. M. (1980). *Judgment and choice: The psychology of decision.* Chichester, UK: Wiley.

Marlatt, G. A. (1985). Relapse prevention: Theoretical rationale and overview of the model. In G. A. Marlatt & J. R. Gordon (Eds.), *Relapse prevention: Maintenance strategies in the treatment of addictive behaviors* (pp. 3–70). New York: Guilford.

Meichenbaum, D. (1977). *Cognitive–behavior modification: An integrative approach.* New York: Plenum.

Nezu, A., & D'Zurilla, T. J. (1979). An experimental evaluation of the decision-making process in social problem solving. *Cognitive Therapy and Research, 3,* 269–277.

Nezu, A., & D'Zurilla, T. J. (1981). Effects of problem definition and formulation on the generation of alternatives in social problem-solving process. *Cognitive Therapy and Research, 5,* 265–271.

Pithers, W. D., Marques, J. K., Gibat, C., & Marlatt, G. A. (1983). Relapse prevention with sexual aggressives: A self-control model of treatment and maintenance of change. In J. G. Greer & I. R. Stuart (Eds.), *The sexual aggressor* (pp. 214–239). New York: Van Nostrand Reinhold.

Schalling, D. (1978). Psychopathy-related personality variables and the psychophysiology of socialization. In R. D. Hare & D. Schalling (Eds.), *Psychopathic behavior: Approaches to research* (pp. 85–106). New York: Wiley.

Tedeschi, J. T., & Lindskold, S. (1976). *Social psychology: Interdependence, interaction, and influence.* New York: Wiley.

Yochelson, S., & Samenow, S. E. (1976). *The criminal personality: Vol. 1. A profile for change.* New York: Aronson.

14

High-Risk Recognition:
The Cognitive-Behavioral Chain

CRAIG NELSON
PAMELA JACKSON

From a relapse prevention (RP) perspective, sexual offenses are neither isolated nor discrete events. They do not just happen. Rather, they are the culmination of a long series, or chain, of events (Marques & Nelson, in press; Nelson, Miner, Marques, Russell, & Achterkirchen, 1988). If offenders are successfully to prevent relapsing into illegal sexual acts, it is assumed that they must first recognize and take responsibility for the sequence of their cognitions and behaviors culminating in sexual offenses (Knopp, 1984). It is only after the antecedents and precipitants of their crimes are identified that offenders are able to plan, practice, and eventually implement adequate coping responses that will preclude the relapse process and sustain a position of abstinence. The purpose of the present chapter is to describe a technique used with participants in the Sex Offender and Evaluation Project (see Marques, Day, Nelson, & Miner, Chapter 22, this volume) to identify the pattern of precipitants that place them at risk for a sexual reoffense. The next chapter (Steenman, Nelson, & Viesti, Chapter 15, this volume) describes how this technique can be extended to plan, develop, and practice coping strategies to avert the relapse process.

High-risk situations, which by definition threaten an offender's sense of control over his sexual behavior, are comprised of both personal and environmental variables, or elements. The idiosyncratic constellations of high-risk elements and the way they interact to comprise high-risk situations must be specifically outlined for each offender. The technique of building cognitive–behavioral offense chains is designed to assist offenders in this process. Once developed, these chains concretely highlight the interactions among various elements and provide offenders with an opportunity to analyze the progression of the precipitants of their illicit sexual acts. In addition, this exercise sensitizes offenders to personal choices culminating in their crimes, strengthening their sense of personal responsibility. Inspecting such chains highlights points for intervention with coping responses that will divert the offense pattern.

BUILDING A BEHAVIORAL CHAIN

An important way offenders learn to identify and recognize high-risk elements is by examining past failures in controlling their sexual behavior (Marques, Pithers, & Marlatt, 1984; Pithers, Marques, Gibat, & Marlatt, 1983). The first step in this process is to construct a simple behavioral chain identifying the major events that precipitated an offender's past rape or molestation. The offender is asked to detail the most important observable events that led to a specific past crime. The emphasis, at this point, is on describing the events in behavioral terms (what happened as opposed to why it happened) and on listing the events in sequence as they occurred. The descriptions include either what the offender said or did and/or what someone else said or did. Such observable events as using drugs or alcohol, arguing with a spouse, losing a job, or having a potential victim behave in some manner that the offender misinterpreted as seductive may be identified at this point. These events served as some of the personal and environmental risk elements that were the relevant antecedents to the crime. The time frame of the events is considered irrelevant. Some events may have occurred in close proximity to one another, others may have been temporally distant. The important characteristic is that the offender views all of these events as having in some fashion promoted the conditions for the offense.

Each offender is required to identify at least seven behavioral events that served as antecedents in order to elicit a range of important contributing events. Without such a requirement, some offenders ignore important precipitants that set the stage for their crimes. For example, an offender may, as a justification for the offense, simply claim that he got drunk. This offers little information as to how the crime came about. Certainly, many people become intoxicated without ever committing a sexual offense, and it is likely that the offender had abused alcohol in the past without sexually abusing someone. What observable events made this situation different or special? The answer to such a question prompts the identification of important risk elements that otherwise remain hidden, and it facilitates the ability to view the offense as an endpoint in a series, or chain, of interconnected events.

In contrast to offenders who may ignore or minimize important antecedents, some offenders overelaborate the relevance of inconsequential events that preceded the crime. In such instances, the offender may produce long, unwieldy lists of relatively benign events that serve only to obscure, rather than highlight, important relationships. Therefore, offenders are asked to limit their lists to no more than ten important precipitating observable events. If an offender claims too many events to fit within this limit, he is asked to select only the most relevant events or attempt to combine related events. In this manner, the most influential observable precursors can be recognized.

In our experience using this technique, it has often been initially difficult for offenders to describe precipitating events in objective, observable terms. Frequently, they attempt to interject cognitions or affects in an effort to explain, justify, or otherwise defend their actions or behavior. For instance, a description such as "the victim made me angry" would be unacceptable at this point. Instead, the offender would be asked to describe what the victim did or said to which he responded angrily. In this manner, they are forced to distance themselves from the events leading up to a rape or molestation and learn to become more objective observers of personal events. This is an important first step in the change process according to cognitive–behavior therapy (Meichenbaum, 1977; Meichenbaum & Cameron, 1982), and it prepares the individual to analyze the environmental and personal determinants of relapse—a fundamental step in preventing its reoccurrence (Brownell, Marlatt, Lichtenstein, & Wilson, 1986).

The preparation of a behavioral chain should be as specific to an offense as possible. If an offender committed multiple crimes, a behavioral chain is separately prepared for each specific offense. Attempts at generalizations are avoided. As described later, generalizations can emerge by comparing the behavioral chains for various offenses.

The focus in building a behavioral chain is on the events preceding the offense as perceived and revealed by the offender. Although the offender's actions that constituted the rape or molestation are important, the focus is on identifying places to intervene in the precipitants and antecedents prior to the offense. In several cases, it was noted that an offender had difficulty determining when an actual offense began. For example, a child molester whose molestation included sexual intercourse described the fondling of the victim's breast and vagina as an antecedent to the crime. Although such fondling undoubtedly served as an antecedent to the intercourse, it in itself is illegal and represented a violation of acceptable behavior. The opportunity to identify and clarify this point aids the offender in adjusting his perception of the limits of acceptable behavior.

The pertinence of each event in the behavioral offense chain can be separately evaluated by determining whether the event increased, decreased, or had no effect on the probability that the offense would later occur. Those events that decreased or had no effect on the likelihood of the eventual crime are deleted from the chain as irrelevant.

Some offenders may claim an inability to remember the important events leading up to their offenses because of either intoxication or the length of time between the offenses and their examination in the behavioral chain. In such instances, offenders are instructed to add details or events that were described in the police reports and court testimony, what others have told them occurred prior to the crime, or what they believed most likely happened.

Figure 14.1 represents an example of a completed behavioral offense chain for a child molester. It identifies several relevant risk factors:

1. This offender with four divorces has a significant history of unsatisfactory relationships with adult women.
2. There are situational stressors in the form of a lost job and a pregnant girlfriend to support.
3. There is access to a potential victim.
4. He learns that the victim has been previously molested and that no actions were taken to report the perpetrator.
5. There is the presence of a disinhibitor in the form of alcohol.
6. Finally, with all of these elements operating, he is in the midst of a high-risk situation in which he finds himself alone with the victim.

A completed behavioral chain will reveal many of the high-risk elements that served to precipitate a sexual offense. However, as can be seen in the above example, many of the pieces needed to complete the picture are still missing. How is it that these events led to a molestation? Why did the offender not respond in some other way to his stressors? The answer to these questions can be found in the offender's interpretations, which gave an idiosyncratic meaning and importance to the various observable elements that ultimately culminated in the molestation.

ADDING INTERPRETATIONS TO THE CHAIN

The second step in this process is to develop a cognitive–behavioral offense chain by adding the cognitions and affects that represent the manner in which offenders interpreted the events that propelled them toward their offenses. From a social learning theory perspective (Mischel, 1973), these salient personal factors include: (1) the subjective value of situational cues that serve as incentives or motivators, (2) the expected outcomes of a variety of different behaviors, (3) the ways in which information is encoded and construed, (4) the self-regulatory rules that evaluate personal behavior, and (5) the knowledge and competencies of the individual.

In order to identify the relevant individual risk factors that compose a high-risk situation, offenders are asked to describe their interpretations of each separate event in the behavioral chain leading to the offense. Offenders are

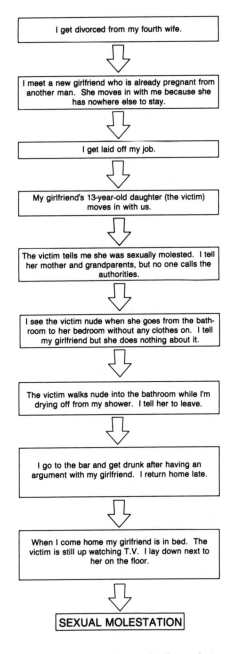

FIGURE 14.1. Behavioral offense chain.

reminded that all events are accompanied by interpretations in the form of cognitive and affective reactions. Some interpretations are so rapid that one might not even be aware of them. Such thoughts are sometimes referred to as "automatic" because of their seemingly involuntary nature (Beck, 1976). Other interpretations, however, may take considerable more reflection. Any event may have a variety of equally plausible interpretations. It is emphasized that personal self-statements interpreting external events will, in large part, determine one's reaction and response (Meichenbaum, 1977).

In recalling pertinent interpretive self-statements for each event, offenders are cautioned not to evaluate the accuracy of the interpretations with the luxury of hindsight. Instead, they are asked to describe how they interpreted or viewed the event at the time it occurred. Each interpretation is described by a self-statement that reflects the personal meaning attributed to the events leading to the offense.

As with the observable events, each identified self-statement is evaluated as to whether it increased, decreased, or had no effect on the probability that the offense would eventually occur. Only those interpretations that increased the likelihood of the crime are retained in the chain, and those that decreased the likelihood or had no effect are deleted.

Sometimes offenders report that they do not recall how they interpreted the event or claim that they had no interpretations or thoughts about it. In such cases, they are reminded that people are constantly interpreting the events around them and that some type of self-statement was inevitable. With this in mind, they are asked to describe how they most likely interpreted the event in light of the fact that it ultimately increased the probability of offending.

By adding interpretations to the behavioral chain, a full picture emerges of how the offense occurred. An ideal, completed cognitive–behavioral offense chain will funnel toward the offense. It can be likened to a roadmap in which each turn and curve in the road moved the offender closer to the offense until the final destination was inevitable. Should the various risk factors fail, as they often do, to fit together to provide an image of this path, it suggests that important and necessary elements are missing. Suggesting that these cognitive–behavioral chains illustrate how events and their interpretations led them to sexual offenses encourages offenders to identify and recognize additional relevant risk elements.

Figure 14.2 represents the addition of the interpretations to the behavioral chain illustrated as Figure 14.1. This cognitive–behavioral offense chain reflects a fairly complete map of the antecedents and precipitants of the offense. It explains how the offender arrived at the point of molesting. The offender's self-esteem, at a particularly low point following his divorce, placed him in an especially vulnerable position. This allowed him to become entangled in yet another dissatisfying relationship. His job loss further exacerbated his low sense

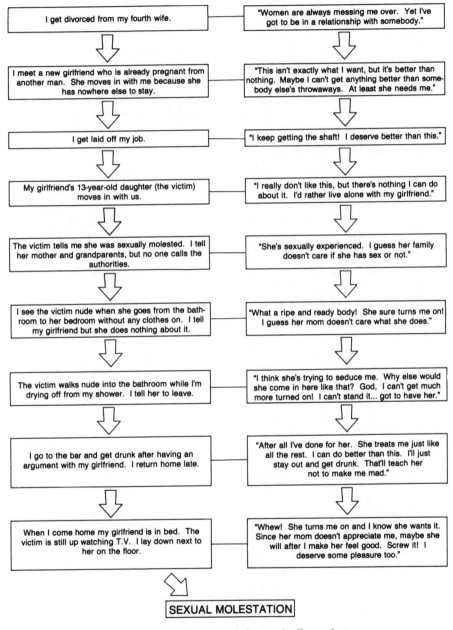

FIGURE 14.2. Cognitive–behavioral offense chain.

of self-worth and fostered a sense that he deserved any pleasure that he could find. The offender placed high stimulus value on the victim when he detected that he was becoming sexually aroused to her. He interpreted her actions as seductive, and he expected that she would be receptive to his sexual advances. Also, he reasoned that there was little chance of aversive consequences resulting from having sex with her, since the previous molesting had not been reported. He was able to justify his actions by interpreting the argument with his girlfriend as a sign that she did not love him and as permission to seek other sources of gratification to which he felt entitled. Finally, his level of intoxication served as a disinhibitor and a justification for relinquishing control over his behavior. Each of the various landmarks of events and cognitions map the path that led him to the molestation. From this cognitive–behavioral chain, many of the high-risk elements as well as the manner in which they interact may be seen.

In addition to identifying the elements that compose high-risk situations, the cognitive–behavioral chain highlights the multiple "apparently irrelevant decisions" (AIDs) that surreptitiously place offenders in high-risk situations and set the stage for their offenses. In the case example, allowing the victim to move into his home, failing to notify the authorities himself of her previous molestation, and returning home intoxicated at a time when he might find the victim alone are some of the AIDs that were identified from the offender's cognitive–behavioral chain. Although AIDs may appear superficially reasonable and defensible, placing them in the context of the cognitive–behavioral offense chain makes their relevance undeniable. In viewing the offense from the perspective of the chain, offenders are confronted with their own responsibility for the choices that culminated in their offenses and for arranging the circumstances that led to their crimes.

An appropriately constructed cognitive–behavioral offense chain will highlight both the specific high-risk elements and the offender's personal responsibility for the past offense. It is assumed that the best predictor of future behavior is the past behavior of the same individual in a similar situation. Therefore, it is reasonable to expect that an identical predicament in the future would again present a high-risk situation that would challenge the offender's ability to cope without relapsing into a reoffense. Although it is possible to develop very specific coping strategies for this particular set of circumstances, it would be naive to believe that this would be adequate to prevent reoffense in the future. It can be anticipated that the future high-risk situations that the offender will need to be prepared to confront will vary in a number of important aspects. However, it is also expected that future high-risk situations will have many elements in common with the past situations that provoked illicit sexual behavior. Therefore, it is necessary to generalize the cognitive–behavioral offense chain so that it includes cognitive themes and classes of events that are common across situations that place an offender at risk.

GENERALIZING THE
COGNITIVE-BEHAVIORAL CHAIN

One way to distill the necessary risk elements with which a sex offender must be prepared to cope in the future is to examine a variety of past situations that resulted in offenses. In a process similar to constructing the initial cognitive-behavioral offense chain, an offender can build an additional chain for each past offense. First, the observable events that served as cues and contingencies to enhance the likelihood of the rape or molestation are described in sequential order. This is followed by adding the relevant interpretations of each event that served as a catalyst to move and channel the offender's behavior toward the rape or molestation. Due to the large number of sexual crimes that some child molesters and rapists have committed (Abel et al., 1987; Groth, Longo, & McFaddin, 1982), it may not be feasible to examine all of the past offenses in detail. However, the construction of cognitive–behavioral offense chains on a representative sample of these crimes may be used. By comparing the chains that are produced for various past offenses, it is possible to understand the types of recurring events and interpretive themes for which coping responses must be developed.

Another technique that can be used to generalize the cognitive–behavioral offense chain is guided relapse fantasies (see Sandberg & Marlatt, Chapter 12, this volume; Marlatt & Gordon, 1985). In this procedure, offenders are asked to imagine circumstances that would likely provoke a relapse into a new sexual offense at some point in the future (Marques et al., 1984; Pithers et al., 1983). Each fantasy is detailed as specifically as possible. It is expected that as offenders progress in treatment, they will reflect their enhanced recognition and awareness of the types of situations that promote their relapses by describing them in greater detail and specificity. As for actual past offenses, complete cognitive–behavioral offense chains can be developed based on these relapse predictions.

By comparing the specific cognitive–behavioral chains for as many past offenses and guided relapse fantasies as possible, one can identify a variety of common characteristics that emerge across the various situations. Through inductive reasoning, it is possible to generate a number of global high-risk elements that characterize the events and interpretations represented in the various chains. An offender can be expected to prepare for only a manageable number of high-risk elements. If there are too many, it may not be reasonable to prepare coping strategies for all of them (Pithers et al., 1983). Overspecific descriptions of high-risk elements multiply the number of narrow, focused, and situation-specific coping strategies that are required. A more general description of high-risk elements, on the other hand, leads to the formulation of a limited number of more universal coping strategies that can be applied in a wider variety of situations that include the elements.

Through the process of examining the cognitive–behavioral chains for a variety of previous molestations and guided relapse fantasies, the offender in the illustrated case was able to identify a number of general elements that present risks for relapse. These included (1) interpersonal stressors that lower his sense of self-esteem, (2) anger-provoking situations, (3) being alone with pubescent females, (4) becoming sexually aroused to a teenage girl, (5) self-statements that reflect a sense that he would not be caught were he to reoffend, (6) the distorted interpretation that a potential victim is trying to seduce him when he becomes sexually aroused to her, (7) distorted self-assurances that a potential victim would not be harmed by the molestation, and (8) the use of such disinhibitors as alcohol. Recognition of these high-risk elements allows a variety of coping strategies to be developed that reduce these elements' potential for promoting relapse and reoffense when encountered in the future.

Properly constructed cognitive–behavioral offense chains for either past offenses or guided relapse fantasies are not viewed as static. Rather, their value rests in the process of their construction. As offenders review their chains, new events may be identified that enhance their recognition of important high-risk elements and the manner in which they interact to precipitate offenses. Whereas offenders may identify observable events that are temporally proximal to the crime upon their first construction of the cognitive–behavioral chain, repeating the exercise frequently elicits increasingly more distal significant events. Such events as an offender's own victimization as a child, early masturbatory practices, or aggressive sexual acts or attempts prior to the first actual offense may be elicited in such reviews of the chains. The construction of cognitive–behavioral offense chains is designed to actively engage and teach the offender to become an increasingly astute and responsible observer of his own past and present behavior.

CONCLUSION

If sex offenders are to successfully avoid relapse in the future, they must be able to identify the salient elements of high-risk situations that increase the likelihood for their reoffending. By identifying relevant events with associated interpretations that served as antecedents to past offenses through the process of constructing cognitive–behavioral chains, the high-risk elements for future offenses become evident. Each element is viewed within the context in which it occurred. The comparison of specific chains for a variety of past offenses and guided relapse fantasies permits the extraction of general high-risk elements for which coping strategies can be planned and practiced. In addition, the development of cognitive–behavioral offense chains encourages offenders to take the perspective of a more objective observer of their own behavior and enhances their sense of accountability for their own actions. It is only after offenders are able to perceive where events may be leading and experience a sense of responsibility for the outcome that effective coping responses will be implemented.

REFERENCES

Abel, G. G., Becker, J. V., Mittleman, M., Cunningham-Rathner, J., Rouleau, J. L., & Murphy, W. D. (1987). Self-reported sex crimes of non-incarcerated paraphiliacs. *Journal of Interpersonal Violence, 2*, 3–25.

Beck, A. T. (1976). *Cognitive therapy and the emotional disorders.* New York: International Universities Press.

Brownell, K. D., Marlatt, G. A., Lichtenstein, E., & Wilson, G. T. (1986). Understanding and preventing relapse. *American Psychologist, 41*, 765–782.

Groth, A. N., Longo, R. E., & McFaddin, T. S. (1982). Undetected recidivism among rapists and child molesters. *Crime and Delinquency, 28*, 450–458.

Knopp, F. H. (1984). *Retraining adult sex offenders: Methods and models.* Syracuse, NY: Safer Society Press.

Marlatt, G. A., & Gordon, J. R. (Eds.). (1985). *Relapse prevention: Maintenance strategies in the treatment of addictive behaviors.* New York: Guilford.

Marques, J. K., & Nelson, C. (in press). Understanding and preventing relapse in sex offenders. In M. Gossop (Ed.), *Relapse and addictive behavior.* Beckenham, Kent, UK: Croom Helm.

Marques, J. K., Pithers, W. D., & Marlatt, G. A. (1984). Relapse prevention: A self-control program for sex offenders. Appendix to: Marques, J. K. *An innovative treatment program for sex offenders: Report to the legislature.* Sacramento: California Department of Mental Health.

Meichenbaum, D. (1977). *Cognitive–behavior modification: An integrative approach.* New York: Plenum.

Meichenbaum, D., & Cameron, R. (1982). Cognitive–behavior therapy. In G. T. Wilson & C. M. Franks (Eds.), *Contemporary behavior therapy: Conceptual and empirical foundations* (pp. 310–338). New York: Guilford.

Mischel, W. (1973). Toward a cognitive social learning reconceptualization of personality. *Psychological Review, 80*, 252–283.

Nelson, C., Miner, M., Marques, J., Russell, K., & Achterkirchen, J. (1988). Relapse prevention: A cognitive–behavioral model for treatment of the rapist and child molester. *Journal of Social Work and Human Sexuality, 7*, 125–143.

Pithers, W. D., Marques, J. K., Gibat, C. C., & Marlatt, G. A. (1983). Relapse prevention with sexual aggressives: A self-control model of treatment and maintenance of change. In J. G. Greer & I. R. Stuart (Eds.), *The sexual aggressor: Current perspectives on treatment* (pp. 214–239). New York: Van Nostrand Reinhold.

15

Developing Coping Strategies for High-Risk Situations

HELEN STEENMAN
CRAIG NELSON
CARL VIESTI, JR.

A major premise of the relapse prevention (RP) approach is that the recurrence of sexual offending can be prevented by recognizing and effectively intervening in the chain of events leading to a reoffense (Marques & Nelson, in press; Marques, Pithers, & Marlatt, 1984; Nelson, Miner, Marques, Russell, & Achterkirchen, 1988; Pithers, Marques, Gibat, & Marlatt, 1983). This chain of events, which is unique for each individual offender, consists of both personal (cognitive and affective) and environmental (behavioral and situational) events. Chapter 14 has already described how these cognitive–behavioral offense chains are constructed and how they are used to identify high-risk elements, or factors that enhance an offender's risk of relapse. High-risk elements, once identified and recognized, serve as danger signals, or red flags, warning offenders of a precarious situation in which the sense of self-control over their sexual behavior may be threatened. This chapter will discuss the identification, planning, and implementation of coping responses to high-risk elements. The preparation of such strategies is an essential step in equipping offenders to utilize more effective behaviors to diminish their likelihood of future relapse/reoffense.

A high-risk situation is hazardous to the degree to which one is unable to handle it without jeopardizing a sense of self-control and increasing the likelihood of reoffense. Therefore, the risk of relapse inherent in any situation is inversely related to an offender's ability to provide adequate coping responses to it. An adequate coping response is defined as an effort initiated by the offender that restores a sense of self-control over his behavior and thinking and a return to a state of abstinence. Adequate coping responses include both overt behavioral acts and cognitive strategies, such as coping self-statements or other thought-regulation techniques. They range in sophistication from simple avoidance and escape strategies to more complex instructional self-statements or facile social skills. The main point is that some response is emitted, regardless of its elegance, which enables the individual to avoid relapse when encountering the high-risk situations that are inevitable (Marlatt & Gordon, 1985).

A major goal for sex offenders in treatment is to learn how to intervene or disrupt the sequence of events leading to offending at the earliest sign of risk (Knopp, 1984). A crucial phase in the behavior-change process of cognitive–behavior therapy is the development of new thoughts and behaviors that are incompatible with the previous maladaptive ones (Meichenbaum, 1977; Meichenbaum & Cameron, 1982). Therefore, the development of adequate coping responses to high-risk elements in the cognitive–behavioral offense chain represents both an important stage of the behavior-change process and the accomplishment of a significant treatment goal for sex offenders.

IDENTIFYING ALTERNATIVE BEHAVIORAL RESPONSES

The first phase in developing coping strategies is to identify specific, alternative responses for each step in the cognitive–behavioral offense chain that the offender can employ to minimize the probability of relapse. Following the schema for the construction of cognitive–behavioral offense chains, there is a listing of alternative behavioral responses to the observable events that promoted the rape or molestation. This is followed, as described in the next section, by an identification of alternative interpretations of these events that could also be used as coping responses.

Offenders are introduced to the idea that, in any given situation, there are a variety of options available for how one may act or behave. Initially, it may be difficult for some offenders to change their belief that only one response is possible in certain situations. However, it is essential that offenders recognize that they have a range of options with which to respond to any given situation. During the initial stage in identifying alternative behavioral coping strategies, offenders are taught that stimulus-control procedures, such as escape and avoidance responses, are almost always available as a method of reducing the danger of high-risk situations. To the degree that the precipitants of an offense include environmental stimuli that serve as cues to deviant sexual thoughts and fantasies, considerable self-control may be gained by simply removing them (Marques et al., 1984; Pithers et al., 1983). Avoidance implies prevention of exposure to a high-risk element. For example, one high-risk element is access to a potential victim. Therefore, a viable response that significantly reduces the potential of an offense in many cases would be staying away from situations in which access to a victim is readily available. For child molesters, this may entail avoiding situations in which children are present, or at least circumstances in which they are in the presence of children without the supervision of a responsible adult. For rapists, on the other hand, such a simplistic response may be less reasonable in many situations. It may not be realistic to expect a rapist to avoid all situations in which he is alone with an adult woman. However, an avoidance response is feasible in more specific high-risk situations, such as access to a victim while in an intoxicated state or after having his anger provoked. For certain offenders, weapons, drugs, alcohol, illicit pornography, or specific locations (e.g., schoolyards, parks, beaches, certain taverns) may all serve as particular high-risk elements that can easily be eliminated through avoidance and escape responses.

The potential for offense may not be recognized until an offender is already in the midst of a high-risk situation. In such instances, leaving the situation through an escape response significantly diminishes the potential for offending. In contrast to avoidance, escape implies leaving a high-risk situation after it has already been encountered. Because avoidance and escape responses require a relatively low level of cognitive sophistication, they are often among the most reliable, immediate, and readily available coping tactics.

Although escape and avoidance responses are highly effective, it is apparent that they may not always be viable options. Three conditions, in particular, appear to impair the value of these responses: (1) if the offender fails to recognize the risk inherent in the situation, (2) if the offender is physically prevented from escape or avoidance, or (3) if the cost of escaping or avoiding the situation appears to outweigh the risk of offending incurred by the predicament. In an incest case, for example, many conditions that preclude effective escape and avoidance responses may be present: (1) initial failure to recognize the offense potential with one's own child, (2) economic limitations on being able to leave or separate from the family in order effectively to escape the risk, (3) inability to afford a babysitter whenever the spouse is not present, or (4) unwillingness to sacrifice the emotional security of the family that separation and divorce would entail. For situations in which escape and avoidance responses may not be viable or the most effective strategies, alternative coping behaviors must be sought. For the example given above, engaging in marital counseling or individual psychotherapy, confiding in the spouse about the urges or fantasies regarding the child and avoiding being alone with the child whenever possible, or actively seeking emotional support from other adults are only a few alternative behavioral responses that might reduce, although not necessarily preclude, the likelihood of an offense.

For each significant event in the behavioral chain leading to a past offense, the offenders are asked to identify as many discrete, specific responses as possible that would decrease the probability of the illicit sexual act. Offenders are encouraged to identify proactive behaviors instead of passive reactions to high-risk elements. In addition to identifying what was not done, offenders are pressed to identify what else they could have done or said. Thus a simple avoidance response, such as staying away from the victim, is not considered complete or adequate. Instead, offenders are asked specifically to describe where they could go or what they could do instead. In addition, they are encouraged to identify as many alternative behavioral responses as possible. Through a problem-solving approach (D'Zurilla & Goldfried, 1971; Goldfried & Davison, 1976), a variety of options are generated, the likely consequences of each examined, and the most useful responses for reducing the likelihood of the offense identified. In this fashion, offenders are encouraged not only to begin to consider coping responses that could be used in similar future high-risk situations but also to gain a greater sense of self-efficacy and responsibility for their own behavior.

IDENTIFYING ALTERNATIVE INTERPRETATIONS

Once direct behavioral coping strategies have initially been identified, offenders are reminded that their responses to events are largely determined by their cognitive interpretations of those events. For example, in the presence of a potential victim the offender may be at risk only if the victim's behavior is interpreted as seductive or if the situation is viewed as providing an opportunity to offend. The offender's interpretations about events, in the form of self-statements, are evaluated in order to determine whether or not to modify them. A key step is for offenders to recall the interpretations they made about events and to note how their interpretations served as antecedents in their past offense patterns. In other words, they must be able to recall a cognition and recognize its determining influence on behavior before it can be changed.

Each self-statement identified in the cognitive–behavioral chain and recognized as a precipitant of the offense is considered and evaluated. Offenders are reminded that for any given set of circumstances there are a variety of ways to construe the events, and they are asked if others are likely to share their interpretations of the situation. For example, would others view a 10-year-old's questions about sex as seductive, or might they consider them a reflection of prepubescent curiosity? Could everyone agree that a girl who is prematurely physically developed is prepared for or desires sexual relations? Would others agree that an attractive female hitchhiker owes sexual favors in return for a ride? The consideration of how others may view the event permits an evaluation of the ways in which interpretations were influenced by the offender's own internal needs, desires, and personal history rather than based on objective events. To emphasize this point, offenders may be provided with the analogy of a camera. Just as a variety of filters may be applied to a camera lens to enhance and diminish particular colors or distort certain features, an individual's personal social learning history and internal state color and distort the interpretation of the world around him.

For each self-statement in their cognitive–behavioral offense chains, offenders are asked to generate several alternative self-statements for interpreting the significant events that served as antecedents to their crimes. In this task, it is important that offenders not seek to modify cognitions that served as danger signals, or red flags. For an offender to deny his sexual arousal in a high-risk situation, for example, serves only to heighten the risk it represents. In such an instance, an alternative self-statement, such as "Even though I am becoming turned on to this kid, it doesn't mean he is being seductive or provocative with me," would be appropriate. Through a problem-solving procedure similar to that employed in examining alternative behavioral responses, offenders are encouraged to identify a variety of alternative interpretive self-statements that reduce the risk potential of the situation. The likely consequences of each of the optional self-statements are determined. Those that decrease the probability of the offense are highlighted as potential coping responses, while those that increase or have no effect on the eventual outcome are discarded.

PLANNING COPING STRATEGIES

The central purpose of RP for sex offenders is to learn to plan and prepare strategies for effectively coping with future high-risk elements in a manner that reduces their danger of reoffending. This requires them to be able to recognize high-risk elements, think of potentially effective coping responses, and implement the coping responses in an effective manner. The ability to identify possible coping responses for past events described in the cognitive–behavioral offense chain does not insure that an offender will be able actually to generate a coping response when a high-risk situation arises in the future. Therefore, the preparation of a few generalized coping strategies can be helpful in enhancing an offender's ability to confront future high-risk situations. For the purposes of this discussion, coping strategies refer to broad and global approaches to managing high-risk elements. Based on such global strategies, specific coping responses to a high-risk situation may be derived.

In Chapter 14 of this volume, Nelson & Jackson described how the cognitive–behavioral chains for various offenses and guided relapse fantasies can be generalized so that high-risk elements common to each offense and fantasy are distilled. By comparing the various chains, a list of high-risk elements that may promote relapse is generated, and general coping strategies can be derived. By examining the similarities of each of the specific alternative behavioral responses and self-statements that could be given in the various chains, common coping strategies emerge. Another technique that is used to identify coping strategies is homework assignments. In one such assignment, for example, offenders are asked to describe for each of their identified high-risk elements five scenarios in which the element is present. They are then asked to describe at least one behavioral coping response and one coping self-statement that would reduce the danger potential in that situation and concomitantly increase their sense of self-efficacy and self-control. Thus for each high-risk element, ten coping responses are identified. By comparing and contrasting the various responses, common strategies and approaches that may be effective across a variety of situations become apparent.

In addition to the escape and avoidance techniques that have already been discussed, a limited list of coping strategies might include (1) avoiding drug and alcohol use, (2) improving stress management through relaxation and self-monitoring techniques, (3) enhancing social skills for developing more satisfactory adult relationships, (4) maintaining self-esteem through positive self-statements, (5) augmenting assertiveness skills, (6) improving or developing anger-management techniques in order to facilitate more satisfactory conflict resolution, (7) increasing victim empathy, and (8) combating distorted attributions to the victim. Also, cognitive coping skills might include thought stopping, identifying and disputing irrational beliefs, cognitive–behavioral rehearsal, and imagery. A complete list of cognitive and behavioral coping strategies is beyond the scope of the present discussion. The important point is that for each high-risk element identified by an offender, a coping strategy is developed to reduce its potential for engendering reoffense.

Regardless of the specific coping strategies developed, offenders may be taught to apply the responses through a type of self-instruction (Meichenbaum, 1977) that walks them through each step of the coping process. Such self-instruction may include steps such as:

1. Identifying the high-risk element present (e.g., "I am finding myself attracted to this cute little boy")
2. Acknowledging the importance of emitting a prepared coping response (e.g., "No matter how cute he may be, the risk of returning to jail isn't worth staying in this situation")
3. Reasserting the sense of self-control (e.g., "Even though I'm getting aroused, I'm still in control of my behavior—it is only my *sense* of control that is decreasing")
4. Selecting and implementing a coping response (e.g., "In these types of situations I need to remind myself that the urge I'm having will go away whether I act on it or not, and I need to get out of here right now")
5. Self-reinforcing effective responses (e.g., "Even though I felt tempted, I did a pretty good job of coping with that situation")

Through such a systematic process, offenders are able to structure their planned coping strategies.

In preparing coping strategies, several points are emphasized. First, it is always easier to intervene earlier rather than later in the cognitive–behavioral chain leading to relapse (Marques et al., 1984; Pithers et al., 1983). Thus offenders are taught to emit coping responses at the first sign of a high-risk element, such as an "apparently irrelevant decision" (AID), rather than to wait until they are experiencing deviant sexual thoughts or urges in the presence of a potential victim (a lapse), a situation from which it will be much more difficult to extricate themselves. Second, it is always easier to cope with a single high-risk element at a time rather than to deal with a fuller constellation of elements that constitute an extremely high-risk situation. Finally, there are no right or wrong coping responses, only more or less effective ones. Therefore, the best coping response is the one that appears most effective for reducing the threat to self-control presented by the high-risk element or situation. Any response by the offender that prevents relapse is considered a successful coping response in the high-risk situation.

PROGRAMMING COPING RESPONSES

Knowing what a coping response should be is one thing; being able to use it when needed is another. If a high-risk element with which an offender is familiar occurs when he is relaxed, thinking clearly, and feeling in control, he may have little difficulty in recalling, selecting, and implementing predetermined coping responses. Unfortunately, many high-risk situations will not occur under such ideal circumstances. In more complex situations, in which competing demands (e.g., intoxication, embarrassment, anger, desire for immediate gratification of impulses) interfere with the execution of new behavioral responses, offenders will likely fall back on habitual response patterns. Due to this tendency, the newly developed coping responses must be overlearned, so that they become "programmed" into the offender's behavioral repertoire. Ideally, such programmed coping responses will become automatic and replace the old, maladaptive behaviors. Intensive practice and behavioral rehearsal will enhance the offender's potential for generalizing the coping strategies, so that they are performed in a variety of moods and situations (Marques et al., 1984; Pithers et al., 1983).

There are many ways to rehearse and program effective coping responses, including (1) repetitive reviews of alternative coping responses to a variety of cognitive–behavioral chains of past offenses and guided relapse fantasies; (2) role-play rehearsals in group and individual psychotherapy sessions; and (3) covert modeling (Kazdin, 1976), in which offenders imagine scenes of themselves successfully coping with various high-risk situations. In addition, offenders are encouraged to practice their coping responses in a variety of real-life situations in which they encounter high-risk elements, even though the potential for reoffending may not be present. In the Sex Offender Treatment and Evaluation Project (Marques, Day, Nelson, & Miner, Chapter 22, this volume), for example, offenders are encouraged to practice their new coping responses and strategies on a daily basis. Although the environment of the project precludes access to potential victims, offenders are encouraged to recognize when many of the elements that compose high-risk situations are present, such as (1) interpersonal stressors, (2) rationalizing their victimization and manipulation of others, (3) lack of meaningful relationships with other adults, (4) deviant sexual fantasies, (5) social isolation, (6) poor social skills, and (7) low self-esteem. The focus on these everyday risk elements as an opportunity to practice newly acquired coping skills, with accompanying feedback from therapists and other offenders, also facilitates the programming of the planned coping strategies.

THE COPING-SKILLS GAME

Previous research using a Situational Competency Test has suggested that the adequacy of a coping response may be less important in preventing relapse than how quickly it can be performed (Chaney, O'Leary, & Marlatt, 1978). In order to program immediacy into the delivery of coping strategies, an exercise that we have come to refer to as the "coping-skills game" has been devised.

In this exercise, an offender is presented with a brief description of a situation that contains a high-risk element. He is then urged to describe a coping response as quickly as possible. If an adequate coping response is produced, a new high-risk element or a new fact is added to the scenario to block or foil the coping strategy. Again, the offender is pushed to provide an immediate description of a coping response to reduce the threat inherent in the situation. The game continues in this manner until either the offender is unable to generate a coping response or no new risk factors can be imagined that would obstruct the offender's plan to cope with the situation. The game is initiated with relatively simple or only slightly risky situations. As it progresses, circumstances are made increasingly complex and dangerous in order to attempt to trap the offender in an extremely high-risk situation. The rules of the coping-skills game permit that only realistic and credible coping responses be given. Fantastic, implausible responses are forbidden and may lead to disqualification. In order to maintain a sense of urgency, a time limit (e.g., 30 seconds) may be used to hasten responses. The exercise may be conducted in either an individual- or group-therapy context. In a group setting, offenders are paired so that one offender presents the high-risk situations and the other defends with the description of coping responses to ward off the potential threat for reoffense. Roles may then be reversed. Matches of the coping-skills game are repeated frequently in order to practice rapidly fashioning coping responses to a variety of high-risk situations. Following each game, the effectiveness of the emitted coping responses is analyzed, alternative coping responses that would also reduce the threat of the situation are identified, the likelihood that the offender would emit such a response in an actual similar situation is determined, whether the offender took the earliest possible opportunity to intervene is examined, and successful responses are reinforced.

Although high-risk elements derived from patterns of past behavior can be anticipated, they will interact in different and unfamiliar contexts, which are impossible to fully anticipate. While coping responses can be planned for the various elements, they can never be expected to cover the potentially infinite number of ways in which two or more high-risk elements may interact with unforeseen situations. Therefore, offenders must ultimately learn to be able to gain agility, ingenuity, and speed in the application of coping skills.

CONCLUSION

From an RP perspective, sex offenders must be able to react to high-risk situations that place them at risk for reoffense with coping responses that will disrupt the relapse process and sustain a state of abstinence from sexual reoffense. In order to accomplish this goal, appropriate ways of handling high-risk elements must be identified, planned, and practiced. One way of identifying coping responses that can be implemented in future high-risk situations is to determine what possible interventions the offender can extrapolate from past offense patterns in order to avoid a rape or molestation. By identifying an alternative response for each step in the cognitive–behavioral offense chain that diminishes the likelihood of the offense, many coping responses are identified. First, behavioral responses to environmental events that served as cues and contingencies for illicit sexual behavior are specified, then alternative interpretations in the form of self-statements that manage the risks more effectively are determined. By examining the similarities across the various coping responses, a set of distinct coping strategies is derived for each offender that can be generalized to a wide variety of situations. Finally, these coping strategies need to be programmed through practice and rehearsal so that they become integrated into the offender's behavioral repertoire. Through this development of coping strategies, the offender gains more competence in managing future high-risk situations.

REFERENCES

Chaney, E. F., O'Leary, M. R., & Marlatt, G. A. (1978). Skill training with alcoholics. *Journal of Consulting and Clinical Psychology, 46,* 1092–1104.

D'Zurilla, T. J., & Goldfried, M. R. (1971). Problem solving and behavior modification. *Journal of Abnormal Psychology, 78,* 107–126.

Goldfried, M. R., & Davison, G. C. (1976). *Clinical behavior therapy.* New York: Holt, Rinehart & Winston.

Kazdin, A. E. (1976). Effects of covert modeling, multiple models, and model reinforcement on assertive behaviors. *Behavior Therapy, 7,* 211–22.

Knopp, F. H. (1984). *Retraining adult sex offenders: Method and models.* Syracuse, NY: Safer Society Press.

Marlatt, G. A., & Gordon, J. R. (Eds.). (1985). *Relapse prevention: Maintenance strategies in the treatment of addictive behaviors.* New York: Guilford.

Marques, J. K., & Nelson, C. (in press). Understanding and preventing relapse in sex offenders. In M. Gossop (Ed.), *Relapse and addictive behaviour.* Beckenham, Kent, UK: Croom Helm.

Marques, J. K., Pithers, W. D., & Marlatt, G. A. (1984). Relapse prevention: A self-control program for sex offenders. Appendix to: Marques, J. D. *An innovative treatment program for sex offenders: Report to the legislature.* Sacramento: California Department of Mental Health.

Meichenbaum, D. (1977). *Cognitive-behavior modification: An integrative approach.* New York: Plenum.

Meichenbaum, D., & Cameron, R. (1982). Cognitive–behavior therapy. In G. T. Wilson & C. M. Franks (Eds.), *Contemporary behavior therapy: Conceptual and empirical foundations* (pp. 310–338). New York: Guilford.

Nelson, C., Miner, M., Marques, J., Russell, K., & Achterkirchen, J. (1988). Relapse prevention: A cognitive–behavioral model for treatment of the rapist and child molester. *Journal of Social Work and Human Sexuality, 7,* 125–143.

Pithers, W. D., Marques, J. K., Gibat, C. C., & Marlatt, G. A. (1983). Relapse prevention with sexual aggressives: A self-control model of treatment and maintenance of change. In J. G. Greer & I. R. Stuart (Eds.), *The sexual aggressor: Current perspectives on treatment* (pp. 214–239). New York: Van Nostrand Reinhold.

16

Coping with Urges and Craving

CAROLYN H. CAREY
ROBERT J. McGRATH

Developing strategies to assist sex offenders in coping with urges and craving is an essential component of relapse prevention with this population. *Urge* is defined here as an impulse or behavioral intention toward a consummatory activity or goal, in this case the act of sexual aggression. *Craving* is the subjective desire for the gratification anticipated from the indulgent behavior.

The sexually aggressive client has engaged in behaviors that, while proscribed, are strongly self-reinforcing, and he therefore typically finds himself vulnerable to desires and impulses to reexperience the "rush" of power and gratification that have become associated with the indulgent act. Because of their intensity, urges and craving may persist even after treatment has been completed. In addition, these impulses and desires are characterized not only by their perceived strength and persistence but frequently by their proximity in time to the sexually aggressive behavior. For these reasons, the deviant urges and craving experienced by sex offenders warrant interventions designed specifically to address their distinctive characteristics, especially their immediacy and intensity.

PRINCIPLES OF INTERVENTION

Treatment strategies for urges and craving are governed by a primary organizing principle: detachment. To detach from an urge is to distance oneself cognitively from a desire or sensation that seems irresistible. For our clients, achieving cognitive and emotional distance from impulses that seem beyond their control is typically a complex process. Therefore, interventions designed to enhance detachment are less like components of a single treatment module than tools to be used throughout the course of treatment.

Three components of the change process assist the sex offender in detaching from deviant urges and craving: naming, reframing, and empowerment.

First, accurately naming an urge is an essential skill for clients. By naming his experience, the offender may invoke a specific coping response rather than struggle with a sense of insufficiency. The principles and techniques of meditation, equally applicable here, emphasize the effectiveness of simply bringing into awareness a particular state of mind: "Each time we acknowledge a state of mind . . . it weakens the state of mind while strengthening the ability to let it go" (Levine, 1979, p. 41). Thus by naming an impulse, the client is better able to disengage from it and treat it as an experience that is transitory and, therefore, within his control.

Detachment from deviant urges and craving is also enhanced by cognitively reframing (i.e., redefining) these impulses as learned, habitual responses to situational stressors rather than as innate, overpowering forces. Thus a theoretical framework that supplies a social learning interpretation of urges and craving changes the meaning of the arousal and enhances the client's confidence that he himself is capable of altering the relapse process.

Empowerment, the third guiding theme of detachment, informs sex offender treatment as a whole. To the extent that sexual aggression can be defined as the sexual abuse of power (Groth & Birnbaum, 1979), our clients' maladaptive attempts to cope with feelings of powerlessness must be addressed if treatment is to be effective. This aspect of treatment is based on the assumption that the human need to feel powerful, to have influence in interpersonal relations with significant others, is essential (Sullivan, 1953). Deviant craving and urges, and the ensuing sexually aggressive behavior, are subjectively experienced as an increase in energy and power and, therefore, as an antidote to prior feelings of powerlessness. This pairing of a rush of power with strongly reinforcing sexual arousal and orgasm, most likely in the absence of sufficient alternative coping strategies, may to a great extent explain the intensity of the urges.

Our clients' experience of the appropriate exercise of power is facilitated by increased self-efficacy (Bandura, 1977), an individual's conviction of being able to perform the behavior required to produce a specific outcome. Self-efficacy in the impulsive client is associated with a sense of confidence in his ability to cope with a high-risk situation and is enhanced by elevating the client to the role of cotherapist in his own treatment. This is achieved by giving him a well-articulated theoretical framework for his behavior and by reinforcing throughout the course of treatment his efforts and successes in naming and coping appropriately with urges and craving.

Thus the principle of detachment, which involves processes of naming, reframing, and empowerment, provides the foundation for treatment strategies designed to assist the sex offender in coping with deviant urges and craving. It is also important when formulating interventions to note that urges and craving appear to be created and maintained by both cognitive and behavioral processes. Prochaska and DiClemente (1983), studying processes of change among people who had quit smoking, found that a combined cognitive–affective reevaluation process bridged the chasm between contemplation of a change and action toward that change, while behavioral strategies, such as stimulus control and counterconditioning, enabled maintenance of the changes achieved during the quitting phase. These findings suggest that for sexually aggressive clients, strategies to cope with urges and craving should comprise a variety of tools that can be employed in different situations at different stages of the change process.

TREATMENT STRATEGIES

Treatment of deviant craving and urges begins with an explanation of the theoretical framework for the relapse process. It is based on a model similar to Marlatt's (1985a) "hypothetical anatomy of an urge to smoke," which posits a classical conditioning paradigm to explain craving and relapse in the treatment of addictive behaviors. The "hypothetical anatomy of an urge to commit a sexual offense," or relapse process, begins with a recognition or reminder of a past or potential victim (conditioned stimulus [CS]), which leads first to sexual fantasy and arousal (craving or conditioned response [CR]) and then to the urge or impulse to commit the act of sexual aggression. This urge is internalized as cognitive distortions in the form of excuses or justifications. Because sexual aggression always involves at least one other person—the victim or victims—an intermediate step is necessary. This step is the grooming, manipulation, or "setting up" of oneself, one's victim, and others in the environment (e.g., family members) to clear the way for acting on the impulse. It should be noted here that urges and craving may occur without specific victim reminders, that is, in high-risk situations for which the client's alternative coping responses are meager or nonexistent.

In terms of the relapse prevention model, the client must learn to discriminate clearly between a lapse and relapse. While the latter refers to the client's return to sexually aggressive behavior (i.e., an actual reoffense), the former describes a single slip, or error, such as indulging in a deviant fantasy after a period of abstinence. A lapse might occur at any point in the relapse process outlined above, short of the act of reoffending. The client should learn to view a lapse not as a sign of failure but as an opportunity to invoke new, adaptive coping strategies.

The remainder of this chapter describes interventions to control deviant urges and craving, giving primary attention to cognitive–behavioral strategies. Biological interventions and environmental manipulations may also be effective methods for helping offenders control their impulses.

Cognitive–Behavioral Interventions

The Relapse Process

The cognitive–behavioral offense "anatomy" described above is presented to our clients early in their treatment as the theoretical framework for their offense, or relapse, process. As a teaching tool, the model considerably enriches their typically scanty understanding of their behavior and begins to provide a vehicle both for achieving detachment from urges and craving and for taking sole responsibility for acting on them. Learning the relapse process and alternative coping responses forms the core of treatment of deviant impulses and desires. We begin the discussion by describing the relapse process and asking group members to generate specific examples of each link in the chain. "Reminders" might include hearing news of one's victim, seeing him/her during a family-therapy session, or remembering the offense while driving to therapy. The "fantasy–arousal" stage of the progression would include any cognitive, affective, or physical aspect of a craving response during which the client has begun to anticipate the positive effects of reoffending. We give considerable attention to the cognitive distortions used by sex offenders, since we see these not only as covert mediators of the sexually aggressive behavior but also as pervasive, habitual components of a maladaptive cognitive style. Excuses, of course, are abundant and diverse: "She must want it because she loves me," "I deserve this," "No one will find out, so it'll be okay," and so forth, with many variations on these and other themes.

The manipulation, or grooming, stage of the relapse process distinguishes this particular pattern from that of most other addictive behaviors. Because sexual aggression always involves a victim, some degree of coercion, control, or manipulation is necessary in order for the offender to act on his impulse. As with cognitive distortions, during the course of treatment we assist clients in identifying their particular methods of controlling, or setting up, their victims. Tactics with victims might range from favoritism to threats of physical harm. Vis-à-vis nonoffending spouses, these might be as crude as sending the wife to the store in order to be alone with the victim or as subtle as quietly discouraging intimacy between mother and daughter. Clients typically find identifying this aspect of their patterns to be both elusive and painful; it seems to be a crucial element in bringing the secret out into the open and in calling the relapse process by its true name.

Awareness of the offense pattern is further underscored at the beginning of each group session when members describe their impulses or lapses of the previous week. We expect that they will have some impulses; our primary concern is that they be honest about these and use appropriate coping strategies when they occur. Thus members are interviewed regarding their lapses, whether (and how far) they proceeded beyond the "reminder" stage, and what coping strategies they used. Verbal reinforcement for adaptive coping responses is offered by both leaders and other group members. Once the dynamics of a client's own relapse process have been discovered, they become useful material for subsequent interventions.

Covert Sensitization

Covert sensitization (e.g., Cautela & Wisocki, 1971) is an aversive countercondi-tioning procedure in which imagined scenes of undesirable behaviors are paired with scenes aversive to the client in an attempt to eliminate the unwanted behavior.

The relapse process described above provides a basic structure for the covert-sensitization procedure. Using a tape recorder, the client relates in detail his own relapse process, proceeding from recognition through fantasy–arousal, excuses, and grooming. Just before describing the offense, he interrupts the sequence with a "punishment scene," such as his arrest or separation from his family. Following numerous pairings of deviant fantasies and punishments, he concludes each tape on a positive note by completing a "reward scene" in which he views himself as a competent and confident individual. For 5 weeks each client prepares two or three 15-minute tapes per week, recording as many different scenes as possible, and presents his tapes in group for feedback, suggestions, and eventual approval.

As a behavioral tool, by pairing a noxious scene with the craving or urge, this approach interrupts the relapse process between the CS (reminder) and the CR (craving) and promotes an avoidance response. As a cognitive intervention, covert sensitization reminds the offender repeatedly of what he had previously "forgotten" or denied, that is, that his sexually assaultive behavior is against the law and warrants severe and disturbing consequences. Clients who have com-pleted this procedure are expected, and report that they do, use these punish-ment scenes continually as a strategy to cope with potential lapses at any point in the relapse process.

Satiation Treatment

During the initial stages of treatment, the client judged to have poor control over his urges can gain immediate control over hypersexuality by satiating his sexual interests. He is instructed to masturbate at a frequency that will signifi-cantly reduce his sex drive and thereby increase his ability to manage his urges and craving. This technique increases detachment by interrupting the offense chain between the CS and CR, thus reducing or eliminating the craving response that had previously been elicited by the sight of a potential victim or other stimulus. In order to prevent reinforcement of deviant interests during this procedure, offenders should be instructed to pair their masturbation and orgasm with nondeviant sexual fantasies.

This form of satiation treatment reduces the sex drive in general rather than deviant sexual interests in particular. The latter is the goal of Marshall's (1979) masturbatory satiation procedure, which can provide long-term behavioral reorientation.

Thought Stopping

Thought stopping (Cautela & Wisocki, 1977) is a useful "first-aid" intervention with potential long-term usefulness in minimizing the extent of lapses by sex offenders. The client generates the deviant thoughts that typically precede or accompany the deviant urges and craving, and the therapist identifies target thoughts. The therapist gives a rationale for the procedure and asks the client to relax with his eyes closed. He then instructs the client to raise a finger to signal the beginning of the deviant thought, at which time the therapist shouts "Stop!" Further instruction and rehearsal assist the offender in utilizing this strategy on his own. This technique may be employed with feelings, images, and behaviors as well as thoughts.

Once mastered, thought stopping may be combined with other behavioral procedures, such as covert reinforcement (Cautela, 1977). For example, immediately following his use of the thought-stopping technique, the offender is told to take a deep breath and relax while exhaling. He is then directed to experience a sense of self-efficacy while imagining himself successfully "escaping" from a high-risk situation, thus gaining control over deviant urges and craving. The client can use this technique effectively to interrupt the relapse process at any point and thereby avoid a potential relapse.

Self-Statements

Self-statements, a lower-order cognitive-restructuring technique, can counteract the self-deprecating effects of a deviant thought that might otherwise cause a downward spiral of guilt, discouragement, and eventual relapse. Many of the self-statements, or slogans, used by members of Alcoholics Anonymous have been adapted for use by persons involved in compulsive sexual behavior (*Hope and Recovery*, 1987). These slogans, although recognized by their authors as appearing "trite and simplistic . . . represent important information and useful instruction in a brief and memorable form" (pp. 99).

One such self-statement, "This too shall pass," corrects the erroneous cognition of many offenders that a craving will inevitably persist and become unbearable unless it is acted on. Application of this self-statement to deviant urges and craving can increase an offender's confidence as he experiences the fading of desires and impulses on which he did not act. Marlatt (1985b) has likened this situation to that of a surfer who rides the crest of a wave (urge) until the crest breaks and the wave of feeling subsides.

This and other self-statements can be augmented by more individually tailored self-statements. For example, offenders can complete the following sentence stems: "A few moments of (e.g., sex, power, pleasure) are not worth (e.g., losing my family, 20 years in jail)."

Self-statements can be typed on a wallet-sized card (a reminder card) to be carried by the offender at all times and referred to during lapses. The reminder card should also contain other useful information, such as telephone numbers of persons to call in a crisis and summaries of the relapse contract, described below.

Relapse Contracts

Pithers, Kashima, Cumming, and Beal (1988) have suggested the use of contracts as a strategy to limit the extent to which an offender will permit himself to lapse. Such a contract, designed collaboratively by the client and therapist, should be tailored to the particular pattern of the offense. For example, the client agrees that before he allows himself to succumb to an urge to masturbate to deviant pornography, he will delay such behavior for at least 20 minutes. If he then indulges in the behavior, he will limit the activity to a single episode. Such a contract gives the offender an opportunity to detach from his urges by, for example, reappraising the lapse process described on the previously discussed reminder cards. The client also agrees to discuss this lapse during the next therapy session.

Biological Interventions

Although the primary emphasis in this chapter is on cognitive–behavioral interventions, the biological correlates of an individual's sexual impulses must also be acknowledged. The intense and compulsive nature of some paraphiliacs' sexual interests may, at least initially, prove too powerful to respond only to cognitive–behavioral or environmental interventions. For this reason, biological interventions may be helpful to hypersexual offenders whose sexual urges and behavior seem beyond their "control." Evidence suggests that treatment of sex offenders with antiandrogen medications such as medroxyprogesterone acetate (MPA/Depo-Provera) lessens sexual libido and reduces the risk of reoffense (e.g., Money & Bennett, 1981).

Wincze, Bansal, and Malamud (1986) have suggested that examination of cue-reactivity research in addictive behaviors may clarify the effects of MPA on sex offenders. Just as the smell and sight of alcohol can trigger a physiological reactivity (salivation) that may lead to relapse among alcoholics, the sight or sounds (recognitions–reminders) of young children may trigger physiological reactivity (sexual arousal) in pedophiles and precipitate a relapse. They found that MPA reduced physiological genital responsivity among their small sample of sex offenders and hypothesized that it therefore assists in preventing relapse by reducing an offender's sexual urges in response to stimulus cues.

Environmental Controls and Interventions

Other chapters in this volume elaborate on the management of environmental and other risk factors. Manipulation of an offender's environment to limit his access to external stimulus cues, and to occupy his time productively, will in itself reduce urges to relapse as well as enhance the efficacy of other interventions.

Environmental interventions acknowledge the importance of the social milieu in facilitating and maintaining treatment changes; these are similar in practice and theory to the Community Reinforcement Approach used in treating alcoholism, pioneered by Hunt and Azrin (1973). They successfully broadened the scope of the traditional, individually oriented approaches to alcohol treatment to include changes in social contingencies—specifically family, employment, and social interactions—that encourage or discourage control of drinking. Such interventions can deter urges and craving by increasing community and family supervision of the offender and by healthy structuring of his activities, which can distract his attention from incipient urges.

Application of these methods to sex offender treatment might include, for example, limiting the offender's employment to those positions in which he would have no access to potential victims. Education of the offender's spouse and significant others should make it difficult for him to set them up or groom them. An incest offender who has reunited with his family can distance himself from his victim by placing a lock on the child's door. Because the disinhibiting effects of alcohol and other drugs can reduce many offenders' control of their impulses and desires, moderation if not abstinence in the use of these substances is essential. Use of pornography that would maintain deviancy should be prohibited. An offender who used a car during his offenses can attach his name to a bumper sticker, exercise limited driving privileges, and keep a driving log.

SUMMARY

The offender's deviant impulses and desires—urges and craving—form the core of the relapse process. Because of the immediate gratification that has been associated with the indulgent act, the client may frequently be overwhelmed by the power of these urges. Treatment strategies, therefore, are based on the principle of detachment, through which the client can externalize and take control of the impulses.

Because of the importance of urges and craving in the relapse process, the client's proficiency in using these strategies will to a large extent determine the effectiveness of treatment. Thus coping with urges and craving can be likened to a performance for which all other sex offender treatment is rehearsal.

REFERENCES

Bandura, A. (1977). Self-efficacy: Toward a unifying theory of behavioral change. *Psychological Review, 84,* 191–215.

Cautela, J. R. (1977). Covert conditioning: Assumptions and procedures. *Journal of Mental Imagery, 1,* 53–64.

Cautela, J. R., & Wisocki, P. A. (1971). Covert sensitization for the treatment of the sexual deviations. *The Psychological Record, 21,* 37–48.

Cautela, J. R., & Wisocki, P. A. (1977). The thought stopping procedure: Description, application, and learning theory interventions. *The Psychological Record, 2,* 255–264.

Groth, A. N., & Birnbaum, H. J. (1979). *Men who rape: The psychology of the offender.* New York: Plenum.

Hope and recovery: A twelve step guide for healing from compulsive sexual behavior. (1987). Minneapolis: CompCare Publications.

Hunt, G. M., & Azrin, N. H. (1973). A community-reinforcement approach to alcoholism. *Behaviour Research and Therapy, 11,* 91–104.

Levine, S. (1979). *A gradual awakening.* Garden City, NY: Anchor/Doubleday.

Marlatt, G. A. (1985a). Cognitive factors in the relapse process. In G. A. Marlatt & J. R. Gordon (Eds.), *Relapse prevention: Maintenance strategies in the treatment of addictive behaviors* (pp. 128–200). New York: Guilford.

Marlatt, G. A. (1985b). Relapse prevention: Theoretical rationale and overview of the model. In G. A. Marlatt & J. R. Gordon (Eds.), *Relapse prevention: Maintenance strategies in the treatment of addictive behaviors* (pp. 3–70). New York: Guilford.

Marshall, W. L. (1979). Satiation therapy: A procedure for reducing deviant sexual arousal. *Journal of Applied Behavior Analysis, 12,* 377–389.

Money, J., & Bennett, R. G. (1981). Postadolescent paraphilic sex offenders: Antiandrogenic and counseling therapy follow-up. *International Journal of Mental Health, 10,* 122–133.

Pithers, W. D., Kashima, K. M., Cumming, G. F., & Beal, L. S. (1988). Sexual aggression: Breaking the addictive process. In A. C. Salter (Ed.), *Treating child sex offenders and victims: A practical guide.* Beverly Hills, CA: Sage.

Prochaska, J. O., & DiClemente, C. C. (1983). Stages and processes of self-change of smoking: Toward an integrated model of change. *Journal of Consulting and Clinical Psychology, 51,* 390–395.

Sullivan, H. S. (1953). *Conceptions of modern psychiatry.* New York: Norton.

Wincze, J. P., Bansal, S., & Malamud, M. (1986). Effects of medroxyprogesterone acetate on subjective arousal, arousal to erotic stimulation, and nocturnal penile tumescence in male sex offenders. *Archives of Sexual Behavior, 15,* 293–305.

17

Relapse Rehearsal

RODERICK L. HALL

THEORETICAL BASE

Within the general relapse prevention model, Marlatt (1985b) conceptualizes relapse rehearsal as an intervention that teaches clients to cope with the slips, or lapses, that they are likely to experience in their efforts to maintain abstinence. The term *relapse rehearsal* is a misnomer, since it actually calls for the client to rehearse coping successfully with a lapse rather than a relapse. *Lapse rehearsal* is perhaps a more valid term. By coping with inevitable lapses—temporary setbacks or failures—the client reduces the probability that the lapse will escalate in to a full-blown relapse, that is, total loss of control and full return to the prohibited behavior. An alcoholic who takes a single drink after a period of abstinence, for example, has experienced a temporary setback, a lapse. This lapse may or may not escalate to the previous pattern of excessive drinking, depending on how effectively the client copes with it. Similarly, a habitual pedophile may or may not engage in sexual activity with a child (full relapse) following active fantasy and masturbation involving children (lapse), depending upon his use of coping skills.

Marlatt (1985a) hypothesizes that the probability of relapse depends mainly on the client's beliefs (attributions) about the cause of the lapse and his emotional reaction to that causal attribution. The client's attributions and associated emotional reaction are collectively referred to by Marlatt as the "abstinence violation effect" (AVE). The AVE, which varies in intensity, occurs whenever the client experiences a lapse in the face of a strong commitment to abstinence. A lapse is more likely to escalate to a relapse when the lapse is followed by an intense AVE. Relapse rehearsal may help to alleviate the AVE, and thereby the probability of relapse, by teaching the client to control factors that are associated with intense AVEs. This, of course, requires knowledge of factors that are associated with increases versus decreases in the AVE.

A strong AVE will occur if the client attributes the cause of a lapse to internal and stable factors that are perceived to be beyond his control (e.g., deficient willpower or motivation). This self-blame and perceived loss of control lowers perceived personal efficacy and motivates the client to obtain relief, often accomplished through some form of cognitive distortion (e.g., rationalization or denial).

In turn, cognitive distortions—which only provide temporary relief from the negative emotional state—impair judgment and decision making, making it easier for the client to seek relief through the very activity that he wishes to avoid. The client makes decisions that seem unimportant to him but that actually move him closer to additional lapses and then a full relapse. These decisions are referred to as apparently irrelevant (Brownell, Marlatt, Lichtenstein, & Wilson, 1986; Marlatt, 1985b; Pithers, Marques, Gibat, & Marlatt; 1983). An example is the habitual pedophile who, in an attempt to cope with disappointment over a lapse into unacceptable fantasy, decides to ease his mind by relaxing at a nearby video arcade, despite the fact that video arcades have been high-risk places for him. Another example is the habitual rapist who decides to relieve the disappointment over a lapse by taking a leisurely drive that just happens to go through an area where he has committed or contemplated rape.

In a manner of speaking, the client sets himself up to experience additional lapses and an eventual relapse. One may reasonably wonder what could possibly motivate the client to seek (though in a disguised manner) the very activity that has led to the negative emotional state in the first place and that he has been working so hard to avoid. Marlatt (1985a) points out that addictive behaviors (which include some abusive sexual behavior) are usually followed by some form of immediate gratification. The client has experienced this gratification in the past in the form of direct sexual pleasure or indirect pleasure in the form of reduction of tension.

Furthermore, the client has almost invariably used the addictive (prohibited) behaviors in stressful situations, due to their demonstrated ability to reduce stress and impart at least a temporary sense of control and personal efficacy. The prohibited behavior (including lapses), then, has a history of working for the client in circumstances that are quite similar to the one he faces after a lapse. In this context, it is understandable that the client will tend to fall back on what has worked for him in the past, especially since he otherwise feels unable to cope (lowered self-efficacy stemming from the AVE).

An example of reliance on the prohibited activity to cope with the negative emotional state associated with an intense AVE is the obese client who feels guilty and depressed (AVE) about eating cheesecake (lapse) and obtains relief from these negative feelings by eating more cheesecake. Similarly, the habitual pedophile who is feeling guilty and anxious about deviant sexual fantasy (lapse) may obtain at least temporary relief by engaging in more deviant sexual fantasy.

In such cases, the prohibited activity is strongly reinforced and is therefore likely to be repeated.

The intensity of the AVE is decreased if the client attributes the cause of the lapse to external and unstable factors that he perceives as controllable. The obese person, for example, may reduce the intensity of an AVE by attributing the cause of his lapse (eating prohibited cheesecake) to the cues associated with a particular high-risk situation (HRS) instead of to a lack of willpower or commitment.

Likewise, the habitual pedophile may reduce the intensity of an AVE by attributing the cause of his lapse (unacceptable sexual fantasy) to a lack of specific coping skills in a specific high-risk situation (HRS) instead of to an underlying character flaw. In this way, the client may avoid generalizing his failure to cope in a particular instance to all high-risk situations. He may also recognize that all hope is not lost, since he could acquire the skills that are necessary to cope with future situations of a similar nature.

Thus a lapse involving a highly habitual (addictive) behavior will almost inevitably lead to a relapse unless the client does something to attenuate the AVE. Attenuation of the AVE can perhaps be best accomplished through monitoring one's cognitive appraisal of the lapse so as to avoid the negative impact of self-blame, guilt, and perceived loss of control. A model of how a lapse escalates to a relapse is presented in Figure 17.1.

THE RELAPSE REHEARSAL PROCEDURE

Preparing the Client to Expect Occasional Lapses

Since the primary goal of relapse rehearsal is to teach clients how to cope successfully with inevitable lapses, the therapist should begin by instructing the client to expect lapses to occur occasionally. In this way, the client can be better prepared to cope with a lapse when it does occur. This orientation encourages the client to view a lapse not as a failure but as an opportunity to apply corrective action, an opportunity to learn ways to prevent additional lapses in similar high-risk situations.

For sexual abusers, the therapist must carefully define the lapse as occasional unacceptable fantasy, not frequent fantasy or even occasional masturbation to unacceptable fantasy. While the frequent occurrence of unacceptable fantasy is not technically a relapse, its presence suggests that the client is approaching relapse. The same conclusion can be made about the client who masturbates to unacceptable fantasy.

Such clients either have not learned requisite self-control and coping skills or are not motivated to use them. In either case, relapse rehearsal is contraindi-

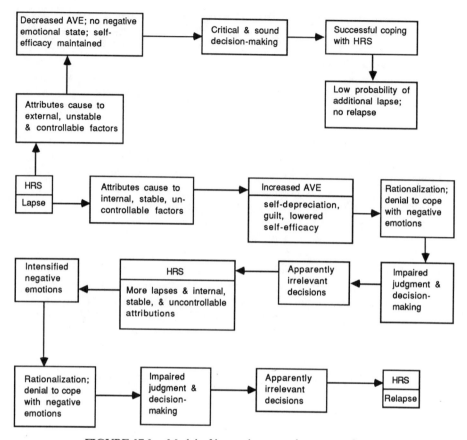

FIGURE 17.1.   Model of how a lapse escalates to a relapse.

cated, because it should only be used with clients who have made substantial behavior change in treatment, who have become skilled in the use of various self-control and coping strategies, and who are in or near the maintenance phase (Brownell et al., 1986) of treatment.

Otherwise, the client may be more likely to use the instruction that he should expect lapses as an excuse for relapse. There is also a possibility that relapse rehearsal may increase rather than decrease unacceptable fantasy in clients already approaching total loss of control (relapse). Furthermore, the client who has not already mastered coping strategies may experience decreased self-efficacy if thrust into high-risk situations with which he is unprepared to cope.

Instructing the Client in the Lapse Escalation Process

After he is oriented to expect occasional lapses, the client is instructed in the process by which a lapse may escalate to a relapse (see Figure 17.1). The client is encouraged to apply the model to himself by describing experiences he has had both before and after actual lapses. The therapist should place particular emphasis on four areas: (1) the causal attributions made after a lapse, (2) the negative emotional state stemming from an AVE, (3) cognitive distortions used to cope with the negative emotions, and (4) the use of apparently irrelevant decisions that gradually lead to additional lapses and eventual relapse (total loss of control). These are key points along the lapse escalation road at which the client can detour by coping effectively, thereby preventing further escalation. The client should be asked to recall situations from his personal experience that relate to each of the four areas specified. He should also discuss the methods used to deal with these situations and their relative effectiveness. Strategies that resulted in the avoidance of a lapse, or those that were effective in averting the escalation of a lapse, should be contrasted with less effective ones. This will teach the client that abstinence will largely depend on his ability to use effective coping strategies in high-risk situations.

Rehearsal of Successful Coping after a Lapse

Once the client understands the lapse escalation process, and how he may effectively cope along the way, he is ready for actual rehearsal. Rehearsal requires the client to fantasize about a lapse occurring in a particular high-risk situation. He is instructed to visualize and experience the emotional reaction to the lapse, especially feelings of guilt, shame, and self-blame. Instead of giving in to these feelings, the client imagines himself coping effectively (using self-control and coping strategies he has learned) and even giving self-reinforcement in the process. As part of the rehearsal, he is encouraged to experience the positive feelings associated with successful coping.

It is important to remember that successful experiences will generally increase the client's sense of personal efficacy, while repeated failures will generally decrease it (Bandura, 1977). To maximize self-efficacy, the client should arrange his high-risk situations hierarchically and begin the rehearsal procedure with those he finds less risky.

The client should rehearse successful coping at each key point along the lapse escalation process. In this regard, it may be beneficial to have the client visualize himself performing imaging techniques as a coping skill itself. For example, the client who fantasizes being very anxious following a lapse may visualize coping with the anxiety through a relaxing image. For example, he may visualize himself invoking images of nature scenes as a means of coping with the anxiety.

Covert modeling may also be useful during rehearsal. This is a technique in which the client is asked to imagine a model engaging in the desired behavior (Meichenbaum, 1977). While its efficacy has not been demonstrated with the sexually abusive client per se, it has been found to be effective in teaching social skills to unassertive individuals (Kazdin, 1974, 1975). Care should be taken to ensure that the client imagines the model coping with the situation, rather than the mastering of it, since clinical literature (Meichenbaum, 1977) suggests that the former procedure may be more effective. Covert modeling may be particularly useful for clients who have difficulty envisioning component steps in coping with a problem or for clients who, for one reason or another, have difficulty envisioning themselves coping in a given situation.

Some clients may have difficulty imagining sufficiently to truly implement the relapse rehearsal procedure. The therapist may wish to identify these clients through use of an imaging scale (Lazarus, 1977). The scale will help to determine the client's overall ability to visualize as well as his ability to create images in specific areas (e.g., self vs. others, past vs. present, and comfortable vs. uncomfortable). Image-building techniques are available for clients who have limited visualization capacity (Lazarus, 1982).

ILLUSTRATIVE EXAMPLE

The example presented is that of a pedophilic client who has completed a year of weekly group, rational–emotive therapy and 6 months of concomitant behavior therapy designed to reduce deviant sexual arousal. The client is skilled in the use of cognitive restructuring, escape–avoidance techniques, relaxation, and imagery designed specifically to cope with deviant urges. An example of the last coping skill is the visualization of a deviant urge as a wave that, if ridden out, is certain to end.

On the basis of self-report and periodic assessment on the penile plethysmograph, deviant arousal is well controlled, and the client is scheduled to begin the maintenance phase of treatment upon completion of relapse rehearsal. He expects to experience occasional lapses and understands how a lapse generally escalates to a full relapse. He has already completed two of five sessions of relapse rehearsal. His fantasy during the third session, in response to instructions to talk out loud, might proceed as follows:

> It is the July 4th weekend, and I am watching television alone at home. I am feeling lonely and am thinking of my ex-wife and daughter, whom I have not seen since I molested my daughter. This is the first July 4th that I can remember spending without them. I remember spending the last July 4th holiday with my ex-wife and

daughter at the beach. The beach scene is so vivid. I can see my ex-wife lying on the sand and my daughter holding onto me while I swim. I feel myself getting sexually aroused and then realize that I am engaging in deviant fantasy. I immediately begin to feel angry and upset with myself that I allowed the fantasy to happen. I am also beginning to wonder whether the progress I thought I was making was just a fluke. I am feeling like a failure right now. But I know that this feeling will pass. I am giving myself permission to feel badly for a while, but I will not make excuses for the slip. It happened, but it doesn't mean that I am a failure or that all of the gains I made in treatment are gone down the drain. It only means that I didn't cope well enough with that particular high-risk situation. Feelings of loneliness have been very risky for me for a long time. They were usually present when I molested my daughter. I have to remember this so that I can anticipate lapses that are likely to follow such feelings. The slip also doesn't mean that I have to act on the fantasy or the urges. Proof of this is the fact that I am not acting on the fantasy right now. Knowing how disappointment over a lapse may lead to apparently irrelevant decisions, I must be vigilant not to do that. It is okay to feel disappointed, but I will not let my feelings get out of hand and make matters worse. I actually have something to be proud of. I am doing okay compared to how I've handled these situations in the past. What I am doing right now is what it's all about—coping with the slip so that it doesn't lead to relapse. I am no longer sexually aroused, and I am beginning to feel less lonely. Instead of sitting at home alone, I'll take my brother up on his invitation to come over to his place for a cookout. Since I just had a lapse, I had better make sure that I am not making an apparently irrelevant decision. Let's see, there will be no children there, and I'll get the opportunity to socialize with family and friends. I go to the cookout, have a good time, and, on the way home, feel especially proud of the way that I handled a situation that would have overwhelmed me just 18 months ago. I can't wait to share my experience in the group and get feedback.

UTILITY OF RELAPSE REHEARSAL
WITH SEXUALLY ABUSIVE CLIENTS

There are no studies that have examined the efficacy of relapse rehearsal as a treatment technique with sexually abusive clients. However, several questions can be raised about the applicability of the technique to these clients.

The first issue concerns differences in how a lapse must be defined for the sexually abusive client versus clients presenting other forms of addictive or self-indulgent behavior. As stated previously, a lapse for the sexually abusive client is defined as an occurrence of unacceptable sexual fantasy—behavior that actually precedes the prohibited activity from which the client is attempting to abstain. It is so defined because of the harmful effects even a single occurrence of sexual abuse (relapse) has on the victim. In contrast, a lapse for an excessive drinker, an overeater, and an excessive smoker is defined as a single occurrence of taking a drink, overeating, or smoking. The lapse in all three cases is a single occurrence of the prohibited activity. The equivalent behavior in the sexual abuser is considered a full relapse.

The potential problem is that, by defining the sexual abuser's lapse as activity that precedes his prohibited behavior, we have in effect created more of an absolute requirement of abstinence for the client. As Marlatt (1985a) points out, the absolute requirement of abstinence may in itself increase the chances that a lapse will escalate to a relapse. This may be due to certain self-fulfilling prophesy effects, the "forbidden fruit" phenomenon, and psychological reactance (Brehm & Brehm, 1981), in which loss of freedom to indulge motivates the individual to regain that freedom. Rehearsing lapse control with the sexually abusive client, then, may accentuate reactance effects and thereby increase rather than decrease the probability of relapse.

A related issue that also raises some question about the applicability of relapse rehearsal to the sexually abusive client is that of commitment and motivation. The relapse rehearsal procedure, indeed the entire relapse prevention model, requires a very high level of commitment and motivation. On what other basis would one be expected to learn and apply such complex and highly intellectual self-control procedures? The sexually abusive client is typically not the most motivated of clients. Most are semivoluntary candidates for treatment, usually coming to the attention of the therapist under legal duress. Many, if not most, are not particularly uncomfortable with their unacceptable sexual behavior. What is most often upsetting to such clients about their proscribed behavior is that others hold them accountable for it. Even when the client's deviant behavior is formally denounced by the legal system, this usually occurs after long periods during which the behavior went undetected. Furthermore, unlike excessive drinkers or smokers, who are bombarded almost daily with reminders about the harmful effects of their prohibited behaviors, the sexual abuser is relatively isolated from such social pressure.

Given the background that the sexually abusive client brings to treatment, one may reasonably ask what it is that motivates the client to learn the self-control and coping skills required in relapse rehearsal. An even more relevant question is what motivation the client has to apply these procedures properly. I submit that the requisite motivation must be internal versus external, at least by the time the client is expected to apply self-control on a daily basis. I submit further that many sexually abusive clients will lack the internal motivation necessary to refrain from using the relapse rehearsal procedure to act out instead of control deviant fantasy. This seems even more plausible in light of the fact that such fantasy cannot be detected except by self-report.

Finally, the use of relapse rehearsal may be differentially effective with some types of sexual abusers. To the extent that it is effective, one might predict that the greatest success will be realized with pedophilic and incest abusers, many of whom readily engage in self-blame and often feel inadequate to cope with high-risk situations. Rapists, however, may be less likely to experience an

AVE following a lapse, due to their general tendency to externalize blame and to hold themselves in relatively high esteem, regardless of the opinions of others. Although the rapist may not be prone to experiencing intense AVEs, one should not assume, contrary to what is predicted by the lapse escalation model in Figure 17.1, that he will be free of errors in judgment and decision making. These should be anticipated, even in the absence of an intense AVE, owing to the rapist's general use of cognitive distortions, such as "superoptimism" and "victim stance" (Yochelson & Samenow, 1976). These thinking errors tend to elevate the rapist's self-efficacy to unrealistic levels, so that he may not be fully aware of risks taken and apparently irrelevant decisions made. Thus, while the cognitive distortions and apparently irrelevant decisions of the pedophilic and incest abuser may more often stem from lowered self-efficacy, those manifested by the more aggressive abuser may more often stem from unrealistically high self-efficacy.

In conclusion, caution should be used in applying relapse rehearsal to treatment of sexually abusive clients. It should only be used with clients who have made substantial behavior change in treatment, who have become skilled in the use of various self-control and coping strategies, and who are in or near the maintenance phase of treatment.

REFERENCES

Bandura, A. (1977). Self-efficacy: Toward a unifying theory of behavioral change. *Psychological Review, 84*, 191–215.

Brehm, S. S., & Brehm, J. W. (1981). *Psychological reactance: A theory of freedom and control*. New York: Academic.

Brownell, K. D., Marlatt, G. A., Lichtenstein, E., & Wilson, G. T. (1986). Understanding and preventing relapse. *American Psychologist, 41*, 765–782.

Kazdin, A. E. (1974). Effects of covert modeling and model reinforcement on assertive behavior. *Journal of Abnormal Psychology, 83*, 240–252.

Kazdin, A. E. (1975). Covert modeling, imagery assessment, and assertive behavior. *Journal of Consulting and Clinical Psychology, 43*, 716–724.

Lazarus, A. (1977). *In the mind's eye: The power of imagery for personal enrichment*. New York: Rawson.

Lazarus, A. (Speaker). (1982). *Personal enrichment through imagery* (Cassette Recording). New York: BMA Audio Cassettes/Guilford.

Marlatt, G. A. (1985a). Cognitive factors in the relapse process. In G. A. Marlatt & J. R. Gordon (Eds.), *Relapse prevention: Maintenance strategies in the treatment of addictive behaviors* (pp. 128–200). New York: Guilford.

Marlatt, G. A. (1985b). Relapse prevention: Theoretical rationale and overview of the model. In G. A. Marlatt & J. R. Gordon (Eds.), *Relapse prevention: Maintenance strategies in the treatment of addictive behaviors* (pp. 3–70). New York: Guilford.

Meichenbaum, D. (1977). *Cognitive–behavior modification: An integrative approach*. New York: Plenum.

Pithers, W. D., Marques, J. K., Gibat, C. C., & Marlatt, G. A. (1983). Relapse prevention
    with sexual aggressives: A self-control model of treatment and maintenance of
    change. In J. G. Greer & I. R. Stuart (Eds.), *The sexual aggressor: Current perspectives
    on treatment* (pp. 214–239). New York: Van Nostrand Reinhold
Yochelson, S., & Samenow, S. E. (1976). *The criminal personality: A profile for change*
    (Vol. 1). New York: Aronson.

18

Cognitive Restructuring

KATURAH D. JENKINS-HALL

Cognitive restructuring is the process of modifying thinking, both its premises and its assumptions (Meichenbaum, 1977). Most cognitive therapies operate on the basic assumption that thoughts cause feelings and feelings cause behaviors. These therapies attempt to incorporate some aspect of challenging, and thereby changing, the misperceptions, stereotypical beliefs, and cognitive distortions that lead to maladaptive functioning. Specifically, the goal of these therapies is to challenge the validity and usefulness of the maladaptive thinking patterns and gradually to substitute more adaptive ones.

According to McMullin (1986), most techniques for cognitive restructuring follow three basic steps:

1. The identification of those thoughts (beliefs, perceptions) that cause negative emotional states and maladaptive behaviors.
2. An objective analysis of those thoughts and beliefs to assess their validity and usefulness.
3. Some intervention designed to change the cognitive misperceptions and distortions to rational, adaptive ones.

COGNITIVE DISTORTIONS OF SEX OFFENDERS

In understanding how sexual deviancy is maintained, one must necessarily examine the cognitions of the sex offender. As stated by Akers (1977), human behavior results from a set of supporting cognitions that define, evaluate, and justify continued performance of the behavior. Criminal behavior, specifically the behavior of sex offenders, is no exception. Historically, others (e.g., Yochelson & Samenow, 1976) have identified patterns of thinking that seem to differentiate criminals from noncriminals and are characteristics of a "criminal personality." These criminal thinking patterns are thought to sustain criminal behavior. Although not all sex offenders can be described as having criminal personalities, many of these patterns identified by Yochelson and Samenow appear relevant. Some of the salient ones are:

Zero state: the view of self-esteem as all or nothing

Pride: a grandiose evaluation of the self; manhood is equivalent to sexuality

Power thrust: a high need for control

Extreme duality of religion: seeing people as good or evil; using religion to further personal goals

Anger: an emotion that is all consuming and often a reaction to fear and depression

Yochelson and Samenow (1976) also discuss automatic thinking errors that criminals make. These errors are also similar to the cognitive distortions found in sex offenders. Examples of automatic thinking errors are:

1. *The victim stance.* Criminals often take the victim stance when a crime is discovered. For example, child molesters will sometimes describe themselves as victims of "seductive" 8-year-olds, or victims of nonresponsive adult sexual partners, or victims of unfair societal laws. Having the offender take full responsibility for the offense is one of the desired goals of challenging this type of cognitive distortion.

2. *Failure of empathy.* Criminals often have difficulty placing themselves in the role of others. Yochelson and Samenow (1976) describe a process in which the criminal's "mind is closed, and he views people as favorably disposed to him, even when they are not . . . if he is really sensitive to others and listens to them, he runs the risk that he will hear ideas opposed to his position" (p. 373). In this regard, the sex offender is often unable to recognize signs of fear, distress, or discomfort in the victim and has difficulty realizing the impact of his behavior on the victim. Only after there is an objective examination of the victim's response, and appropriate challenging of the offender's distortions, is he able to admit to possible negative reactions from the victim. Even then, there may still be a lack of emotional identification with the victim's response.

3. *Failure to recognize injury to others.* Related to the lack of empathy, the criminal does not view himself as injuring others. He may feel that his behavior is perfectly justifiable and that he is an innocent victim of unjust laws (Yochelson & Samenow, 1976). It is not uncommon to hear from pedophiles that their love of and sexual attraction to children is perfectly normal and that they could be happy if society accepted their behavior.

4. *Ownership.* The criminal often functions as if others are his property. This "if I want it, it's mine" mentality is often seen in the rapist who targets a victim ahead of time, "claims her," and systematically plans how to overtake her.

5. *Superoptimism.* The criminal engages in a type of grandiose thinking that serves to shut off his fear response. He is usually sure that the crime can be executed without being caught. The rapist may manifest this type of thinking when, after his offense, he asks the woman if he can give her a lift home or date her in the future. Child molesters often long to reestablish relationships with their victims after the child reaches the age of consent. The anticipated response of the victim is glamorized.

The above thinking errors represent a *general* style of erroneous thinking that most sex offenders share. Sex offenders also engage in cognitive distortions—deviant cognitions that are more specifically related to their preferred deviant activity. These types of distortions can be extremely complex and organized on a number of levels designed to justify, excuse, and allow for the practice of deviant behavior (Akers, 1977). The distortions differ with the type of offense. The following is a list of common cognitive distortions made by incest offenders, pedophiles, exhibitionists, and rapists, respectively:

Incest offenders
- It's better to molest your own child than to commit adultery.
- The child treated me more like a husband than her own mother did.
- She was really not blood kin, just another woman in the home.
- She was so promiscuous that I had to satisfy her needs rather than let some punk get her pregnant.
- I've taught her everything else, why not about sex?

Nonincest offenders (pedophiles)
- Some little girls (boys) are very sexually seductive/promiscuous.
- Children can make their own decisions about sex.
- I'm not hurting the child, just showing love.
- If I didn't penetrate, I really didn't hurt him/her.
- The child didn't resist so he/she must have wanted it.

Exhibitionists
- If they see how well developed I am, they'll want to have sex with me.
- They can't resist looking at me, so they want me to expose myself.
- If they look at me, they want me sexually.
- I'm not harming anyone by exposing myself as long as I don't touch the person.

Rapists
- Women who dress or act a certain way deserve to be raped.
- I can rape her, and she'll still like me afterward.
- If she resists, she's just playing hard to get.
- When she said "no," she really meant "yes."
- She enjoyed the act as much as I did.

Some researchers and clinicians have attempted to objectively measure these types of cognitions as an indicator of treatment change. Examples of two such assessment inventories are the Pedophile Cognition Scale (Abel & Becker, 1984) and the Rape Myth Scale (Burt, 1980). The Pedophile Cognition Scale is a primary tool used to identify and restructure deviant cognitions in one therapy component of the Center for Prevention of Child Molestation (CPCM), an outpatient treatment program for sex offenders in which cognitive restructuring is used as a tool for relapse prevention (Jenkins-Hall, Osborn, Anderson, Anderson, & Shockley-Smith, Chapter 23, this volume). This scale will be discussed below.

COGNITIVE RESTRUCTURING TECHNIQUES

McMullin (1986) discusses a number of different approaches to cognitive restructuring. These techniques, known generally as "countering," involve having the client generate truthful, realistic thoughts that go against the irrational thoughts in which they engage. Selected counters, chosen for their relevance in the model of cognitive restructuring that the CPCM uses with sex offenders, include:

1. *Alternative interpretation.* The client is taught that his initial interpretation of a given situation may not be the most accurate. He is asked to generate a list of alternative explanations.
2. *Utilitarian counters.* The client is asked to examine his thinking in terms of whether it assists or impedes the achievement of the desired goal.
3. *Objective counters.* The client is assisted in examining the logic behind certain types of thinking.
4. *Disputing and challenging.* This type of countering is perhaps one of the hallmarks of rational–emotive therapy (RET), an approach that is amply described in the literature (Ellis & Grieger, 1977; Ellis & Harper, 1976). The client is asked to identify certain types of irrational thinking and underlying beliefs, which are disputed and challenged as they occur in therapy.

Most programs now attempt to incorporate some of the above methods of restructuring into their treatment of sex offenders. One approach involves the use of a method of restructuring that combines 1 and 2 above. In a group setting, the client is asked to identify his self-statements about a given situation and his interpretations of the events. Then group members are polled in order to assess whether they share the client's interpretations. Next, the question of whether the client's interpretation leads him closer to or away from reoffense (relapse) is raised. Finally, group members are asked to generate alternative interpretations.

I have observed that heterogeneous groups (child molesters and rapists) facilitate the generation of alternative interpretations. For example, in one group session, a child molester described a situation in which he was working in a garage and a 5-year-old boy walked up to him and playfully punched him in the groin area. His interpretation of this event was that the child was sexually curious about his genitals and was perhaps seeking sexual contact. During his description of his interpretation of the events, a rapist in the group indicated that his immediate interpretation would have been that the child was deliberately trying to cause him great bodily pain. Both of these interpretations were extreme and erroneous, but they provided rich material for the therapy session.

At the CPCM, the methods described in 1 and 4 above are primarily used. Cognitive restructuring is introduced to clients as a part of RET, a major treatment component directed at challenging deviant cognitions, teaching assertiveness and communication skills, and addressing social adequacy with adults. After the client has learned to distinguish rational from irrational thinking and has some familiarity with underlying irrational belief systems that perpetuate irrational–deviant cognitions, he learns the basics of cognitive restructuring through a four-step process. These steps are described in detail by Lange (1986).

In Step 1, the client identifies his internal dialogue in terms of his specific thoughts in a given situation. These thoughts are grouped in categories of thoughts about himself, about others, and about the situation. For example, a child molester who finds himself with a child who had walked up to him and hugged him might think about himself: "I am really turned on by this kid. I wish I could find a way to be alone with her." His thoughts about others might be: "She is flirting with me. She likes me. She wants me sexually." His thoughts about the situation might be: "What an ideal situation. No other adults are around, so I may not get caught. The child won't resist, so no crime will be committed." The client is asked to list as many of these types of thoughts that come to mind.

In Step 2, the client labels his irrational thoughts as either catastrophic, absolutistic, or as rationalizations. He then chooses, from the following list, those irrational beliefs that support his thinking (Lange, 1986):

1. *Fear of rejection.* I must be liked and respected by everyone, and it is awful if I am not.
2. *Fear of failure.* I must be thoroughly competent and adequate at everything I do.
3. *Fairness.* People and things should always turn out the way I want them to.
4. *Blame/punishment.* If I am rejected, if I fail, someone deserves to be strongly blamed or punished.

5. *Rumination.* If something seems threatening or fearsome, I must become terribly occupied with it.
6. *Perfect solutions exist.* It is awful, horrible when I don't find quick and good solutions to my problems.
7. *Avoidance.* It is easier to avoid difficulties and responsibilities than to face them.
8. *I'm not responsible.* People and external things make me feel and act the way I do. I have little ability to direct and control my feelings and behavior.
9. *Past conditions.* Because something once influenced your life, it has to keep determining your feelings and behavior today.
10. *Detachment.* You can achieve happiness by passively and uncommittedly "living." (p. 68)

In the example given for Step 1, the client is mainly using rationalization, and the underlying irrational beliefs are low frustration tolerance, the belief that he should have whatever he wants when he wants it, fear of rejection, and the belief that everyone must love and accept him or life will be unbearable.

In Step 3, two essential questions are asked to challenge the irrational–deviant thinking: (1) What is true about the thoughts, and (2) what is not true. Continuing the above example:

It is true that the child hugged the client.
It is true that the client responded sexually.
It is not true that the hug was sexually motivated.
It is not true that the client must act on his sexual desires.
It is not true that because an adult is not around, the act will not be reported.
It is not true that if he is not caught no crime was committed.

In Step 4, the client substitutes rational thoughts for irrational ones. This step is perhaps the most difficult one to learn. The client becomes better at this as therapy progresses and his thinking becomes more rational. Rational thoughts are phrased in terms of realistic preferences. An example of a rational substitution for the above situation might be:

I *am* sexually attracted to this child. I would prefer that the child was sexually attracted to me, *but she is not.* The fact that she is not does not mean that I am being rejected personally. It is *not* awful that I cannot meet my sexual needs immediately with this child, and the world will not end if I am not immediately satisfied. Also, it would be better if I could commit this crime with no negative consequences. But even though another adult is not present, a crime is being committed, and the child may report the crime. Worse, she may suffer long-term consequences if I commit this crime.

The client is guided through the process of rational thinking by the therapist until he demonstrates his ability to carry out the process independently. During the learning of the four-step restructuring process, the client is presented with a list of common deviant cognitions in which sex offenders engage. This is done by administering the Cognition Scale (Abel & Becker, 1984). The client is asked to read the statement and indicate his degree of agreement on a 5-point scale on which 1 = strongly agree and 5 = strongly disagree. Following are sample items from that scale:

1. If a young child stared at my genitals it means that the child likes what he/she sees and is enjoying looking at my genitals.
2. A man (or woman) is justified in having sex with his (her) children or step-children if his wife (husband) doesn't like sex.
3. A child 13 or younger can make her (his) own decision as to whether she (he) wants to have sex with an adult. (p. 1)

The client's ratings are reviewed during the group session. When the ratings reflect deviant cognitions, the client's thinking is critically examined, and the client is asked to challenge the cognition using the four-step process. Therapists use this opportunity to instruct and educate clients regarding childhood sexuality, response of victims, the ability to consent, and other relevant issues that the client may use to construct more rational thinking.

COGNITIVE RESTRUCTURING AS A COPING SKILL IN RELAPSE PREVENTION

As described by Marlatt (1985), a major component of relapse prevention requires that the client learn adaptive coping skills to deal effectively with high-risk situations. Cognitive restructuring is one of several coping skills a sex offender might use when confronted with high-risk situations or deviant urges (George & Marlatt, 1986).

When confronted with a high-risk situation, a client who has received training in cognitive restructuring generally becomes aware of his thoughts in that situation. Although he may not actively classify his thoughts as thoughts about himself, the situation, and others, he may actively identify the underlying irrational beliefs. Based on his acquired insight into his thinking processes, he immediately begins to challenge what is true and not true about his thinking. He then begins to consciously attempt to think more rationally in the situation. A client must be highly proficient in the use of cognitive restructuring for this to be used as a coping strategy in a high-risk situation. Even with maximum proficiency, the client may need to rely on other coping strategies in addition to cognitive restructuring. When confronted with a high-risk situation, such as a voyeur watching a young girl sit casually with her underwear showing, the client can attempt to use cognitive restructuring while watching the potential victim. He can repeat to himself "It is not true that the girl is coming on to me" when the obviously more adaptive response would be to leave the room.

A client may also use cognitive restructuring to deal with deviant urges as they occur. The following is an example used in instructing CPCM clients in dealing with deviant urges (Jenkins-Hall, 1987; Lange, 1986):

Initial thought: I feel this overwhelming urge to touch a child whenever he is around me.

Step 1. Identify the internal dialogue. What are you thinking about yourself? What are you thinking about the victim?
  1. I must give in to the urge to touch this child (absolutistic).
  2. I *have to* satisfy my sexual desires right now (absolutistic).
  3. I will go crazy if I don't act on this urge (catastrophic).
  4. This is out of my control (rationalization).

Step 2. Identify the underlying irrational beliefs.
  1. I have little ability to direct and control my feelings and behaviors.
  2. I must have what I want when I want it or else the world is unfair.

Step 3. Challenge any irrational thinking or rationalized thinking in Steps #1 and #2 by identifying what is true and what is not true.
  1. It's true that I have this urge.
  2. It's true that it is uncomfortable not to give in to the urge.
  3. It's not true that I will go crazy if I don't give in to the urge, in fact, the urge will pass.
  4. It's not true that I must satisfy my sexual desires right now.

Step 4. Substitute specific rational thoughts to counter those thoughts that were disruptive.
  1. I would like to be able to give in to my sexual desires at every urge, but it would not be terrible if this didn't happen.
  2. I can control my behavior through rational thinking, and I am committed to not behaving impulsively when I have an urge.

Whether used as an independent technique in rational–emotive therapy or as a part of the comprehensive therapeutic approach such as relapse prevention, cognitive restructuring is a valuable skill for sex offenders to learn. It allows for a systematic approach to deal with the deviant–distorted cognitions that seem so germane to all types of sexual deviations. Although use of this approach is becoming increasingly widespread, caution should be taken not to use this as an exclusive approach with sex offenders. In addition to deviant cognitions, focus should also be placed on such factors as decreasing deviant sexual arousal, increasing adaptive coping skills for high-risk situations, empathy toward victims, and appropriate adult behaviors.

REFERENCES

Abel, G. G., & Becker, J. V. (1984). *Adult cognition scale.* (Available from G. G. Abel, Behavioral Medicine Institute, 3193 Howell Mill Rd. NW, Ste. 202, Atlanta, GA 30327)

Akers, R. L. (1977). *Deviant behavior: A social learning approach* (2nd ed.). Belmont, CA: Wadsworth.

Burt, M. R. (1980). Cultural myths and supports for rape. *Journal of Personality and Social Psychology, 38,* 217–230.

Ellis, A., & Grieger, R. (Eds.) (1977). *Handbook of rational emotive therapy.* New York: Springer.

Ellis, A., & Harper, R. A. (1976). *A new guide to rational living.* Englewood Cliffs, NJ: Prentice-Hall.

George, W. H., & Marlatt, G. A. (1986). *Relapse prevention with sexual offenders: A treatment manual.* Unpublished manuscript, Florida Mental Health Institute, Tampa.

Jenkins-Hall, K. D. (1987). *Conventional follow-up for rational emotive therapy: A treatment manual.* Unpublished manuscript, Florida Mental Health Institute, Tampa.

Lange, A. (1986). *Rational emotive therapy: A treatment manual.* Unpublished manuscript, Florida Mental Health Institute, Tampa.

Marlatt, G. A. (1985). Relapse prevention: Theoretical rationale and overview of the model. In G. A. Marlatt & J. R. Gordon (Eds.), *Relapse prevention: Maintenance strategies in the treatment of addictive behaviors.* (pp. 3–70). New York: Guilford.

McMullin, R. E. (1986). *Handbook of cognitive therapy techniques.* New York: Norton.

Meichenbaum, D. M. (1977). *Cognitive–behavior modification: An integrative approach.* New York: Plenum.

Yochelson, S., & Samenow, S. E., (1976). *The criminal personality: Vol. 1. A profile for change.* New York: Aronson.

B · GLOBAL INTERVENTIONS

19

Lifestyle Interventions: Promoting Positive Addictions

J. KEVIN THOMPSON

In recent years, treatment approaches for sexual offenders have become multi-faceted in nature (George & Marlatt, 1984; Pithers, Marques, Gibat, & Marlatt, 1983). Included in the complex inventory of techniques designed to promote and maintain therapeutic gains are numerous procedures that target general lifestyle areas. Inherent in the logic of applying lifestyle modification procedures to the sexual aggressive is the belief among researchers and clinicians that an unbalanced lifestyle leads to a subjective sense of being out of control (Marlatt, 1985). In turn, the individual may seek the release of accompanying anger or hostility via maladaptive means.

Of greater relevance for this chapter, however, is the role of positive lifestyle interventions in the prevention of or rapid recovery from lapses and relapses. Generally, in cases of effective initial treatment, the individual experiences a sense of deprivation when the maladaptive focus of tension reduction is removed from his repertoire. Concomitantly, if an unbalanced lifestyle is present, the tandem pairing of these possible lapse–relapse precipitators may produce an individual at great risk for repeat offenses. Therefore, the careful implementation and monitoring of a client's compliance to positive lifestyle behaviors is an integral aspect of treatment (Pithers et al., 1983).

There are multiple considerations in the integration of such procedures with sexual offenders. This chapter focuses on the specific lifestyle interventions that appear feasible for this difficult patient sample. Initially, definitions of relevant techniques and *positive addiction* are offered, followed by a brief review of the research literature. Specific details for using these procedures constitute the bulk of the chapter, followed by recommendations for future research. It should be noted that very little controlled research has been conducted with these procedures on samples of sexually aggressive individuals. Therefore, many of the guidelines offered here are extrapolated from the literature on relapse prevention with addictive disorders, such as smoking, drinking, and eating (Brownell, Marlatt, Lichtenstein, & Wilson, 1986).

DEFINITIONS OF LIFESTYLE INTERVENTIONS AND POSITIVE ADDICTION

There are many aspects of a person's lifestyle that can be detrimental or positive, depending on the individual's specific level and/or mode of engaging in the behavior. The most basic lifestyle behaviors include biological necessities, such as eating or sleeping. At the next level are those activities that are not inherently necessary but do promote physical and psychological health. In this category, one might include adequate exercise, freedom from stress, and relaxation. At the next level are personal preference activities, which might include hobbies and interpersonal relationships. Examples of these behaviors would include reading, writing, constructive hobbies (e.g., building furniture), group social activities (e.g., church, bowling leagues), and interactions with family members or significant others. There are other activities, but the foregoing serve to illustrate and define the general category of lifestyle interventions.

As mentioned earlier, the essential purpose of these activities is for them to serve as behaviors that are incompatible with the problematic, sexually aggressive response. Additionally, the logic is that these behaviors are potentially as rewarding as the maladaptive response under treatment and that they may thus come to elicit a positive hedonic reaction in the individual. Thus, in countering the "negative addiction" that has led the client to seek socially undesirable reinforcement, the repeated use of these prosocial activities will eventually lead to a state of "positive addiction."

Unfortunately, the term *positive addiction* has been used in a confusing manner by various researchers and theoreticians (Glasser, 1976; Thompson & Blanton, 1987). In one sense, it connotes the same level of compulsive dependence on an activity for gratification that negative addictions require. As discussed by various authors, however, the excessive reliance on an apparently positive activity may, in fact, lead to detrimental consequences. For instance, Yates, Leehey, and Shisslak (1983) were the first researchers to note the similarities between "obligatory" runners and individuals with anorexia nervosa. Although the issue is far from settled with regard to the potential negative aspects of excessive exercise behavior, it is generally believed that a positive addiction may not always be so positive (Thompson & Blanton, 1987).

Peele (1981) posits a continuum from daily routines to dependencies, compulsions, and, finally, addictions. Therefore, for our purposes it may be more precise to label our techniques as attempts to augment positive lifestyle behaviors, thus avoiding the confusion of the term *positive addictions*. In fact, of the activities generally subsumed under the heading of lifestyle modifications, exercise is probably the only activity that reasonably lends itself to possible addiction.

OVERVIEW OF RESEARCH
ON LIFESTYLE INTERVENTIONS

To date, researchers have not carried out controlled investigations of lifestyle interventions versus other treatments on populations of sexual offenders. However, an active area of investigation with obvious relevance to these individuals is that of lifestyle interventions with addictive behaviors (Brownell et al., 1986; Marlatt, 1985). Most of this research has targeted exercise training and some form of relaxation training.

For instance, retrospective evidence supports the possibly salutary effect of meditation on alcohol and drug use (Benson & Wallace, 1972; Shafii, Lavely, & Jaffe, 1975). Beginning an exercise program has also been associated with cessation of smoking (Koplan, Powell, Sikes, Shirley, & Campbell, 1983). Shiffman (1982) also noted that exercise was a major coping response for those smokers who avoided relapse.

Marlatt and colleagues have been involved with a systematic examination of the role of exercise and relaxation as treatments for heavy drinkers. In the first study, these researchers compared three relaxation groups (progressive muscle relaxation, meditation, and bibliotherapy) with controls. All three groups were found to reduce their drinking levels to a degree significantly below that of the control subjects (Marlatt & Marques, 1977; Marlatt, Pagano, Rose, & Marques, 1984). Marlatt (1985) concluded that "taking regular time-out periods to relax, even if only for short periods each day, is associated with significant reductions in drinking rates" (p. 327).

In a second study, Murphy, Pagano, and Marlatt (1986) compared the effect of aerobic exercise (running) and meditation on alcohol consumption in male college students. Subjects in the exercise group were assigned an individually tailored running regimen, and meditation subjects were trained in a mantra-based relaxation technique. Subjects in both groups met three times a week for sessions led by trained instructors. The results indicated that only the subjects who received the aerobic exercise treatment differed significantly from controls in reducing their alcohol consumption.

Although there is little literature on lifestyle modifications and positive therapeutic outcome with sexual offenders, experts in this area agree that this component is an important ingredient in any comprehensive program (George & Marlatt, 1984; Pithers et al., 1983). Controlled experimental analyses with sexual offenders will most likely continue to be problematic, given the difficulty of acquiring a sufficiently large subject population and the urgency of providing the most efficacious treatment to those patients under investigation. Therefore, research in the addictive disorders will continue to provide useful information regarding specific lifestyle interventions that may be integrated, in methodology and content, into ongoing programs of relapse prevention for sexual aggressives. However, researchers involved with the treatment of this population might consider regression analyses to pinpoint lifestyle strategies most connected with positive posttreatment outcome.

IMPLEMENTATION OF LIFESTYLE
INTERVENTION STRATEGIES

The general lifestyle modification procedures described above should be implemented with an idiographic approach. Each individual is unique in his previous history of exercise behavior, ability to relax, interest in specific hobbies, interpersonal contacts, and other aspects of lifestyle. Financial concerns are also important, and possibly limiting, factors for some individuals. Age and physical ability may interact with financial concerns to preclude some lifestyle interventions.

In order to maximize the potential usefulness of these procedures, the therapist must work closely with each person to identify optimal interventions. A careful interview that focuses on a large number of lifestyle areas is a beginning method of determining possible intervention avenues. Patients should be encouraged to recall any premorbid activities and interests that may be relevant. The therapist should be directive and engaging with a difficult client, suggesting various activities that the client may have taken part in but forgotten. Along the lines of George and Marlatt (1984), clients may also be asked to self-monitor pleasant events to provide information about individually specific lifestyle elements that lend themselves as interventions.

Although the selection of activities is necessarily idiosyncratic to each individual, general issues of eating, exercising, relaxing, hobbies, and adaptive social involvements should receive examination. The specific guidelines for implementing these procedures have been covered extensively by Marlatt and colleagues (George & Marlatt, 1984; Marlatt, 1985). However, each deserves some comment with regard to the specific population of sexual offenders.

The issues of food consumption and sleeping habits may initially appear to be minor ones to both therapist and client. If the presentation is couched in terms of a general regulatory model emphasizing that adequate and regular food consumption and sleep are necessary for health, which, in turn, increases the chance that one can control destructive impulses (anger, irritability, sexual urges, etc.), these issues become more obviously relevant. If patients are required to self-monitor other facets of lifestyle interventions, the inclusion of nutritional and sleeping information may be easily added to recording chores.

Exercise tasks can be adapted to the interests of the individual and are not necessarily limited to running. Important in this area is providing adequate instructional information, including specific details about performing the activity, warm-up, optimal work-out intensity, and so forth. For instance, in a series of studies on running compliance conducted by Martin et al. (1984), subjects received specific instructions regarding footwear, warm-up, running style, breathing, cool-down, and other aspects of the activity. If the activities are somewhat complex to the novice, such as weightlifting or calisthenics, the importance of adequate instructional guidance is heightened. Finally, if possible, activities should be conducted in groups and led by experienced therapists.

A variety of relaxation methods are available, and patients may be allowed to experiment with different versions. Some may prefer the more active progressive muscular relaxation, while others may select a more passive meditation procedure. In any case, insession training is necessary, along with gradual generalization to the extralaboratory setting. Home practice should be encouraged and monitored on self-recording forms.

The selection of hobbies and interpersonal activities may require some inventiveness by both parties. However, some hobbies (e.g., woodworking, photography, reading) are reasonable from a financial viewpoint. Augmenting interpersonal activity levels may require various types of assistance from the therapist, from the location of adaptive social outlets (e.g., bowling leagues, singles' groups, church groups, neighborhood organizations) to training in social skills (which may involve role-playing or other active interventions).

In sum, the collaboration between therapist and patient should yield lifestyle-intervention strategies that provide a high probability of usefulness in relapse prevention. The issue of compliance is, of course, the crucial concern. If patients do not follow through by implementing strategies, there is no adequate test of their efficacy. Encouragement may work with highly motivated clients, but more stringent measures, such as contingency contracting or reinforcement programs, are likely to be necessary. Financial incentives or reward systems may be effective in this regard (Epstein, Wing, Koeske, Andrasik, & Ossip, 1981; Epstein, Wing, Thompson, & Griffin, 1980; Lichtenstein, 1982). Again, if possible, the initial implementation of and patient participation in these strategies should be conducted under the supervision of trained therapists.

CUE-CONTROLLED UTILIZATION OF STRATEGIES

Training of patients in lifestyle intervention strategies is only the first step in their appropriate utilization. From a pragmatic viewpoint, the salutary effects of lifestyle modifications may have an effect on the general function of the client. In a base-rate sense, they lead to a greater sense of balance, control, and so forth, which enhances the possibility of relapse prevention. However, these strategies can also be used as immediate deterrents to maladaptive responses. The distinction can be readily understood if one considers the general practice of running each afternoon following work versus deciding to jog given the immediate recognition of an unacceptable, problematic impulse, thought, or situation. In the latter case, the individual is showing greater control by using certain cues to engage in a behavior that is incompatible with the occurrence of a lapse or relapse.

Research has recently identified several predictors of lapse and relapse, although, again, the bulk of these data come from studies of addictive disorders. Brownell et al. (1986) offer a review of these factors, several of which are relevant to lifestyle interventions. For instance, considerable data support the contention that negative emotional factors, such as stress, depression, and anxiety, lead to lapse and relapse (Cummings, Gordon, & Marlatt, 1980; Shiffman, 1982). Interpersonal conflict and lack of interpersonal support have similarly been related to a failure to maintain treatment gains in weight control and smoking cessation (Brownell, 1984; Brownell et al., 1986; Cummings et al., 1980). Specific environmental stimuli, such as social events or cues, have also been related to lapse and relapse. Shiffman (1982) found that eating and drinking situations were associated with relapses in smokers, and Mermelstein and Lichtenstein (1983) found that environmental cues associated with the consumption of alcohol, such as celebrations, were predictive of alcohol lapses.

Thus these interpersonal and environmental factors should be closely monitored for each patient. Perhaps, in a retrospective sense, patients may be able to identify events that were problematic in the past, and this information could be used to predict future events that might foretell lapses. In addition, subjects might self-monitor situational factors and emotional states, along with using specific lifestyle intervention strategies. The therapist might then be able to pinpoint specific problem areas and suggest solutions. Furthermore, stress-inoculation procedures might prove useful, that is, re-creating specific emotional states or situations in session, with the client practicing coping procedures. In fact, if relaxation or exercise training is taking place in groups, therapists might consider inducing negative mood states (via imagery or verbal scenarios) and then requiring subjects to engage in the coping strategies.

SUMMARY

Although generally regarded as an integral aspect of the treatment of sexual offenders, lifestyle interventions have received limited research attention. Much of the theory and methodology behind the use of these procedures with sexual aggressives comes from corollary research with the addictive disorders. While accepting the inherent difficulties of conducting controlled research in populations of sexual offenders, researchers and clinicians should strive to investigate lifestyle interventions with this clinical group. Nonetheless, they should remain cautious about adopting these procedures simply because they appear to be effective with addictive disorders. Nonetheless, the similarities between these disorders and the urgent necessity for constructing optimal intervention plans argue for the current movement toward comprehensive programs that contain lifestyle modification techniques.

REFERENCES

Benson, H., & Wallace, R. (1972). Decreased drug abuse with transcendental meditation: A study of 1862 subjects. In C. J. Zarafonetis (Ed.), *Drug abuse: Proceedings of the international conference* (pp. 369–376). Philadelphia: Lea & Febiger.

Brownell, K. D. (1984). Behavioral, psychological, and environmental predictors of obesity and success at weight reduction. *International Journal of Obesity, 8,* 543–550.

Brownell, K. D., Marlatt, G. A., Lichtenstein, E., & Wilson, G. T. (1986). Understanding and preventing relapse. *American Psychologist, 41,* 765–782.

Cummings, C., Gordon, J. R., & Marlatt, G. A. (1980). Relapse: Prevention and prediction. In W. R. Miller (Ed.), *The addictive disorders: Treatment of alcoholism, drug abuse, smoking, and obesity* (pp. 291–322). New York: Pergamon.

Epstein, L. H., Wing, R. R., Koeske, R., Andrasik, F., & Ossip, D. J. (1981). Child and parent weight loss in family-based behavior modification programs. *Journal of Consulting and Clinical Psychology, 49,* 674–685.

Epstein, L. H., Wing, R. R., Thompson, J. K., & Griffin, W. (1980). The effects of contract and lottery procedures on attendance and fitness in aerobic exercise. *Behavior Modification, 4,* 465–479.

George, W. H., & Marlatt, G. A. (1984). *Relapse prevention with sexual offenders: A treatment manual.* Unpublished manuscript.

Glasser, W. (1976). *Positive addictions.* New York: Harper & Row.

Koplan, J. P., Powell, K. E., Sikes, R. K., Shirley, R. W., & Campbell, C. C. (1982). An epidemiologic study of the benefits and risks of running. *Journal of the American Medical Association, 248,* 3118–3121.

Lichtenstein, E. (1982). The smoking problem: A behavioral perspective. *Journal of Consulting and Clinical Psychology, 50,* 804–819.

Marlatt, G. A. (1985). Lifestyle modification. In G. A. Marlatt & J. R. Gordon (Eds.), *Relapse prevention* (pp. 280–348). New York: Guilford.

Marlatt, G. A., & Marques, J. K. (1977). Meditation, self-control, and alcohol use. In R. B. Stuart (Ed.), *Behavioral self-management: Strategies, techniques, and outcomes* (pp. 117–153). New York: Brunner/Mazel.

Marlatt, G. A., Pagano, R., Rose, D., & Marques, J. K. (1984). Effect of meditation and relaxation training upon alcohol use in male social drinkers. In D. H. Shapiro & R. Walsh (Eds.), *The science of meditation: Theory, research and experience* (pp. 120–165). New York: Aldine.

Martin, J. E., Dubbert, P. M., Katell, A. D., Thompson, J. K., Raczynaki, J. M., Lake, M., Smith, P. O., Webster, J. S., Sikora, T., & Cohen, R. E. (1984). Behavioral control of exercise in sedentary adults: Studies 1 through 6. *Journal of Consulting and Clinical Psychology, 52,* 795–811.

Mermelstein, R. J., & Lichtenstein, E. (1983, April). *Slips versus relapses in smoking cessation: A situational analysis.* Paper presented at the meeting of the Western Psychological Association, San Francisco.

Murphy, T. J., Pagano, R. R., & Marlatt, G. A. (1986). Lifestyle modification with heavy alcohol drinkers: Effects of aerobic exercise and meditation. *Addictive Behaviors, 11,* 175–186.

Peele, S. (1981). *How much is too much?* Morristown, NJ: Human Resources Institute.

Pithers, W. D., Marques, J. K., Gibat, C. C., & Marlatt, G. A. (1983). Relapse prevention with sexual aggressives: A self-control model of treatment and maintenance of change. In J. G. Greer & I. R. Stuart (Eds.), *The sexual aggressor: Current perspectives on treatment* (pp. 214–239). New York: Van Nostrand Reinhold.

Shafii, M., Lavely, R., & Jaffe, R. (1975). Meditation and the prevention of alcohol abuse. *American Journal of Psychiatry, 132,* 942–945.

Shiffman, S. (1982). Relapse following smoking cessation: A situational analysis. *Journal of Consulting and Clinical Psychology, 50,* 439–440.

Thompson, J. K., & Blanton, P. (1987). Energy conservation and exercise dependence: A sympathetic arousal hypothesis. *Medicine and Science in Sports and Exercise, 19,* 91–99.

Yates, A., Leehey, K., & Shisslak, C. M. (1983). Running—An analogue of anorexia? *New England Journal of Medicine, 308,* 251–255.

20

How to Handle the PIG

G. ALAN MARLATT

A story is told in India about the best way to control a poisonous snake. A peasant who first found the snake decided the best way to control it and avoid harm would be to tie it up in a strong wicker box until it starved and died. After the snake was imprisoned in this way for a day or two, the peasant grew curious about its current state. Was the snake alive or dead? He could not tell just by looking at or listening to the box—it gave off no clues. Finally, his impatience grew so strong that he could stand it no longer. He carefully untied the ropes around the box and lifted the lid just a crack to take a quick peek at the snake. Without warning, the snake sprang forth, biting the man and injecting him with deadly venom. At the funeral, one of the peasant's friends remarked, "In retrospect, I don't think that shutting the snake up in the box was the best way to control it. He should have gotten to know the snake and his habits. If he had become friends with it instead of locking it up like it was a deadly enemy, the snake would not have bitten him."

For the purposes of this chapter, let us imagine the snake is another animal, the PIG (perhaps a dangerous wild boar). As described in Chapter 3, the PIG is an acronym for the "problem of immediate gratification," which refers to the desire for gratification associated with sexual craving and urges. This chapter outlines methods sex offenders can use to better understand and cope with the PIG. These methods include observing the PIG and its habits, developing a sense of detachment and objective labeling of the PIG's craving and urges, and mastering coping strategies to better handle it. The underlying theme of this approach is illustrated in the story about the snake in the box. Attempts to control the snake (or the PIG) by sheer restraint or overcontrol (e.g., tying it up with ropes of willpower) often backfire. Rather, one should get to know the beast and its habits so that effective coping can be mastered. As the Zen teacher Shunryu Suzuki once wrote: "To give your sheep or cow a large, spacious meadow is the way to control him" (1970, p. 31). The same goes for snakes and pigs.

AWARENESS OF THE PIG AND HOW IT OPERATES

The first task in coping with the PIG is to become familiar with its behavior: how it manifests itself in craving and urges, what makes it hungry, and how it is gratified. In presenting these ideas to clients, it is helpful to objectify the PIG. Imagining the problem of immediate gratification as a PIG may help clients grapple with this otherwise vague motivational construct. Most people have a stereotyped negative image of pigs. They see them as greedy animals, fat and dirty swine rutting about in the mud (a stereotype that is probably unfair to the pig as an animal but that seems to fit the concept of PIG as we have discussed it in this context). The PIG craves food and sex and gives into its urges with abandon. Each indulgence in gratification makes the PIG grow fatter. Never fully satisfied, the PIG is hungry again soon after each meal or sexual act; the more it has, the more it wants. Its appetite is insatiable; its cravings can never be fully gratified.

What brings the PIG into action? What makes the PIG hungry—what stimulates its appetite in the first place? Getting to know the PIG and its habits is the first step in controlling its behavior. In Chapter 3, it was stressed that the PIG is frequently stimulated into action by external cues (conditioned stimuli and discriminative stimuli). Exposure to stimuli associated in the past with sexual gratification is particularly powerful in arousing its hunger (e.g., the sight of children playing in a park makes the pedophile "hungry" for sex). Negative emotional states, such as feeling depressed, rejected, jealous, or angry, are also known to whet the PIG's appetite. The PIG's craving is particularly voracious if it first experiences a negative emotional state and is then exposed to an arousal-enhancing cue or provocative stimulus (as in the case of Bob X., described in Chapter 3).

Offenders in treatment need to be taught the emotions and cues that stimulate the appetite of their own PIGs. Assessment of the triggering cues is relatively straightforward for many offenders. Assessment techniques described in Part II of this volume may be helpful in this regard. Asking the offender to self-monitor sexual urges and craving on an ongoing basis is one useful procedure; the therapist must take care to identify the external cues that elicit these responses. Objective measures of sexual arousal (such as the penile strain guage) can also be used to monitor arousal to various stimuli (e.g., photographs of children). Descriptions of past offenses or ongoing sexual scenarios are often helpful in the assessment process. It is important for the therapist to point out both the discrete cues that elicit craving and the emotional state or mood in which these cues are experienced. In getting to know the PIG and its ways, we must find out what "turns on" the PIG.

COPING WITH THE PIG

The following steps are recommended in teaching clients to cope with the PIG:

1. Clients are taught to recognize the PIG when it first is experienced, most often as increased craving (desire for sexual gratification) and urges (impulsive intentions to act out sexually).
2. Once cravings and urges are recognized, the client needs to execute an effective coping response to ward off the PIG before it gains control.
3. Lifestyle balancing procedures can be acquired to reduce the PIG's overall influence.
4. Additional clinical interventions, including aversion and extinction procedures, may be necessary with some clients.

Each of these steps is detailed briefly in the following paragraphs.

Recognizing the PIG

The goal here is to teach the offender to recognize the earliest indicators of sexual arousal as soon as they are perceived (i.e., when the PIG first shows itself), usually as increased desire (craving) or sudden urges. As soon as the PIG is recognized, the client should attempt to identify the triggering cue or stimulus (e.g., sight of an attractive sexual object). Awareness of the background mood state (e.g., negative emotional state) may also be helpful in this regard. The triggering cue should be labeled as an *early warning signal* (e.g., a railway-crossing sign that reads STOP, LOOK AND LISTEN) calling for an appropriate coping response (e.g., stop the car before it crosses the railway tracks). In cognitive–behavioral terms, the stimulus for the PIG needs to be restructured, or reframed, as a discriminative stimulus designating the need for a coping response.

The critical message that needs to be impressed on the client is that once the PIG is recognized and the stimulus identified, fast action is called for. The longer the delay in exercising a coping response, the greater the probability the PIG will grow in size and strength. Research on motivation and the goal gradient effect (also known as the delay-of-reinforcement gradient) shows that the reinforcing effect of a reward (e.g., a food goal for a hungry rat) increases as a function of proximity to the goal (Kimble, 1961). The closer the animal is to the goal, the more motivated it becomes (rats run faster the closer they are to the goal reward). In terms of the present metaphor, the PIG grows fatter and more difficult to stop as the individual approaches the sexual target. Conversely, the PIG is easier to handle when it first appears as an initial urge (when it is still a PIGlet, so to speak).

One problem many clients face in learning to recognize the PIG is that they fail to identify it as a response triggered by external cues and high-risk situations. Instead of seeing the urge as externally mediated, they overidentify with the urge and see it as coming from inside themselves, sometimes as a result of willpower failure. Clients who give into or identify with an urge often believe the urge will continue to grow until it becomes impossible to resist. To see the urge as a conditioned response, on the other hand, is to recognize that this response will arise and then subside and pass away on its own. Giving into the urge at the peak of its intensity feeds the PIG; conversely, active coping and not giving in starves the PIG.

Developing a sense of *detachment* is an important step to follow after the PIG is first recognized. Instead of identifying with the urge (e.g., "I really want to touch that girl's bottom"), the client learns to monitor the urge or desire from the point of view of a detached observer (e.g., "I am experiencing an urge to touch that girl"). By externalizing and labeling the urge and "watching" it come and go through the eyes of an observer (much as a meditator learns to passively observe ideas, feelings, and images as they pass through the mind), the client will have a decreased tendency to identify with the urge and feel overwhelmed by the PIG. Some clients, particularly those who have difficulty recognizing the emergence of urges or craving, may benefit from meditation or mindfulness training to enhance their sense of awareness of mental and physical events. Meditation strategies for use in relapse prevention programs have been described elsewhere (Marlatt, 1985; Marlatt & Marques, 1977).

Coping Strategies

Effective coping strategies fall into two major categories: behavioral coping and cognitive coping. Before being taught these coping strategies, many clients need to learn that *willpower* alone is not an effective way of coping. For most people, willpower connotes "resistance to temptation" or some "willful" attempt to inhibit the problematic behavior. This exercise of "power" is akin to the Indian's attempt to control the poisonous snake by keeping it tied up in a box. Tests of willpower usually end in defeat. It may be helpful to reframe "willpower" as the client's *motivation* to change. Motivation alone is insufficient, however, because it sheds little light on the *means* used to achieve the goal. Clients need both the motivation (will) to change and the means (coping) to achieve the goal and master the PIG.

Behavioral coping strategies include avoidance or escape from the high-risk situation (e.g., sexual cues) and/or the performance of alternative behaviors that reduce the intensity of the PIG. The simplest strategy is *planning ahead* to avoid potential high-risk situations. To avoid relapse set-ups, clients need to ascertain their own high-risk situations and attempt to avoid them whenever possible. Keeping away from temptation, whenever possible, lessens the risk that the PIG will be activated by sexual cues. Not all temptations can be avoided, of course. Once in a high-risk situation, *escape* is often the best coping strategy; for example, doing something else, such as going for a walk, taking an alternative route, or calling a friend and arranging a place to meet. The third behavioral coping strategy, engaging in alternative activities to reduce or to substitute for sexual desire, will be described below in the section on lifestyle balancing procedures.

Cognitive coping strategies include self-talk and the use of motivational imagery. Self-talk may involve an internal monologue in which the client reminds himself of the consequences of giving in to the PIG. Reminding oneself of the negative costs of indulgence helps bring these delayed consequences into the foreground. Because of their temporal delay, such negative consequences, regardless of their magnitude, have less deterrence value in comparison to the immediate reinforcement associated with the PIG. Motivational research shows that the *immediacy* of the reinforcement has the greatest effects on performance, even when the payoff is relatively small in comparison to the strength of the delayed costs. Bringing imagined consequences to mind when faced with temptation, on the other hand, increases their motivational saliency and controlling impact. Participants in Alcoholics Anonymous speak of "thinking through the drink" as an effective cognitive coping skill. The alcoholic, when tempted to drink, does a cognitive "fast-forward" maneuver and imagines what would happen *after* the drink was consumed, *after* he became intoxicated, *after* his family found out, and so on down the line. Recovering sexual offenders may find this to be a useful technique as well; clients who "think through" the sexual act and its various consequences may be more able to keep the PIG from growing fatter.

Imagery is another effective cognitive coping strategy. One useful imagery technique is to imagine oneself coping effectively in high-risk situations associated with potential relapse (for details, see Hall, Chapter 17, this volume). There is another imagery technique that is helpful in countering the belief that an urge will increase in intensity unless it is indulged in. This procedure, called *urge surfing* (Marlatt & Gordon, 1985), may help the client perceive an urge as a response that grows stronger at first, peaks, and then subsides, much like an ocean wave. The wave analogy is a useful externalization technique and facilitates detachment from the experience of the PIG. Here the client is told to imagine himself as a person learning to surf. The urge is described as a wave and the client's goal is to learn to keep his balance, to ride the wave without being "wiped out" by its strength. Other similar imagery techniques to enhance self-efficacy and facilitate coping can be constructed. Macho clients may take to a gunfighter image in which the urge is defined as an enemy, a threat to their life and well-being. As soon as the gunfighter recognizes the urge target, he shoots it with an active response. The urge is annihilated with the "bullet of awareness."

Lifestyle Balancing

A lifestyle short on pleasurable activities or rewarding experiences enhances feelings of deprivation. Deprivation makes the PIG grow hungrier and harder to deal with. To lessen this sense of deprivation, clients need to develop other sources of gratification to rebalance their overall lifestyle. If illicit sexual activity is the primary or only source of pleasure in a client's lifestyle, the PIG will always be lurking at the door, hungry and demanding. In addition to acquiring the basic coping skills described in the foregoing section, clients will benefit from a restructuring of their daily activities to increase the number of "wants" (pleasurable and rewarding activities) in order to balance the "shoulds" (the demanding and obligatory activities). Because the topic of a balanced lifestyle is covered in detail elsewhere (Chapter 5 in Marlatt & Gordon, 1985), only the highlights will be covered here.

For many clients, developing alternative pleasurable activities will placate the PIG's hunger. Sexually addicting behaviors can be replaced in some instances as the client learns new forms of gratification, sometimes called "positive addictions" (Glasser, 1976; Thompson, Chapter 19, this volume). These behaviors are thought to be "addictive" if failing to continue in the behaviors results in a feeling of deprivation or discomfort. The most frequently described positive addictions are exercise (particularly aerobic activities) and relaxation (especially meditation). The benefits of exercise as an effective lifestyle change technique in the behavioral-medicine literature have been reviewed by others (e.g., Martin & Dubbert, 1982). Relaxation and meditation also have advantages in this regard, since they enable the client to reduce tension and stress (including sexual craving) and to develop a sense of detached awareness that facilitates urge coping. For a general overview of the meditation literature, including clinical applications with addictive behaviors, the reader is referred to Shapiro (1980) and Shapiro and Walsh (1984).

The PIG's appetite may also be sated by activities other than illicit sexual behavior. Substitute forms of indulgence may be called for, including other more appropriate sexual outlets (e.g., intercourse with a consenting adult, masturbation to adult stimuli, which might result adventitiously in orgasmic reconditioning) or related sensual experiences (e.g., receiving a massage, "pigging out" on one's favorite foods, treating oneself to a favorite drink, reading erotic literature, or watching a *x-rated* movie). Masturbation to adult-oriented stimuli has been found in one study to decrease sexual arousal to deviant stimuli (Kremsdorf, Holmen, & Laws, 1980). One must be on guard here to choose alternative sensual experiences that do not feed the PIG, that is, do not play into and increase fantasies of illicit sexual acts that may spill over into overt behavior.

Aversion and Extinction Techniques

If clients are continuing to have problems with the PIG, despite efforts at the self-control training described above, additional behavioral-therapy procedures may be implemented. One method that has been used in the treatment of sex offenders is *aversion therapy* (Quinsey & Marshall, 1983). To continue the metaphor af this chapter, aversion methods can be viewed as attempts to poison the PIG. Through the association of provocative sexual cues (presented in pictorial form or imagined by the client) with aversive consequences (e.g., nausea, pain, or anxiety), an attempt is made to transform craving into aversion. The effectiveness of aversion therapy in the treatment of sexual offenders has yet to be firmly established in the experimental literature, however. Most authorities believe that aversion may have a temporary suppression effect on sexual craving and urges. Aversion may be more effective if combined with cognitive–behavioral self-control methods. Aversion methods include the use of either real aversive agents (including emetic substances, electric shock, and noxious odors) or imagined aversive consequences (as in the use of covert-sensitization-methods).

One final technique involves *extinction* (attempts to starve the PIG). As already noted, each time an offender gives in to an urge for illicit sexual activity, the PIG is fed (reinforced) and increases in power. An extinction method that has received attention in the field of addictive behaviors is *cue exposure* (Hodgson & Rankin, 1982). Based on classical conditioning theory, cue exposure is based on the assumption that direct exposure to addiction cues (e.g., liquor, cigarettes, or sexual stimuli) elicits conditioned craving responses. According to this theory, if these craving responses are not reinforced by giving into the urge, they should eventually subside through the mechanism of extinction. Just as Pavlov's dogs showed a gradual reduction in conditioned salivation in response to repeated presentations of a stimulus that no longer signaled that food was forthcoming, so it is that the addict's conditioned urges will gradually subside if they are not reinforced by the sexual act. Alternatively, cue exposure may be effective because it enhances self-efficacy; clients may feel more confident that they can be exposed to addictive cues without losing control. Most current work with cue exposure has been conducted with smokers and drinkers, and little is known about its efficacy in the treatment of sexual offenders. The procedure is similar, however, to various stimulus-satiation programs in which illicit erotic scenarios are repeated over and over in an attempt to weaken their influence

(Marshall, 1979). Future treatment programs may find that a combination of cue-exposure and cognitive urge-control techniques is an effective way of coping with the PIG (Cooney, Baker, & Pomerleau, 1983).

CONCLUSION

The PIG is such a pervasive concept in the treatment of addictive behaviors that a newsletter devoted entirely to this topic is published. Entitled *The Problem of Immediate Gratification,* this newsletter is published by a psychologist in Texas.[1] It seems fitting to close this chapter with a quote from a recent issue:

> The PIG is our way of labeling the phenomenon by which a small but immediate gratification exerts more control over behavior than does a large but delayed one. In fact, in a choice among assured, familiar outcomes of behavior, the PIG's prey choose the less rewarding over the more rewarding alternatives. By trading the large, but delayed, gratifications of life for small ones, addicted persons are incompetent hedonists. So whether you have noble goals or seek life's sensual pleasures, you would do well to take George Bernard Shaw's advice (from *Man and Superman*), "To choose the line of greatest advantage instead of yielding in the direction of least resistance." (Vol. 2 [3], pp. 2-3)

REFERENCES

Cooney, N. L., Baker, L., & Pomerleau, O. F. (1983). Cue exposure for relapse prevention in alcohol treatment. In R. J. McMahon & K. D. Craig (Eds.), *Advances in clinical behavior therapy* (pp. 194–210). New York: Brunner/Mazel.

Glasser, W. (1976). *Positive addiction.* New York: Harper & Row.

Hodgson, R. J., & Rankin, H. (1982). Cue exposure and relapse prevention. In W. M. Hay & P. E. Nathan (Eds.), *Clinical case studies in the behavioral treatment of alcoholism* (pp. 207–226). New York: Plenum.

Kimble, G. A. (1961). *Hilgard and Marquis' conditioning and learning.* New York: Appleton-Century-Crofts.

Kremsdorf, R. B., Holmen, M. L., & Laws, D. R. (1980). Orgasmic reconditioning without deviant imagery: A case report with a pedophile. *Behaviour Research and Therapy, 18,* 203–207.

Marlatt, G. A. (1985). Lifestyle modification. In G. A. Marlatt & J. R. Gordon (Eds.), *Relapse prevention: Maintenance strategies in the treatment of addictive behaviors* (pp. 280–348). New York: Guilford.

Marlatt, G. A., & Gordon, J. R. (Eds.). (1985). *Relapse prevention: Maintenance strategies in the treatment of addictive behaviors.* New York: Guilford.

[1]For information on this newsletter, contact Dr. Bill Dubin, Addiction Control Clinic, 4005 Spicewood Springs, Austin, TX 78759.

Marlatt, G. A., & Marques, J. K. (1977). Meditation, self-control, and alcohol use. In R. B. Stuart (Ed.), *Behavioral self-management* (pp. 117–153). New York: Brunner/ Mazel.

Marshall, W. L. (1979). Satiation therapy: A procedure for reducing deviant sexual arousal. *Journal of Applied Behavior Analysis, 12,* 10–22.

Martin, J. E., & Dubbert, P. M. (1982). Exercise applications and promotion in behavioral medicine. *Journal of Consulting and Clinical Psychology, 50,* 1004–1017.

Quinsey, V. L., & Marshall, W. L. (1983). Procedures for reducing inappropriate sexual arousal: An evaluation review. In J. G. Greer & I. R. Stuart (Eds.), *The sexual aggressor* (pp. 267–292). New York: Van Nostrand Reinhold.

Shapiro, D. H. (1980). *Meditation: Self-regulation strategy and altered states of consciousness.* New York: Aldine.

Shapiro, D. H., & Walsh, R. N. (Eds.). (1984). *Meditation: Classic and contemporary perspectives.* New York: Aldine.

Suzuki, S. (1970). *Zen mind, beginner's mind.* New York: Weatherhill.

21

Enhancing Offender Empathy for Sexual-Abuse Victims

DIANE HILDEBRAN
WILLIAM D. PITHERS

THERAPEUTIC IMPORTANCE OF VICTIM EMPATHY TO RELAPSE PREVENTION

As a cognitive–behavior therapy program, relapse prevention provides the sex offender with a systematic process for appraising his thinking and behavior. It also offers the client tools with which he can control his deviant urges. The cognitive tools, though they are ample as resources for recognizing and avoiding the relapse process, will not in themselves serve as motivators for circumventing the relapse process.

When we modified relapse prevention for use with sex offenders (Pithers, 1982; Pithers, Marques, Gibat, & Marlatt, 1983), we initially recommended introducing relapse prevention concepts during the first therapy session. Currently, however, we advocate that relapse prevention not be discussed with clients until after they have developed empathy for sexual-abuse victims. While the early introduction of relapse prevention facilitated offenders' comprehension of their relapse processes, it often impeded emotional acknowledgment of the harm their acts had inflicted on others. Offenders gained an intellectual understanding of the precursors that had led to victimizing others, and they developed an awareness of what they needed to do to refrain from abusing again, but they lacked the emotional recognition of the victims' trauma that could energize a dedication to implementing what they had learned.

Offenders must develop emotional motivation, as well as cognitive understanding, in order to feel committed to utilizing the behavioral-management tools they have been offered. Victim empathy is an essential, noncognitive component of relapse prevention that has the potential for shifting the offender's worldview enough to lead him to use the tools relapse prevention has given him.

The sex offender in a relapse prevention treatment program is heavily exposed to cognitive tools for controlling his addictive impulses. Every facet of his thinking is continually challenged in order to shift awareness so that he will recognize each element of his individual relapse process. With recognition, he learns what must be done to abstain from the relapse process or interrupt it once it has begun. The offender who has authentically invested himself in treatment *knows* how to avoid reoffending.

Unfortunately, however, the resolve to avoid reoffending can itself be a purely cognitive phenomenon, based as it is on evidence that his next sexual offense will bring catastrophic consequences to himself and thus dash his hopes for a normal life. Resolve based on logic (e.g., identification of obvious consequences) has a tendency to break down in the face of the ingrained urges seen in sexual offenders. Thus purely cognitive resolutions often dissolve in the presence of powerful emotional needs and high-risk situations.

Urges to reoffend can be elusive and irresistible for the offender. Regardless of how conscientiously he has pursued new behavioral choices, he will forever have the memory of pleasure derived from each element of his relapse process. The memory of that pleasure remains as a seductive invitation to reenter the relapse process, particularly during occasions when he begins to feel out of control. When the offender perceives himself as being so out of control that no way of regaining some perspective seems to exist, the deterring motivation of avoiding personal loss no longer exists.

Research examining the influence of punitive sanctions for criminal behavior has demonstrated repeatedly that imposition of even the most severe consequences fails to deter offenses (Schwartz, 1968; Schiff, 1971). Thus recognition that sexual-offense convictions are likely to lead to prolonged incarceration is unlikely to have a significant impact on the incidence or repetition of such crimes. However, if a treated sex offender who had previously considered victims as objects to be used has acquired empathy and compassion for sexual-abuse victims, the likelihood of his enacting fantasies might be diminished.

Even with the earliest and least serious lapses, intentional interruption of familiar patterns involves sacrifice, renunciation of that which in the past was associated with at least momentary pleasure. The sense of sacrifice will encourage such cognitive distortions as "I deserve this one fantasy; I know I can engage in it and not let it lead to the next one." Just as close proximity to alcohol encourages the alcoholic to decide that "it's just one beer," the sex offender, in the initial stages of his relapse process, shifts into that part of his consciousness that wants to reoffend.

Victim empathy has the potential to block this shift in consciousness. Because it is not limited to the individual's cognitive understanding, it is possible for empathy to continue to restrain the offender when he no longer logically recognizes that a specific chain of events is predictable and will almost surely lead to reoffending. Empathy for his victim can provide emotional identification with his/her vulnerability and fear. An empathetic connection with a potential victim motivates the offender to set in motion all of the mechanisms he has learned to keep from reoffending.

Victim empathy gives him the pivotal reason for not reoffending, for, with empathy, he can no longer remain unaware of his victim's pain. Unless he experiences this shift of consciousness, he will manage to dismiss the logical consequences of moving further into the relapse process. The further into the process he moves, the less he can count on logic to pull him back.

SOURCES OF RESISTANCE

Men in treatment show enormous resistance to opening themselves to developing empathy for their victims. Usually the resistance is due to two phenomena.

First, offenders are reluctant to relinquish fantasies that are frequently the most reliable and available sources of pleasure they have known. Real victim empathy creates a shift in perception whereby nonrecognition of another's pain, even in one's fantasies, is no longer possible. Offenders must face giving up a major aspect of their lives without certainty that other sources of gratification will be attainable. Allowing that shift requires quite a bit of emotional growth in men who, for the most part, have lived self-absorbed lives.

Second, sex offenders tend to be men who are emotionally underdeveloped. When they begin to understand the pain, fear, and vulnerability their victims have experienced at their hands, they are connecting with emotions they have, more often than not, spent lifetimes suppressing. These are the very feelings offenders have convinced themselves they will not be able to bear.

Many offenders are both drawn to and terrified of emerging feelings. Though they are hungry for comfort and affirmation, they tenaciously defend against any experience of their victims' (and their own) anger, fear, and sense of violation. If the rapist or child molester is to put himself in touch with his victim's experience of these feelings, he will at the same time be acknowledging his own experience of them, not an easy task for someone who may have decided that negative emotions will destroy him.

Because of the power of these emotions, access to them within himself can be the prerequisite to victim empathy. And, ironically, empathy for his victim can be the key to unlocking acceptance of his own emotional vulnerability. In order to help the offender integrate his feelings for himself with his developing feelings of empathy for his victim, group sessions should be accompanied by individual therapy. Just as empathy is not a purely cognitive experience, an individual's opening himself to empathy is not always undertaken deliberately; it may instead be a spontaneous or idiosyncratic reaction to new information about what it feels like to be a victim. Individual therapy can provide a sense of safety that will enable him to embrace what may feel like profound vulnerability.

The offender who risks vulnerability deepens his commitment to treatment. Unless this deepening is experienced, there is a tendency for him to involve himself only superficially in the process of change. Empathy is the vehicle for penetrating shallow levels of treatment and authentically engaging the offender. The goal of preventing another victimization gives him an increased sense of purpose, a higher level of motivation to be authentic. It is important to remember that such a commitment to future potential victims must be experienced on the empathetic level. Intellectual espousal alone dissipates as soon as the offender encounters inevitable frustrations in treatment or upon his return to society.

TREATMENT PROCEDURES
TO ENHANCE VICTIM EMPATHY

In the inpatient treatment unit of the Vermont Treatment Program for Sexual Aggressors, victim empathy is developed through group therapy and reinforced by individual therapy. Each group consists of eight men who meet once weekly for 2 hours. Men are informed at the beginning of the group that only those members who show progress in this area will be able to move on to the next phase of treatment, which concentrates on identifying precursors to their sexual offenses.

Each victim empathy group is comprised of both pedophiles and rapists. This mix creates an environment in which each man is in the company of his peers (men with similar offenses) as well as persons who tend to show special abhorrence of his offense because they have not experienced the urge to engage in the same behavior. The rapist is quick to verbalize contempt for "someone who would do that to children," and the pedophile is appalled at "using force to get sex." Group members with dissimilar offenses will provide realistic rather than sympathetic feedback, thus making it less likely that offenders will be able to find support for denying or justifying their actions. In addition, a mixture of the verbal aggressiveness frequently found in rapists and the sensitivity common to pedophiles can yield a powerful group dynamic.

Content is initially introduced to the group through reading assignments. We have used a variety of written materials, including selections from such books as *I Never Told Anyone* (Bass & Thornton, 1983), *Kiss Daddy Goodnight* (Armstrong, 1978), *Betrayal of Innocence* (Forward & Buck, 1978), and *Father's Days* (Brady, 1979), which are compilations of articles and poems by women survivors of childhood and adult sexual abuse. Group members are instructed to read specific selections, concentrating their reactions on the authors' feelings, then comparing the authors' experiences to those likely encountered by their victims. They are required to prepare reports describing what they have read and concluded. Men with inadequate reading skills are required to complete the assignment by listening to audiotapes of the victims' recollections.

At the following group session, the offenders read their summaries aloud, describe the relevance of the readings to their own victims, and respond to comments of other group members. The reading and reviewing process allows the men an opportunity to approach the subject at an unhurried pace. The men's initial reactions reveal a sensitivity that appears to startle them. Their sharing of reactions is low key and involves little confrontation with each other.

Subsequent group sessions increase the intensity of their reactions quite a bit. Men view a series of video productions highlighting emotional damage to victims of sexual abuse and various coping mechanisms of survivors. One film deals with child sexual abuse, one with rape, and a third with victims' struggles to recover.

Unlike the reading assignments, which can be absorbed at a fairly gentle pace, the videos contain a number of rather jolting scenes that penetrate even the most apathetic or defensive offenders. It is at this point that members of the group begin to deeply experience some unsettling insights into what it feels like to be a victim of sexual abuse. In these videos, offenders witness victims relating the open-ended quality of their pain. Rape victims tell of their inability to feel safe again. Victims of child sexual abuse convey the loss of their childhood and the damage done to their ability to form adult relationships.

Seeing the faces while hearing the recollections of survivors is startling to offenders. Typical reactions from child molesters are "It's hard to believe it, but I never really thought of them (15–16-year-old males) as anyone's sons; I can see that they were kids just like my own boy" or "I didn't think it would hurt her (a 6-year-old); she had already been abused by someone else." Rapists are shocked by the permanence of rape victims' fears. What to treatment staff might seem like the most obvious evidence of trauma is new insight to many offenders.

After considerable discussion of the videos, members are asked to write an account of their offense from the perspective of one of their victims. Group members are generally required to write about their most recent victim because (1) later victims often appear to have been more severely abused than earlier ones, and (2) the recency of the abuse may enhance the offender's ability to revivify the victim's affect within himself. Each offender is then required to read his account before the group. Afterward, the offender may either remain in his victim's role or return to his own role as the abuser while he responds to questions and confrontations from the group. These sessions are often highly emotional for many group members. Typically, each offender requires 2 hours of group time to complete the reading and review process. We recommend videotaping sessions for later feedback to each offender.

Men resist this assignment in a number of ways. Some come to group with incomplete work, complaining that "It was too hard to think about." They have a great deal of difficulty opening themselves to the pain suffered by their victims. It seems easier for offenders to admit responsibility for their crimes than for them to tolerate the feelings evoked by identifying with their victims. A straightforward "yes, I did it" does not necessarily require self-reflection. Empathy, however, puts them back in touch with considerable emotional turmoil. It is at this point that parallel individual therapy can encourage the offender to probe and endure the difficult emotions. Frequently, if offenders have not previously discussed their own sexual abuse, they do so at this point.

Men in our groups have shown a variety of distancing styles. Most commonly they avoid detailing events and emotions. Two months of manipulation may be depicted in one or two sentences. Imprecise definitions of emotion also permit distancing. Speaking as the victim, they may say that they feel simply "hurt" or "confused." Other offenders distance themselves from the experience by speaking in the past rather than the present tense. Some describe the victim as participating in the abuse, with loving feelings toward the offender. Victim rage may be altogether misread as some other, less threatening emotion. Others report an inability to discern any emotional reaction from the victim.

Another mechanism for avoiding the core experience of the victim is that of turning his/her statement into a piece of theater. Offenders who do this are quick to point out that, indeed, the story is sordid but "that's how it happened." There is a sensational quality to these stories that is enhanced by the offender's badly overacted, starring role. In his fascination with his role in the drama, the writer loses track of the effect of the offense on the victim. He distances himself by obsessing about the details of his performance while superficially attending to the victim's feelings. Each form of resistance is confronted by other group members, who tend to identify the distortions of others more easily than they do their own.

After reviewing these victim accounts, some group members acknowledge the superficial quality of their attempts and the need to produce new efforts, this time with greater attention to details of both the event and its effects on the victim.

An offender who is resistant to acknowledging and experiencing his victim's emotions is asked to follow the reading of his victim's perspective by engaging in a more active role-play. The offender is asked to act out the concrete details of the offense. If he feels self-conscious, he is first requested to play himself in reenacting the offense. After the mood of the scene has been established, he is asked to switch roles and take the part of his victim. He may require some prodding to stay in character, because, after all, this is exactly what he has worked to avoid. Another group member is requested to play the abuser. Again, we recommend that these sessions be videotaped for later review with the offender.

As he develops the role-play, group members are invited to ask him questions, to be answered as the victim would answer. He is asked to describe at each moment leading up to the victimization how he, as victim, feels emotionally, how his body feels, what he wants, why he is not trying to escape, and so forth. He may be asked, as a child victim, "How does it feel to have your body respond to someone who is abusing it?" or "How does it feel to know this person you trust is using you?" or, as an adult victim, "How does it feel knowing you have no control over what he does to you?" It is not uncommon for a man to be able to respond throughout a 2-hour group in the person of either a male or female victim. The offender is often as surprised as anyone in the group to find himself identifying with victim feelings that he had previously refused to believe were present.

Breakthroughs in this experience provide the offender with at least a partial experience of his victim's pain. In addition, he has the opportunity to experience his victim's rage, something many offenders have, until this point in treatment, steadfastly denied. He gets a taste of the sense of unfairness the victim experiences, not only the initial violation but also from the need to justify and defend himself/herself to law enforcement officials and perhaps to family members and friends. Pedophiles begin to understand the helplessness and betrayal experienced by child victims, and rapists gain new insight into the fear and powerlessness felt by rape victims.

In the final phase of victim empathy groups, the offenders may meet with adult survivors of rape and child sexual abuse. The offenders are usually shocked to discover that these individuals have volunteered to meet with them not in order to assail them but rather to protect others from suffering the trauma of sexual abuse. Great care is exercised in separate preparatory meetings with both the victims and offenders to insure that the meeting will be therapeutic for both groups of individuals. Both groups are informed that the victims will have control of the session. Offenders who have not, by this time, demonstrated empathy for victims are excluded from the meeting. Typically, these sessions leave both groups drained but with a sense of hope that the future can be different from the past.

CONCLUSION

Offenders who have completed the victim-empathy groups describe the groups as being the most difficult aspect of their therapy. At times, they experience self-hatred as they are affected, perhaps for the first time, by the emotional weight of the damage created by their acts. Group members often express disdain for offenders who are unable, or unwilling, to permit themselves to endure the pain of their victims. For those individuals who have demonstrated the strength to face the true consequences of their behaviors, the memory of the experience is never far away.

REFERENCES

Armstrong, L. (1978). *Kiss daddy goodnight.* New York: Pocket Books.

Bass, E., & Thornton, L. (Eds.). (1983). *I never told anyone.* New York: Harper & Row.

Brady, K. (1979). *Father's days.* New York: Seaview.

Forward, S., & Buck, C. (1978). *Betrayal of innocence.* New York: Penguin.

Pithers, W. D. (1982, August). *The Vermont Treatment Program for Sexual Aggressors: A program description.* Waterbury: Vermont Department of Corrections.

Pithers, W. D., Marques, J. K., Gibat, C. C., & Marlatt, G. A. (1983). Relapse prevention with sexual aggressives: A self-control model of treatment and maintenance of change. In J. G. Greer & I. R. Stuart (Eds.), *The sexual aggressor: Current perspectives on treatment* (pp. 214–239). New York: Van Nostrand Reinhold.

Schiff, A. F. (1971). Rape in other countries. *Medicine, Science and the Law, 11,* 139–143.

Schwartz, B. (1968). The effect in Philadelphia of Pennsylvania's increased penalties for rape and attempted rape. *Journal of Criminal Law, Criminology, and Police Science, 59,* 509–515.

IV

PROGRAMS

The following three program descriptions are long and complex and cannot be briefly summarized. However, some guidance for the reader is necessary for proper examination of these program statements.

The three programs were selected for inclusion because they are representative of the two major ways that relapse prevention may be implemented with sex offenders. The Marques and Pithers programs use RP as a core, unifying concept throughout, and all adjunctive therapeutic activities are organized around it. The Jenkins-Hall program, on the other hand, uses RP as one treatment component in addition to rational–emotive therapy and behavior therapy. This use of RP as a maintenance strategy is consistent with its original use.

The programs were not selected because they are representative of RP-based programs in the United States; indeed, they are highly unrepresentative. Most treatment programs, whether state supported or fee for service, could not afford to include the rich mix of activities, the expensive staff, or the scope of treatment seen in these programs. All of the programs were funded to meet special needs of various governing bodies, not to serve the needs of all potential clients in their respective locales. The Marques program is funded by special appropriations from the California State Legislature for determining if sex offenders can, in fact, be successfully treated in confinement. The Pithers program is similarly funded by the Vermont Department of Corrections and is deeply involved with its probation and parole system. The Jenkins-Hall program is funded by a grant from the National Institute of Mental Health. It is actually a research project, a controlled group outcome study comparing a sophisticated cognitive–behavioral program that contains RP with another, less intricate program. Thus none of the programs represent the "real world" of doing RP with sex offenders.

The generalizability of the results obtained from these programs is further limited by their selection procedures. Many program directors would argue, and I would not disagree, that any client who voluntarily presents for treatment should be accepted. Operating in this fashion, over the long run we would find out what sort of persons can and cannot be treated. But the inclusionary criteria of the programs described here exclude many clients, often those who are most dangerous and most in need of treatment. This is simply a fact of life in public service. External funding agencies have a single question: Can sex offenders be effectively treated? Their goals are a reduction in recidivism statistics, fewer arrests, and fewer reoffenses. Thus program directors in this situation must favor those clients who have the best chance of succeeding in treatment.

The generalizability of findings is further limited by the nature of the client pool for the three programs. Marques's and Pithers's programs draw exclusively from a confined, criminal justice population. Jenkins-Hall's draws heavily from the probation and parole system; a large number of other clients who have been somehow involved with that system; and self-referrals who also are usually under some pressure to seek treatment. In no way, therefore, can the clients in these programs be seen as representative of the total, available population of sex offenders in the United States. These clients are the persons who failed, not succeeded, in deviant careers. Most sex offenders are never apprehended, so client characteristics and data obtained from those who have been may be quite different.

Why, then, you might ask, were these programs singled out for attention? The answer is quite simple. These are the three programs known to me that place the greatest stretch on the concepts of RP and associated therapies applied to sex offenders. They accurately represent what might be done if rich resources were available to design and implement a treatment program. In a practical sense their limitations are overridden by their testing of a rich variety of therapeutic activities on a fairly typical sample of sex offenders. The subsequent application of these activities in more realistic, community-based settings will inform us of the ultimate utility of using RP with sex offenders.

22

The Sex Offender Treatment and Evaluation Project: California's Relapse Prevention Program

JANICE K. MARQUES
DAVID M. DAY
CRAIG NELSON
MICHAEL H. MINER

In the early 1980s, the California State Legislature passed a law that repealed existing statutes providing for the commitment of mentally disordered sex offenders to state hospitals and required that convicted sex offenders be delivered to the Department of Corrections after sentencing (California Laws, 1981). Although this legislation eliminated the direct commitment of these offenders to state hospitals, it did allow for the voluntary transfer of certain sex offenders to the Department of Mental Health for inpatient treatment during the last 2 years of their prison terms. The state hospital program for these offenders was to be "established according to a valid experimental design in order that the most effective, newest and promising methods of treatment of sex offenders may be rigorously tested." Subsequent legislation limited the experimental program to 50 beds and required that formal evaluation reports be submitted biennially to the legislature until its termination in 1991 (California Laws, 1982).

In 1985, the Department of Mental Health initiated the Sex Offender Treatment and Evaluation Project, a clinical research program designed to meet the two goals specified in the legislative mandate: (1) the development and operation of a small, innovative treatment unit for sex offenders, and (2) the evaluation of the effectiveness of the treatments provided in the experimental program. In this chapter, the project's design, treatment model, and evaluation methods are presented, and the results of the first 30 months of operation are described.

PROJECT DESCRIPTION

In order to achieve the treatment and evaluation goals specified by the legislature, two separate but interrelated projects are conducted under the direction of a project director in Sacramento. The treatment project, housed in a 46-bed unit at Atascadero State Hospital, is staffed by a treatment director, 1 psychiatrist, 3 clinical psychologists, 3 clinical social workers, 6 social work associates, 2 rehabilitation therapists, and 28 nursing personnel (most of whom are psychiatric technicians). This team is responsible for the assessment and treatment of project participants during their inpatient stay. The evaluation project, located in the department's central office in Sacramento, is staffed by research professionals and assistants who are responsible for the screening and selection of participants and for measuring program fidelity and treatment outcome.

Design

The treatment program's effectiveness will be measured by comparing the postrelease activities of three matched groups of subjects:

1. *Treatment group.* This is the experimental group, consisting of sex offenders who have volunteered to participate and are randomly selected for the treatment project at Atascadero State Hospital.

2. *Volunteer control group.* This group is composed of sex offenders in prison who volunteer but are not randomly selected for treatment (a control for the factor of voluntarism). These offenders are matched to the treatment group members on the basis of type of offense, criminal history, and age.

3. *Nonvolunteer control group.* This is a second matched control group, consisting of prisoners who qualify for the project but do not volunteer to participate.

Subjects

The study participants are male inmates in the custody of the California Department of Corrections who have been convicted of one or more violations of penal code sections pertaining to rape and child molestation. Inmates who have offended only in concert (e.g., gang rape) or only against their biological children (incest) are not included. The study is also limited to those who: (1) are between 18 and 30 months of their release from incarceration, (2) are between 18 and 60 years of age, (3) have no more than two prior felony convictions, (4) acknowledge commission of the offense(s) for which they are incarcerated,

(5) do not have pending felony warrants or holds, (6) have an IQ over 80, (7) can speak English, (8) do not have a psychotic or organic mental condition, (9) are not so medically debilitated as to require skilled nursing care, and (10) have not presented severe management problems in prison.

Procedure

Participants are involved in four phases of the project: subject selection, treatment, aftercare, and follow-up.

Subject Selection Phase

Selection of participants begins with the identification and screening of subjects in the custody of the Department of Corrections. Project staff regularly visit the 14 institutions that house sex offenders and review the prison records of potential subjects to determine which inmates meet the project's eligibility criteria. Screened inmates are then scheduled for an interview session in which the project is explained in detail and the informed consent of volunteers is obtained. A brief mental status interview is also conducted by a licensed clinician at this time, in order to detect any undocumented organic, psychotic, or other disqualifying conditions present in the volunteers.

After inmate screening is completed, evaluation project staff match pairs of candidates within the volunteer pool on the variables of age of subject, type of offense(s) committed, and criminal history (number of prior felony convictions). Assignment of one member of each pair to the treatment group and one member to the volunteer control group is then made on a random basis. Finally, members of the third group, the nonvolunteer control group, are selected and matched from a pool of inmates who learned of the project but did not elect to participate.

Treatment Phase

During this phase, treatment group members participate in an intensive relapse prevention (RP; Marlatt & Gordon, 1985) program at Atascadero State Hospital for approximately 2 years ($R = 18$–30 months). As applied with project participants, RP provides a framework within which a variety of behavioral, cognitive, educational, and skill-training approaches are prescribed to teach offenders how to recognize and interrupt the chain of events leading to reoffense (Marques, Pithers, & Marlatt, 1984; Nelson, Miner, Marques, Russell, & Achterkirchen, 1988). The focus of both assessment and treatment procedures is on the specification and modification of the steps in this chain, from broad characterological factors and cognitive distortions to more circumscribed skill deficits and deviant sexual arousal patterns.

Assessment

The hospital program begins with an orientation and assessment period, during which the offender is assisted in making the transition from prison to hospital and completes an extensive battery of pretreatment measures. The assessment techniques include standardized tests, structured exercises, and direct behavioral measures designed to accomplish three tasks:

1. *Analysis of high-risk situations.* The core of the RP assessment process is the identification of the circumstances that threaten the offender's sense of self-control and increase the probability of relapse. Assessment techniques used to identify high-risk situations include structured exercises designed to analyze the chain of events preceding prior offenses, guided relapse fantasies (in which the offender imagines and describes future situations that could provoke relapse), and self-monitoring (of fantasies, urges, or other precursors). The analysis of offense chains begins with the offender's starting at the crime and moving back in time, identifying each significant step preceding the offense. This is first done for events and behaviors; then the affective components and cognitive steps (decisions and interpretations) are added. Each step is also evaluated to determine its relative importance in moving the offender toward the commission of an offense. Although this process is considered an assessment technique, it should be emphasized that the construction, analysis, and revision of the cognitive–behavioral chain leading to relapse is an ongoing process that continues throughout the RP program.

2. *Assessment of coping skills.* Because a given situation is high risk only to the extent that the offender has difficulty coping with it, several assessment procedures are used to determine the areas of strength and weakness in his coping abilities. Again, the analysis of the sequence of events preceding past or fantasized relapses is a primary source of information, since coping failures are integral parts of these offense chains. The subject's coping repertoire is also assessed by self-efficacy ratings, a procedure in which the offender is presented with a list of common high-risk situations and is asked to rate each according to how difficult it would be to cope with without offending or moving closer to an offense. Finally, project staff have developed a behavioral assessment tool based on the Situational Competency Test from the field of alcoholism (Chaney, O'Leary, & Marlatt, 1978). In this procedure, the subject describes how he would respond to various high-risk situations faced by sex offenders (see Miner, Day, & Nafpaktitis, Chapter 10, this volume).

3. *Identifying specific determinants and early antecedents.* The comprehensive assessment of sex offenders requires that the relative importance of various common determinants of sexual deviance be determined. First, each treatment group member receives a thorough assessment of his sexual arousal patterns in the project's sexual behavior laboratory. In this procedure (e.g., Laws

& Osborn, 1983), a variety of deviant and nondeviant stimuli (slides, audiotapes, and videotapes) are used to identify the offender's sexual arousal profile and to measure his ability to exert self-control over his sexual responses. These behavioral data, supplemented by self-report measures such as the Multiphasic Sex Inventory (Nichols & Molinder, 1984), assess the role of deviant sexual arousal and interests in the subject's offense chain.

Other common determinants are addressed in the intake assessment battery by measures of sexual knowledge and attitudes, hostility, social skills, attitudes toward women, and cognitive distortions. Finally, the role of more general characterological and lifestyle factors is determined by a variety of standard psychological inventories, offender autobiographies, and measures of empathy, self-esteem, and locus of control.

Treatment Program

Based on the assessment results, a structured program is prescribed specifically to address the offender's identified precursors of relapse. The primary treatment structure is the core relapse prevention group, which meets for 5 hours each week throughout the program. This highly structured group is the setting in which the cognitive–behavioral offense chains are constructed and used to integrate other program components into a system specifically designed to enhance control and prevent relapse for each individual offender.

The core RP group provides a familiar and secure environment in which participants can openly confront the personal, social, and sexual difficulties that place them at risk for reoffending. Group size is from six to eight offenders, most of whom will stay in the same group throughout their hospitalization. Each group's leaders are the participants' primary clinician (either a clinical psychologist or a psychiatric social worker) and one of their sponsors (licensed psychiatric technicians).

It is in this treatment activity that the major tenets of the RP model (Marlatt, 1985)—such as "apparently irrelevant decisions" (AIDs), high-risk elements and situations, adequate coping responses, lapses, the "abstinence violation effect" (AVE), and the "problem of immediate gratification" (PIG)— are presented and personalized for each individual participant. The group is designed to teach the offender two broad sets of skills, those needed to avoid a first lapse and those designed to reduce the probability that a lapse (if one occurs) will lead to a full relapse. More specifically, the goals of the core RP group are to have the offender (1) recognize the decisions and conditions that place him at risk for reoffending; (2) plan, develop, and practice a range of coping responses to his identified high-risk elements and situations; (3) restructure his interpretation of urges; (4) develop strategies for reducing the likelihood that a lapse will result in a full-blown relapse; (5) increase his empathy toward victims and modify the cognitive distortions that are likely to facilitate future victimization; (6) make lifestyle modifications designed to promote continued abstinence; and (7) learn that the prevention of relapse is an ongoing process in which he must take an active and vigilant role.

In order to maintain consistency across the various core RP groups, all group leaders follow a highly structured treatment manual, which specifies insession goals and methods as well as homework assignments for learning key RP concepts and strategies. The manual organizes the group's content into modules and its structure into a quarterly system. Each quarter includes three treatment modules: an introductory module, a basic module, and a specialty module.

The introductory module (approximately 1 week) is designed to orient new members, assess ongoing members' treatment goals and progress, and introduce or review key RP concepts. This module is followed by one of the two basic modules, either the cognitive–behavioral offense chain or the decision matrix. The basic modules take from 4 to 8 weeks and are repeated in alternating sequence throughout the program.

The cognitive–behavioral offense chain module consists of identifying the relevant events and cognitions that served as antecedents for group members' past offenses. The point in the chain to be defined as a lapse for a particular offender is also identified in this module. A variety of coping responses are then formulated for each link in this chain, and those most likely to interrupt the chain are practiced. Cognitive–behavioral chains for the instant offense, past offenses, or guided relapse fantasies may be prepared by each offender during this module.

The decision matrix module concentrates on specifying the positive and negative consequences (both immediate and delayed) of either committing or abstaining from a sexual offense. Decision matrices may be prepared for past offenses, guided relapse fantasies, or the participants' expectations at the present time. Decision matrix exercises are also used to assist the offenders in making decisions about other problem situations and behaviors that occur in the hospital.

After the goals of the basic module are attained, the remainder of each quarter is devoted to one of eight specialty modules: autobiographies; guided relapse fantasies; enhancing victim empathy; dealing with deviant sexual urges, thoughts, and fantasies; lifestyle modification; coping with high-risk elements; miscellaneous RP topics (e.g., testing the limits, positive outcome expectancies, coping with the AVE, and preparing a maintenance manual); and coping with negative emotional states. The group is designed so that participants are exposed to each of these specialty modules at least once during the inpatient phase of their treatment.

In addition to this intensive RP training, treatment group subjects participate in a wide range of other treatment activities designed to modify various determinants of sexual offending. The project's specialty groups focus on the specific knowledge, attitudes, and skills that the offender needs in order to identify and cope with potential high-risk situations. All offenders are required to attend the following groups: sex education, human sexuality, relaxation training, stress management, and social skills. A prerelease class designed to prepare the offender for "life on the streets" is also mandatory for participants. Other specialty groups (e.g., the substance-abuse group) are provided by the project on a prescriptive basis, depending on the needs of the individual offender. In order to maintain consistency and fidelity in the application of treatment services, all group activities follow treatment manuals that describe the major goals and treatment procedures for each session. Most specialty groups also require participants to complete behavioral homework assignments between the sessions.

Each treatment group member participates in at least 1 hour of individual psychotherapy per week with the clinical psychologist or psychiatric social worker who conducts his core RP group and 1 hour of individual counseling with each of the two nursing staff who cofacilitate this group. Thus each participant receives, weekly, at least 3 hours of individual treatment devoted to addressing unique issues and concerns that have arisen in the group sessions; applying individualized treatment techniques that are not suitable for group intervention; and assisting the participants in integrating their various treatment experiences into a cohesive, individualized program. The orientation of the individual sessions is consistent with the cognitive–behavioral and RP perspectives of the project.

In addition to the group and individual treatment activities, each group member participates in approximately 6 hours of structured leisure activities and 4 hours of rehabilitation therapy each week. Individual behavior-therapy sessions in the sexual behavior laboratory are also offered to offenders who show deviant sexual arousal patterns. The most frequently used intervention in the lab is olfactory aversion, although masturbatory satiation and orgasmic reconditioning treatments are also available.

Since control subjects are in correctional settings that allow them to reduce their sentences by earning work credits, similar work opportunities, credits, and compensation are provided for treatment group participants. In all, most participants have a 30-hour work assignment and take part in 13 to 20 hours of program activities per week.

The primary evaluation project tasks during the treatment phase involve the measurement of treatment process and intreatment changes. For the core RP group, measures focus on whether the group is indeed teaching its members the RP model. Other intreatment changes are measured globally by readministration of the pretreatment assessment battery described above and by pre–post changes in variables relevant to speciality groups (e.g., Situational Competency Test scores before and after the substance-abuse group) or individual treatment components (e.g., sexual arousal patterns before and after behavior therapy). In addition to allowing evaluators to measure intreatment changes and determine the outcomes of various interventions, these assessment data help identify the major predictors of community success and recidivism among treated subjects.

Before discharge, treatment group members also complete the Sex Offender Situational Competency Test, self-efficacy ratings for a number of high-risk situations, and assignments measuring their mastery of the RP model. In the exit interview, conducted by evaluation project staff, participants are asked to evaluate their treatment experiences and to describe their postrelease situations, including work, housing, social supports, and anticipated high-risk situations. They are also given a program evaluation form to complete, anonymously, and mail to the project director. Finally, participants are trained in the randomized response technique (Fox & Tracy, 1986) and use this procedure to provide data on their history of sexual deviance. Randomized responding, a statistically based technique designed to ascertain group differences while protecting the identity of individual subjects, is used to supplement official criminal records in determining offense rates.

Volunteer control group members receive no treatment services from the project during the treatment phase, but those consenting are interviewed by evaluation project staff just before their release from prison. These individuals are paid to participate in a 90-minute session in which they (1) are interviewed about their postrelease situations, (2) complete self-report measures of their deviant sexual interests and the cognitive distortions associated with sexual offending, (3) provide self-efficacy ratings for various high-risk situations, and (4) answer questions regarding prior crimes using the randomized response technique.

Members of the nonvolunteer control group, since they did not consent to be a part of the project, do not participate in any assessment or treatment activities during the treatment phase.

Aftercare Phase

California sex offenders are routinely placed on parole for a period of at least 1 year following their release from incarceration. For treatment group members, attending two sessions a week in the Sex Offender Aftercare Program (SOAP) is a condition of parole for the first year. SOAP services are provided either by state aftercare programs or by private clinicians, depending on the needs of the offender and the availability of state providers in his community. Aftercare clinicians are individually trained by project staff to provide an extended version of the RP program that is tailored to meet the needs of the paroled offender. Sessions focus on "boosting" treatment effects; that is, enhancing the participant's understanding of RP concepts, practicing the skills learned in the program, and testing nondeviant lifestyles. Most SOAP sessions are individual;

however, providers with ongoing sex offender groups may have project participants for one group and one individual session per week. Depending on the
treatment needs of the offender, aftercare may also include family interventions,
drug testing, laboratory assessments of sexual arousal, and/or behavior-therapy
booster sessions (e.g., having the offender self-administer a dose of ammonia if
he becomes inappropriately aroused).

Treatment progress is monitored during the aftercare phase by monthly
contacts between project staff and SOAP providers as well as by written quarterly reports. In addition, providers are obligated to notify the Department of
Corrections in the event of treatment failure or violation of other conditions of
parole. During this period members of the two control groups are also on parole,
which may be revoked (thus returning them to custody) if its conditions are
violated.

At the end of the 1-year aftercare period, evaluation project staff meet
individually with members of the treatment and volunteer control groups and
collect information on the offender's life situation, use of alcohol and other
drugs, and perceived self-efficacy. Also in this session, specific questions about
whether the subject has reoffended during the aftercare period are asked, using
the randomized response technique. Volunteer controls are paid for their
participation.

Follow-Up Phase

This phase, which overlaps the aftercare phase, lasts for 5 years following the
release from incarceration of all study participants (treatment, volunteer control,
and nonvolunteer control subjects). In this period, information is gathered on a
periodic basis from the Department of Justice concerning contacts between
participants and the criminal justice system. When documented contacts do
occur, local criminal justice agencies are asked to provide data on the nature
and context of the offense, victim characteristics, and other pertinent variables.

FINDINGS

Results of Subject Selection

Since the project began in 1985, information on the sex offender population
incarcerated in California's correctional system has been reviewed on a quarterly basis, and staff have regularly visited the institutions that house potential
participants. The number of sex offenders in prison during the project period
has averaged 5,250, but only 10% of these men met the stated eligibility criteria.
The most common reason for ineligibility was that the offender's remaining
sentence exceeded 30 months. The next most common reason for disqualifica-

tion was a remaining sentence of less than 18 months, followed by low IQ (below dull normal), incest offense only, denial of offense, psychosis, pending warrant or hold, severe medical condition, inability to speak English, three or more prior felony convictions, offense committed in concert, age over 60, organicity, and history of severe management problems in prison.

In the process of evaluating offenders for eligibility, project staff review the prison records of each with respect to social and demographic characteristics, criminal histories, and instant offenses. In order to describe the eligible offender pool and the differences between volunteers and nonvolunteers, data from the records of 168 volunteers and a sample of 268 nonvolunteers were analyzed. As classified by instant offense, this pool of eligibles consisted of 135 rapists (31%) and 301 child molesters (69%). Nearly all (98%) of the rapists' victims were female, but 2 of these offenders assaulted males and 1 assaulted victims of both sexes. Among the child molesters, 192 had only female victims, 77 had only male victims, and 32 had both male and female victims. Thus these offenders can be divided into four groups based on their offenses and the sexes of their victims: rapists, heterosexual child molesters, homosexual child molesters, and bisexual child molesters.

Statistical comparisons of the demographic characteristics of the four offense groups revealed the following significant differences: (1) Rapists were younger, more ethnically diverse (i.e., nonwhite), and less likely to be employed at the time of their offenses than were child molesters; (2) heterosexual and bisexual child molesters were more likely to be married than were the other two groups, and (3) homosexual child molesters had higher IQ scores (or estimates) than did the other three groups.

Criminal history and offense characteristics of the four groups differed significantly as follows: (1) Rapists were least likely to have been previously treated under the provisions of California's Mentally Disordered Sex Offender (MDSO) statute, were most likely to victimize strangers and to use violence in their offenses, and were more often intoxicated at the time of their crimes than were the child molesters; (2) homosexual child molesters most often had prior MDSO commitments and "acquaintance" victims (as opposed to strangers or family members); and (3) heterosexual and bisexual child molesters were more likely to have victimized their families.

Thus far, approximately 25% of the eligible offenders have volunteered to participate in the project. Comparing the volunteers with the nonvolunteers revealed no significant differences with respect to any social–demographic variable except age, with volunteers being younger than nonvolunteers. No differences were found with respect to criminal history variables, but there were significant tendencies for homosexual and bisexual child molesters to be over-represented among the volunteers and for the volunteers to have been less violent in offending.

Characteristics of the Treatment Group

During the first 30 months of the project (through December 1987), 77 subjects (60 child molesters and 17 rapists) were assigned to the treatment group and admitted to Atascadero State Hospital. Nine participants (6 child molesters and 3 rapists) dropped out of the program during this period, and 3 subjects (1 child molester and 2 rapists) were involuntarily returned to the Department of Corrections because they created severe management problems during their hospital stays.

For the analyses presented in this chapter, the treatment group has been defined as those participants who had been admitted to the program through the end of 1987. The 6 individuals who withdrew or were involuntarily returned to the custody of the Department of Corrections within their first year of treatment have been excluded. In the next section, the demographic and clinical characteristics of this treatment group will be described.

The treatment group defined above included 71 men: 30 heterosexual child molesters, 17 homosexual child molesters, 8 bisexual child molesters, and 16 rapists. Of the child molesters, 87% were white, 7% were black, 4% were Hispanic, and 2% were other minorities. Among rapists, however, only 43% were white, while blacks comprised 38%, Hispanics 13%, and other ethnic groups 6% of the total. The mean ages were 35.6 for child molesters and 29.5 for rapists. The heterosexual child molesters were more likely to be married (67%) than the other three groups (23% of the homosexual child molesters, 50% of the bisexual child molesters, and 25% of the rapists). More (73%) child molesters were employed at the time of offense than were rapists (47%).

Although several treatment group members had no prior criminal histories, over two-thirds (69%) of the rapists and a majority (59%) of the homosexual child molesters had at least one prior felony conviction. Fewer offenders in the other two groups had previous felony convictions (37% of the heterosexual child molesters and 25% of the bisexual child molesters). When only prior sex crimes were considered, the homosexual child molesters had the most extensive histories, with 71% having a prior arrest and 53% a prior conviction for a sex offense. In contrast, less than half of the other two groups had prior sex-crime arrests, and less than a third had prior convictions for sex offenses.

Eighty-eight percent of the rapists in the program reported both a history of substance abuse and the use of alcohol or drugs at the time of their offenses. A lower proportion (69%) of the child molesters reported a history of substance abuse, and 51% stated that they were drinking or using drugs when they committed their offenses.

In terms of *DSM-III* or *DSM-III-R* diagnoses (American Psychiatric Association, 1980, 1987), nearly all (93%) of the heterosexual child molesters and all of the homosexual child molesters were given an Axis I diagnosis of Pedophilia.

Sixty-three percent of the rapists had an Axis I diagnosis of Aggressive Sexuality, while another 31% had an Axis I diagnosis of Sexual Sadism. Thirty-four subjects also had a secondary Axis I diagnosis, usually indicating substance abuse or dependence. A majority of the child molesters were not diagnosed on Axis II, but three-quarters of the rapists were, most often as Antisocial Personality Disorders. Intelligence, as measured by the WAIS-R (Wechsler, 1981), did not differ significantly across the four offense groups, with all means for full-scale IQ between 95 and 100.

According to the norms of Nichols and Molinder (1984), the treatment group's scores on the Cognitive Distortion and Immaturity Scale of the Multiphasic Sex Inventory (MSI) indicated that 22% of the heterosexual child molesters, 29% of the bisexual child molesters, 38% of the rapists, and 63% of the homosexual child molesters viewed themselves as victims. The difference between the heterosexual and homosexual child molesters was significant. Responses to the MSI Justification Scale indicated that 42% of the group showed at least a "marked justification" of their sexual deviance. Although more (48%) of the heterosexual child molesters and fewer (29%) of the bisexual child molesters were classified as using "marked justification," this difference was not significant.

Finally, the perceived locus of control scores (Nowicki & Strickland, 1973) of treatment group members did not vary significantly by offense type. Over half (54%) of the child molesters and nearly three-quarters (73%) of the rapists scored above the mean for incarcerated offenders reported by Nowicki (1983) and therefore would be typed as "external" compared with this population.

Treatment Process and Outcome Data

In the following sections, the evaluation data collected in the project's first 30 months of operation are summarized. First, the intreatment changes associated with the core group, various speciality groups, and behavior therapy are described. Next, data from the prerelease assessments are presented, including changes in psychological test data from admission to discharge and client evaluations of treatment. Finally, some preliminary follow-up data are summarized.

Intreatment Changes

Core RP Group

The project's group activities, including those of the core group, follow an academic schedule, with each year divided into quarters. During the 1-week break between quarters, participants complete two instruments designed to measure their progress in mastering the RP model. The first of these, the Test of Basic Relapse Prevention Concepts, was developed on the premise that participants must be grounded in the model's lexicon before they can apply it to their own treatment. Subjects who score at least 80% on this test pass and need not take it again; those who score under 80% repeat the test until they reach criterion. Thus, at any test administration, the testees include recently admitted participants and those who have previously failed to reach the criterion. Thirty-four percent of the subjects passed the Test of Basic Relapse Prevention Concepts on the first administration, 58% of those taking it a second time passed, and all of those taking it a third time passed.

The second mastery test assesses the participant's ability to reproduce the conceptual structure of the cognitive–behavioral chain leading to relapse (Nelson et al., 1988). This concept serves to unify and focus treatment interventions made during the program and thus is a necessary framework for structuring individual programs. Thirty-nine percent of the subjects completed this task successfully on their first attempt, 88% of those who tried a second time succeeded, and all others succeeded on their third try.

Specialty Groups

Sex-education group. The sex-education group is designed to provide subjects with basic knowledge of anatomy, physiology, and the nature of the sexual response. To date, 46 subjects have completed this group. The results of a test for mastery of the material indicated that most offenders have gained and retained the information presented. Since the project began, 5 subjects have failed the posttest. These subjects were either readministered the test, which they subsequently passed, or repeated the group and then passed the test.

Human-sexuality group. This group differs from the sex-education group in that its purpose is to help participants gain a better understanding of their attitudes toward sexuality and women and to modify extreme attitudes, such as viewing women solely as sex objects or as subservient to men. This group was evaluated using two self-report instruments: the Attitudes Toward Women Scale (Spence & Helmreich, 1972) and the Thorne Sex Inventory (Thorne, 1966).

Pre–post comparisons of the mean scores on the Attitudes Toward Women Scale revealed that, although they differed in the predicted direction, the difference was not significant. The relevant scales of the Thorne Sex Inventory, as reported by Thorne (1966), failed to yield acceptable reliabilities for our sample, so two rational composites of six items each were constructed using the original item pool. The first composite measured attitudes toward and acceptance of sexuality, and the second, attitudes toward and acceptance of homosexuality. Reliability coefficients for both composites were quite high (*alphas* = 0.82 and 0.84). A multivariate analysis of variance with repeated measures on these composites indicated that completion of the human-sexuality group was associated with greater acceptance of and more positive attitudes toward both sexuality in general and homosexuality.

Relaxation and stress-management groups. Before being assigned to the stress-management group, participants complete the relaxation group, in which they learn and practice several standard relaxation procedures. The only effectiveness measure used in this group was heart rate, taken before and after each session. Comparisons showed that the group sessions were effective in reducing heart rates of participants.

Patterned after Meichenbaum's (1985) approach, the stress-management group is designed to help participants control those environmental stimuli that they can control and minimize the upset caused by those stressors in life that they cannot change. Given these two goals, the evaluation of the impact of this group was approached in two ways. First, the Hassles Scale (Kanner, Coyne, Schaefer, & Lazarus, 1981) was used to measure the number of stressors that an offender perceived in his environment and to obtain his estimates regarding the subjective intensity of these perceived hassles. Pre–post comparisons of the means for the number of hassles reported by patients did not show a significant difference; however, the reported intensities of the hassles significantly decreased on the posttest.

The second evaluation strategy was to present subjects with active stressors and measure their physiological responses to them before and after completion of the group. Two tasks were selected: the Breakout Video Game, an eye–hand coordination task used extensively in stress research (McKinney et al., 1985), and a guided imagery relaxation task (Nathan & Charlesworth, 1980). The physiological measure used was digital skin temperature. To date, few subjects have been assessed using this strategy. For those who have been, some increase in ability to control physiological response to stress was exhibited, but this effect was not strong enough to support the conclusion that it was due to the stress-management group.

Social-skills group. Relapse prevention requires that offenders develop the skills necessary to cope effectively with high-risk situations when they occur. One set of skills considered particularly relevant for sex offenders is that of appropriate social behaviors. The project's 3-month social-skills training group is designed to help subjects learn how to function better in social situations, interact with others in less self-destructive ways, and develop better and more fulfilling relationships. The impact of this group was assessed by measures of (1) perceived skill and anxiety in a number of different areas as measured by the Social Reactions Inventory (SRI; Curran, Corriveau, Monti, & Hagerman, 1980); (2) self-reports of subjects' appraisals of their skill and anxiety during a set of seven role-play situations; and (3) ratings, by two independent raters, of participants' skills in these situations.

On the SRI, social anxiety scores decreased and skill scores increased significantly after completion of the group, but the self-report data from the role-play assessments showed only one significant change (decreased anxiety in one of the seven situations presented) and one marginally significant change (an increase in perceived skill in one situation). Observer ratings of behavior in the role-play situations were aggregated into rational composites measuring manifest self-esteem, problem solving, and assertiveness. The ratings of problem-solving behaviors exhibited in the role-plays increased significantly pre–post, and for assertive behaviors the increase was marginal.

   Substance-abuse group. Subjects who either have a history of alcohol or drug abuse or for whom these substances were contributing factors in their offense(s) are assigned to the substance-abuse group. This group uses the relapse prevention techniques developed for substance abusers (Marlatt & Gordon, 1985). In the group sessions, participants identify the factors involved in their abuse of alcohol and drugs, explore the cognitive–behavioral chains that lead them into situations in which the use of these substances becomes inevitable, and practice the necessary coping skills to successfully conquer high-risk factors and interrupt the cognitive–behavioral chain.

   Impact of the substance-abuse group was assessed by pre–post changes on self-efficacy ratings and on performance on the Situational Competency Test (Chaney et al., 1978). Altogether, 20 self-efficacy ratings were obtained on situations varying along the six dimensions described by Chaney and Roszell (1985). Overall, subjects had significantly higher self-efficacy ratings after completing the group. On the Situational Competency Test, subjects were asked how they would respond to 12 situations that are high risk for alcohol and drug abusers (Chaney et al., 1978). Responses were scored in three ways: latency of the response, duration of the response, and independent ratings of the response's effectiveness in coping with the situation presented. Pre–post comparisons revealed that, while latency did not change significantly, both response duration and rated effectiveness of the subjects' coping responses increased significantly after completion of the group.

Behavior Therapy

Of the 44 participants recommended for behavior therapy, 9 (8 child molesters and 1 rapist) completed this treatment component by the end of 1987. Olfactory aversion (Laws, Meyer, & Holmen, 1978) was the treatment most frequently used. Analyses of pre–post changes in laboratory assessment data showed that arousal to deviant stimuli was significantly reduced after treatment, while arousal to nondeviant (consenting adult) stimuli did not change significantly.

Prerelease Assessments

As described above, participants completing the hospital phase of the program are readministered the pretreatment assessment battery, including both physiological and psychometric measures. They also complete tests of their mastery of RP concepts, evaluate their treatment experiences, complete the Sex Offender Situational Competency Test, provide self-efficacy ratings for various high-risk situations, and give estimates regarding their prior sexual deviance using the randomized response technique. Although insufficient data are available on the latter three measures, prerelease assessment results on the other measures have been analyzed and are summarized below. Unless otherwise noted, the analyses included data from all 28 of the treatment group members who have completed the hospital program.

Physiological data. Because deviant sexual arousal is considered to be a critical risk factor for sex offenders, all participants (even those not receiving behavior therapy) are reassessed in the project's sexual behavior laboratory prior to discharge. These assessment data, along with the corresponding pretreatment data, were analyzed for the discharged subjects. A complex analysis of variance with repeated measures revealed several interesting findings. First, arousal to particular types of stimulus categories appeared to differentiate the various types of offenders. As a group, subjects who had molested boys were aroused by stimuli depicting male adults and children, while those who had molested girls were aroused by stimuli depicting female adults and children. The profiles for rapists did not appear to distinguish them from the other offense groups. Second, levels of deviant arousal decreased across all subjects from the initial to the prerelease assessments. Third, arousal to nondeviant (consenting adult) stimuli also decreased pre–post, except among subjects who participated in behavior therapy.

The finding that deviant arousal decreased across all subjects, not just those receiving behavior therapy, may be due to a number of factors, such as habituation effects, demand characteristics, or small sample size (allowing large decreases in a few subjects to create a significant pre–post effect). Another possibility, which is theoretically most appealing, is that even though all subjects did not receive the behavioral intervention, all were involved in an intensive cognitive–behavioral treatment program. Since sexual arousal, like other autonomic responses, has a strong cognitive component (Annon, 1974; Kaplan, 1974), one might expect that treatment-induced changes in the subjects' perceptions of children, women, appropriate sexual expression, and self-control capabilities would be reflected in their physiological arousal profiles.

Although these assessment data must be regarded as tentative because of the small number of subjects, they do suggest that treatment group members with deviant arousal at admission show significant reductions in this arousal and that, overall, the patterns of sexual arousal among participants at discharge are nondeviant.

Test data. In addition to physiological data, the overall effectiveness of the treatment program for the discharged participants was evaluated by two sets of test data: pre–post comparisons on various psychometric tests and measures of the subjects' ability to apply the RP model to their own behavior. First, in order to tap progress in accepting responsibility for offending, two measures were selected from the Multiphasic Sex Inventory (Nichols & Molinder, 1984), the Cognitive Distortion and Immaturity Scale and the Justification Scale. On both measures, subjects' scores were significantly lower at posttest, indicating a shift toward accepting responsibility for their crimes and away from excusing their deviance or blaming it on the victim. Also, the locus of control scores (Nowicki & Strickland, 1973) of treated subjects became more internal, suggesting a move toward personal responsibility.

Other pre–post comparisons of psychometric data revealed that completion of the treatment program was associated with significant decreases in depression as measured by the Depression Inventory (Beck, 1967) and with significant increases in scores on the Self-Esteem Scale (Rosenberg, 1965). Empathy Scale (Mehrabian & Epstein, 1972) scores also changed in the predicted direction, with subjects scoring as significantly more empathic following treatment.

In addition to psychometric tests, the prerelease assessment battery includes measures of mastery and application of the RP model. Just prior to discharge, each participant completes two assignments: an individualized cognitive–behavioral chain detailing events leading to his instant offense and a decision matrix comparing both immediate and delayed consequences of reoffending or abstaining. These documents are used both for evaluating the subject's understanding of the model and for structuring his RP program for the aftercare phase of treatment.

The assignments are evaluated by the participant's primary clinician, who rates them with respect to completeness on a 7-point scale from "inadequate" (1) to "complete" (7). The clinicians evaluate the cognitive–behavioral chain in terms of how well it presents the subject's step-by-step progression toward his instant offense; they evaluate the decision matrix in terms of the extent to which the subject has presented all of the salient positive, negative, short-term, and long-term consequences of either reoffending or remaining abstinent.

In general, the clinicians' ratings have indicated that subjects have gained at least a minimal ability to describe the behaviors and cognitions that led them to commit sex crimes. All of the released participants' cognitive–behavioral chains were rated at the midpoint or above, and 50% received ratings above 6, indicating that omissions from the chain were relatively unimportant. The mean rating for the chain assignment was 5.4. Subjects' decision matrices were less complete than their behavior chains, with a mean rating of 4.1. Twenty-seven percent of the subjects received ratings of less than 4 on the matrices, and almost two-thirds (64%) received ratings from their clinicians indicating that they had omitted important positive or negative consequences.

Client evaluations. Treated subjects are asked to complete a client evaluation form when they leave the hospital program. This instrument was constructed in three parts, the first of which is a set of five overall evaluation ratings on 4-point scales from "not at all" to "very much so." Subjects are then asked to rank-order each of the treatment activities they have experienced from most to least important in helping them to avoid relapse. Finally, subjects can suggest ways of improving the program. In order to encourage participants to make honest appraisals of treatment, responses were voluntary and anonymous.

Twenty-three of the 28 released subjects completed and returned the forms. In response to the Part-1 item "Did the program help you feel more self-confident and in control of your life?", 87% said "very much so" and 13%, "moderately so." Similarly, in response to "Did the program help you understand why you offended?", 83% endorsed "very much so" and 17%, "moderately so." On the item "Do you think the program will help you avoid offending again?" nearly all (96%) said "very much so" and 4%, "moderately so." On the item "Does the treatment model, relapse prevention, seem like a useful approach for sex offenders?", 74% responded "very much so" and 26%, "moderately so." Finally, to the question "Have you generally been satisfied with the treatment provided?", 61% replied "moderately so" and 39%, "very much so."

In Part 2, the rank-order task, the core RP group was rated as the most important component in helping the participant avoid relapses followed by, in descending order, individual therapy (with the subject's primary clinician), individual counseling (with nursing staff), and behavior therapy in the sexual behavior laboratory. The lowest rankings were given to the substance-abuse group and "other activities," including work assignments and noncompetitive sports.

When asked for suggestions for improving the program, subjects most often made recommendations about the groups, for example, that they be more structured, presented in a different order, standardized across therapists, or voluntary. Other popular suggestions included more program structure and activities, fewer work assignment hours, more social activities, and more consistency and fairness in the rules on the treatment ward. Finally, a few subjects were concerned with the overall treatment orientation, with one suggesting more emphasis on insight and confrontation of denial and two suggesting a more individual focus that would allow participants to work at their own speed.

Follow-Up Data

Treatment Group

By the end of 1987, 36 subjects originally selected for the treatment group had been released to the community. Of these, 28 were discharged from the treatment program and 8 were released from prison after having been returned (either voluntarily or involuntarily) to the custody of the Department of Corrections. The subjects who completed treatment had a mean length of stay of 20.8 months ($R = 12.6-29.8$ months). Four of the 8 subjects who were released from prison were in the treatment program for less than 12 months, while the remaining 4 were in treatment for a mean of 14.78 months ($R = 12.6-18.1$ months) before their return to prison. Subjects with stays of less than 12 months, and their matched controls, were excluded from this analysis.

The mean time at risk in the community for the 32 treatment group participants was 6.5 months ($R = 1.5-12.4$ months) as of the cutoff date. Official records indicated that 1 of these participants had been returned to prison for violation of parole. There was no record of any arrests for sex crimes, and none of the aftercare providers reported suspected reoffenses.

Volunteer Control Group

Thirty-two members of the volunteer control group had been released from prison as of the cutoff date. The mean time at risk for these subjects was 4.5 months ($R = 0.1-12.4$ months). For these subjects, official records indicated that 2 had been returned to prison for violations of parole. No arrests for sex crimes were recorded.

Nonvolunteer Control Group

As treatment group participants are released to the community, matched subjects are selected from the pool of individuals who qualified for the project but did not volunteer. As of the cutoff date, 18 of the persons so matched had been released from prison, with a mean time at risk of 6.9 months ($R = 1.8-12.4$ months). Of these subjects, 3 had their paroles revoked and were returned to prison. Again, there was no record of any arrests for sex crimes.

SUMMARY AND CONCLUSIONS

The Sex Offender Treatment and Evaluation Project is a clinical research program specifically mandated by the California State Legislature. The project, which began in 1985, consists of a treatment component (an intensive, 2-year relapse prevention program for sex offenders) and an evaluation component (a comparison of the outcomes of treated subjects with those of two matched control groups). At this time, 28 offenders have completed the treatment program. Although prerelease data indicate that the RP program is producing expected treatment effects, sufficient follow-up data are not yet available to determine if treatment is successful in reducing recidivism among these offenders.

REFERENCES

American Psychiatric Association. (1980). *Diagnostic and statistical manual of mental disorders* (3rd ed.). Washington, DC: Author.

American Psychiatric Association. (1987). *Diagnostic and statistical manual of mental disorders* (3rd ed., rev.). Washington, DC: Author.

Annon, J. S. (1974). *The behavioral treatment of sexual problems* (Vol. 1). Honolulu, HI: Enabling Systems.

Beck, A. T. (1967). *Depression: Clinical, experimental and theoretical aspects.* New York: Hoeber.

California Laws. (1981). Chapter 928, codified as *California Penal Code* Sections 1364 and 1365.

California Laws. (1982). Chapters 1529 and 1549, amending *California Penal Code* Sections 1364 and 1365.

Chaney, E. F., O'Leary, M. R., & Marlatt, G. A. (1978). Skill training with alcoholics. *Journal of Consulting and Clinical Psychology, 46,* 1092–1104.

Chaney, E. F., & Roszell, D. K. (1985). Coping in opiate addicts maintained on methadone. In S. Shiffman & T. A. Willis (Eds.), *Coping and substance use* (pp. 267–293). New York: Academic.

Curran, J. P., Corriveau, D. P., Monti, P. M., & Hagerman, S. B. (1980). Social skill and social anxiety. *Behavior Modification, 4,* 493–512.

Fox, J. A., & Tracy, P. E. (1986). *Randomized response: A method for sensitive surveys.* Beverly Hills, CA: Sage.

Kanner, A. D., Coyne, J. C., Schaefer, C., & Lazarus, R. S. (1981). Comparison of two modes of stress measurement: Daily hassles and uplifts versus major life events. *Journal of Behavioral Medicine, 4,* 1–39.

Kaplan, H. S. (1974). *The new sex therapy: Active treatment of sexual dysfunctions.* New York: Brunner/Mazel.

Laws, D. R., Meyer, J., & Holmen, M. L. (1978). Reduction of sadistic sexual arousal by olfactory aversion: A case study. *Behaviour Research and Therapy, 16,* 281–285.

Laws, D. R., & Osborn, C. A. (1983). How to build and operate a behavioral laboratory to evaluate and treat sexual deviance. In J. G. Greer & I. R. Stuart (Eds.), *The sexual aggressor: Current perspectives on treatment* (pp. 293–335). New York: Van Nostrand Reinhold.

Marlatt, G. A. (1985). Relapse prevention: Theoretical rationale and overview of the model. In G. A. Marlatt, & J. R. Gordon (Eds.), *Relapse prevention: Maintenance strategies in the treatment of addictive behaviors* (pp. 3–70). New York: Guilford.

Marlatt, G. A., & Gordon, J. R. (Eds.). (1985). *Relapse prevention: Maintenance strategies in the treatment of addictive behaviors.* New York: Guilford.

Marques, J. K., Pithers, W. D., & Marlatt, G. A. (1984). Relapse prevention: A self-control program for sex offenders. Appendix to: Marques, J. K. *An innovative treatment program for sex offenders: Report to the legislature.* Sacramento: California State Department of Mental Health.

McKinney, M. E., Miner, M. H., Ruddell, H., McIlvain, H. E., Witte, H., Buell, J. C., Eliot, R. S., & Grant, L. B. (1985). The standardized mental stress test protocol: Test-retest reliability and comparison with ambulatory blood pressure monitoring. *Psychophysiology, 22,* 453–463.

Mehrabian, A., & Epstein, N. (1972). A measure of emotional empathy. *Journal of Personality, 40,* 525–529.

Meichenbaum, D. (1985). *Stress inoculation training.* New York: Pergamon.

Nathan, R. G., & Charlesworth, E. A. (1980). *Stress management: A conceptual and procedural guide.* Houston: Stress Management Research Associates.

Nelson, C., Miner, M., Marques, J., Russell, K., & Achterkirchen, J. (1988). Relapse prevention: A cognitive–behavioral model for treatment of the rapist and child molester. *Journal of Social Work and Human Sexuality, 7,* 125–143.

Nichols, H. R., & Molinder, I. (1984). *The Multiphasic Sex Inventory manual.* (Available from Nichols and Molinder, 437 Bowes Drive, Tacoma, WA 98466)

Nowicki, S. (1983). Manual for the adult Nowicki–Strickland locus of control scale. Unpublished manuscript.

Nowicki, S., & Strickland, B. (1973). A locus of control scale. *Journal of Consulting and Clinical Psychology, 40,* 148–154.

Rosenberg, M. (1965). *Society and the adolescent self image.* Princeton, NJ: Princeton University Press.

Spence, J. T., & Helmreich, R. (1972). The Attitudes Toward Women Scale: An objective instrument to measure attitudes toward the rights and roles of women in contemporary society. *Psychological Documents, 2,* (Ms. No. 153).

Thorne, F. C. (1966). The Sex Inventory. *Journal of Clinical Psychology, 22,* 367–374.

Wechsler, D. (1981). *WAIS–R manual: Wechsler Adult Intelligence Scale–Revised.* New York: Psychological Corporation.

23

The Center for Prevention
of Child Molestation

KATURAH D. JENKINS-HALL
CANDICE A. OSBORN
CARMEN S. ANDERSON
KENNETH A. ANDERSON
CAROL SHOCKLEY-SMITH

OVERALL STRUCTURE

The Center for Prevention of Child Molestation (CPCM) is an outpatient treatment facility supported by a grant from the National Institute of Mental Health (NIMH) to perform assessment, treatment, and outcome research on adult sex offenders. The project is housed at the Florida Mental Health Institute, University of South Florida, Tampa. The major goals of the project are to evaluate, treat, and prevent relapse in outpatient child molesters seen in a community setting.

Specifically, the project tests the effectiveness of a variety of assessment and treatment approaches, using a two-group research design. The experimental group receives 20 weeks of rational–emotive therapy (RET; Walen, DiGiuseppe, & Wessler, 1980), focused on cognitive-restructuring, self-efficacy (Bandura, 1977), and social-adequacy skills, paired with two types of behavior therapy (BT; Laws, Meyer, & Holmen, 1978; Laws & Osborn, 1983; Maletzky, 1973, 1974, 1980), focused on decreasing deviant sexual arousal; this is followed by 20 weeks of relapse prevention (RP; Marlatt & Gordon, 1985), focused on long-term self-management and adaptive coping skills in high-risk situations. The comparison group receives 20 weeks of RET alone, followed by 20 weeks of a more conventional follow-up (CF; Jenkins-Hall, 1987a; Lange, 1986) during which clients practice daily applications of RET principles and deal with issues

268

relevant to community adjustment. RET, RP, and CF are all conducted in a group-therapy format. Clients then participate for a minimum of 6 months in weekly or biweekly sessions of individual therapy. After this initial individualized follow-up, clients are seen at least monthly for an indefinite period of time.

All clients are evaluated prior to treatment, at the end of each 20-week treatment phase, and every 6 months thereafter on a number of self-report and penile plethysmographic measures of sexual arousal.

Three problems have been targeted for attention by this program: deviant sexual cognitions/rationalizations, deviant sexual arousal, and a strong tendency toward relapse. The major hypothesis is that the treatment approach of the experimental group will adequately address these three problem areas common to most sex offenders.

Participants

Eligible participants must be male child molesters who meet the following criteria: (1) They are aged 18 to 70, (2) they possess at least low average intelligence, (3) they are able to read and write, (4) they are nonpsychotic, and (5) they admit to sexual or presexual behavior with a child. Incest offenders are included in the study if they have also offended outside the home or admit to more generalized sexual attraction to children.

Based on the above admission criteria, we are currently treating 65 clients, of whom approximately 85% are white, 10% are black, and 5% are Hispanic. Most of our clients (75% to 80%) have low incomes and are single, separated, or divorced. About 52% molested females; 40%, males; and 8%, both. The vast majority (90%) did not use force during commission of the offense.

Referrals

Clients are referred to the CPCM from a variety of community sources. We have targeted the Florida Department of Corrections (Probation and Parole) as a key referral source from which we actively recruit. Approximately 40% of our clients come from this source and are mandated to successfully complete a sex offender treatment program as a condition of probation or parole. Another 45% are referred by private mental health practitioners, attorneys, and community mental health centers. The remaining are self-referred. The rate of referrals to the CPCM averages about 8 to 12 per month, a rate that has remained steady since January 1987. Although this rate is low, an extensive amount of public-relations work is involved in maintaining it. This includes regular contact with referral sources through seminars, lectures, and other training activities, periodic mailings of program information, and good relations with the media.

Staffing

The project is staffed by a project director, clinical director, project administrator–laboratory coordinator, three group therapists, two clinical assistants, three research assistants, and a secretary. All group and individual therapies are conducted by persons with at least master's degrees in psychology or counseling and experience in working with clients involved in the criminal justice system. Therapists are supervised by the clinical director, who is a licensed clinical psychologist. The psychophysiological assessments are conducted by research assistants with at least bachelor's degrees; these research assistants are supervised by the laboratory coordinator, a master's-level researcher with expertise in the use of penile plethysmography. All staff members are carefully selected and undergo extensive training in relevant treatment procedures and approaches.

PRETREATMENT–BASELINE ASSESSMENT

Upon referral to the CPCM, the client undergoes an initial screening interview to ascertain his eligibility. If he is deemed grant-eligible, a comprehensive intake interview is conducted by an assigned therapist. During the intake process, he undergoes psychophysiological evaluations of sexual arousal and computerized assessment of psychosexual attitudes, beliefs, and behaviors. After the completion of assessment, he is assigned to a therapy group and proceeds with the treatment program.

Screening Interview

The screening interview has a dual purpose: to determine grant-eligibility and to gain informed consent for participation in the various treatment components. The interview begins by determining such information as the client's age, level of education, and ability to read and write. The client is then informed about the CPCM's policies regarding confidentiality. Because Florida has a mandatory child abuse reporting law, the client is carefully instructed about the limits of confidentiality. The client is instructed to withhold specific, incriminating details of an offense that has not already been discovered by the authorities. (If such details are given, the information is forwarded to the Department of Health and Rehabilitative Services for investigation.) The client is then asked to describe briefly the circumstances surrounding his referral in order to ascertain whether the offense was against a child or an adult, whether it was against a relative or a nonrelative, and whether it has come to the attention of the authorities. Next, a modified mental status examination is conducted and a brief psychological history is taken in order to rule out organicity and the presence of severe mental impairment as well as to assess whether the client is stable enough to undergo outpatient treatment. Any recent history of suicidal gestures, assaultive behaviors, or severely impaired judgment that would render the client a danger to himself or others would militate against acceptance. Whether the client needs other supportive services (e.g., alcohol treatment, inpatient care) is then determined. If supportive services are needed, appropriate referrals are made. If there is a question about intellectual or personality functioning at this stage, the interview proceeds but a referral is made to the clinical director for more comprehensive psychological assessment.

After it has been determined that the client meets the criteria for admission, a complete explanation of the program is given through a structured informed consent form. This consent form addresses each assessment and treatment procedure, its risks and benefits, the length of treatment, the voluntariness of participation, the limits of confidentiality, and other elements of the program. After the client has read the consent form and fully understands its contents, he signs the agreement to participate in treatment. If the client is on probation or parole, he also signs a waiver to release information to his probation officer regarding his attendance and progress. Such information is released on a monthly basis.

Comprehensive Intake Interview

Subsequent to the screening and acceptance process, the client then begins the comprehensive intake interview, an extensive, five-part questionnaire consisting of 284 questions. This questionnaire is designed to obtain information on the client's history of sexual deviancy (e.g., age of onset; age group, race, and gender of victims; number of victims, number of offenses; sexual and emotional responses to victims; sexual development; past and current deviant and nondeviant sexual fantasies). Demographic and other background information is also obtained (e.g., family history, medical history, past psychological treatment, educational and vocational background, military history, and nonsexual offense history).

In addition, the client completes several computerized questionnaires designed to measure his sexual attitudes, knowledge, and experiences; frequency of and desire for a broad range of deviant and nondeviant behaviors; and cognitive distortions common to adult sex offenders. Therapists also complete questionnaires regarding the client's current level of psychological functioning.

The major assessment inventories used by the CPCM are (1) the Multiphasic Sex Inventory (Nichols & Molinder, 1984), a measure used to classify offenders on the basis of sexual beliefs, knowledge, and attitudes; (2) treatment-specific goal attainment scales (George & Marlatt, 1986; Jenkins-Hall, 1987a; Lange, 1986), which are designed to assess the mastery of treatment goals of each group session; (3) the Sexual Deviance Card Sort (Abel, 1979; Brownell & Barlow, 1976; Laws, 1986a), a procedure used to assess the relative attractiveness of various sexual practices; (4) daily self-report rating forms, on which clients indicate the frequency of deviant and nondeviant sexual fantasies, masturbation, and hands-on activities; (5) the Adult Cognition Scale (Abel & Becker, 1984), a measure of the extent to which clients agree with common deviant cognitions; (6) self-efficacy scales (Laws, 1986b), a measure of the extent to which clients believe they could resist temptation to offend in high-risk situations; (7) the Significant Other Rating Scale (Jenkins-Hall, 1987b), a measure of the client's adjustment within the community; (8) Symptom Checklist-90 (SCL-90; Derogatis, Lipman, & Covi, 1973), a general measure of psychiatric symptoms on which the client rates himself; and (9) the Brief Hopkins Psychiatric Rating Scale (Derogatis, 1978), another measure of psychiatric symptoms on which the therapist rates the client's current level of functioning.

Upon completion of the intake and evaluation process, a comprehensive treatment plan is developed by the clinical staff in order to address the client's specific problem areas that may warrant additional consideration as he undergoes the more structured treatment services of the CPCM.

Psychophysiological Assessment

The psychophysiological assessment at the CPCM consists of two primary components: the pedophile slide assessment (Laws & Osborn, 1983) and the pedophile audiotape assessment (Abel, Becker, Murphy, & Flanagan, 1981; Avery-Clark & Laws, 1984). The client undergoes this assessment on several occasions. He is assessed at intake, at the end of the first component of therapy (RET), at the end of the second component of therapy (RP or CF), and then at 6-month intervals during long-term follow-up.

The client's level of sexual arousal is measured by a device called a penile strain gauge or transducer (Bancroft, Jones, & Pullan, 1966; Pithers & Laws, 1989). This is a small, mercury-filled, rubber loop that the client places around his penis. As the client produces an erection, the strain gauge expands and sends a signal to a computer, which tracks and records the amount of change that has occurred. Changes in erection response are reported as some value between zero and 100% of full erection.

The "laboratory" at the CPCM contains four subject booths. Each booth is 4' × 6' and contains a television monitor, a slide-projection screen, a self-report device, and an interface panel for the penile strain gauge and communication equipment. The self-report device is a slide potentiometer, which allows the client to continuously indicate his subjectively perceived level of arousal throughout the stimulus presentation. Slides are projected into the booth through a hole, 3 inches in diameter, cut in the wall above the door. Audiotaped stimulus presentations are received through a headset. The control area of the laboratory contains the master unit of the communication system, a computer system for each booth, and a sink area for cleaning and sterilizing the penile strain gauges.

The computer system for each booth consists of an interface device that converts and amplifies the signal from the penile strain gauge, a computer that tracks and records the signal and controls the presentation of slides, a printer that produces a hard copy of the client's responses, an audiocassette player for presentation of audiotaped stimuli, a videocassette player for presentation of videotaped stimuli, and a television monitor.

The communication system was custom designed to meet several requirements. The system allows the laboratory staff (1) two-way communication with each booth, (2) presentation of audiotaped stimuli to each booth, (3) presentation of the audio portion of videotaped stimuli to each booth, and (4) monitoring of client verbalizations. The master unit allows independent access to each booth. Each booth contains a set of headphones with a boom microphone, as does the master unit of the communication system.

Pedophile Slide Assessment

The slide assessment (Laws & Osborn, 1983), which consists of 36 slides presented for 2 minutes each, is designed to determine the sex and age of the client's preferred sexual target. The slides are nude photographs of male and female children and adults. The client is instructed to look at each slide and imagine, as clearly as possible, that he is involved in sexual activity with the person in the slide. To ensure that the client is attending to the slides, he is also informed that he will occasionally be asked to describe the slide he has just seen. In addition, the client is asked to indicate his perceived level of sexual arousal throughout the stimulus presentation with the self-report device.

The slides are divided into approximate-age categories based on Tanner's (1962) developmental scale of secondary sexual characteristics. Tanner's Category 1 includes children through approximately age 7. This age range was too broad for our purposes, so we developed Category 0 to separate those clients who preferred extremely young children.

Category 0 includes slides of children aged 0 to 4; Category 1, aged 5 to 7; Category 2, aged 8 to 11; Category 3, aged 12 to 14; Category 4, aged 15 to 17; and Category 5, aged 25 and above to clearly distinguish them as adults.

To ensure reliability in measurement, the client is presented three slides per category for each sex. The slides are presented in a predetermined, randomized order. His responses to each category are averaged and then plotted graphically to display his sexual arousal pattern.

Pedophile Audiotape Assessment

This assessment (Abel et al., 1981; Avery-Clark & Laws, 1984) is designed to determine the sexual attractiveness of aggression against children. It consists of 14 audiotapes, each 3 minutes in length. The tapes include descriptions of various sexual situations that vary according to the amount of aggression described. The client is instructed to listen to each tape and try to imagine, as clearly as possible, that he is involved in the activity being described. Again, to ensure that he is attending to the tapes, he is informed that he will occasionally be asked to describe the tape he has just heard. In addition, he is asked to indicate his perceived level of sexual arousal throughout the stimulus presentation with the self-report device.

Two parallel versions of these 14 tapes are presented alternatively during each successive reassessment. Each version of audiotapes is presented in a predetermined, randomized order. The client's responses are presented graphically to display his sexual arousal pattern.

The audiotapes are divided into the following seven categories for each sex:

1. *Fondling.* The perpetrator fondles a child who complies with the activity.
2. *Mutually consenting.* The perpetrator has sexual intercourse with a child who complies with the activity.
3. *Nonconsenting.* The perpetrator has sexual intercourse with a child who resists. The perpetrator uses verbal threats of physical harm to gain the child's compliance.
4. *Rape.* The perpetrator has sexual intercourse with a child who resists. The perpetrator uses physical force to gain the child's compliance.
5. *Sadism.* The perpetrator has sexual intercourse with a child who resists. The perpetrator uses excessive physical force to gain the child's compliance.
6. *Physical assault.* The perpetrator beats and tortures the child with no sexual activity.
7. *Mutually consenting adult.* The perpetrator has consensual sexual intercourse with an adult.

All audiotapes are recorded in a male voice and are presented in a monotonous, fast-paced, standardized manner to ensure that any response that occurs is to the content of the audiotape rather than to extraneous factors.

Prior to beginning each phase of treatment, the results of the psychophysiological assessment are reviewed with the client by his primary therapist and the laboratory coordinator. During this review it is not uncommon for a client to make significant progress toward accepting responsibility for his sexually deviant behavior when confronted with such concrete evidence of his arousal patterns.

Periodic Measurement

All clients (experimental and comparison groups) undergo periodic measurement of their sexual arousal during the treatment phases. During these measurements, or probes, the client is presented with four 3-minute, audiotaped descriptions of sexual activity, two deviant and two nondeviant. All stimuli used for probes contain descriptions of consensual sexual activity. The content of the stimuli presented is individualized for each client. His responses to these audiotapes are plotted graphically to produce a record of his progress in therapy.

TREATMENT COMPONENTS: PHASE 1

Rational–Emotive Therapy

The first phase of treatment at the CPCM involves the use of rational–emotive therapy (Ellis & Grieger, 1977; Ellis & Harper, 1976; Wessler & Wessler, 1980). In this component of therapy, clients are taught the fundamentals of RET in order to provide the cognitive strategies that will facilitate (1) the challenging of their deviant justifications to engage in sex offending, (2) the developing of a systematic means of cognitive restructuring of deviant thinking that leads to sexual deviant urges and behaviors, and (3) the learning of communication and assertion skills necessary for successful adult relationships. The ultimate goal is to supply the client with skills that are generalizable to his everyday life in order to prevent a relapse to deviant sexual behavior. RET is offered in the first phase of treatment because of its straightforward and pragmatic approach. It appears to be highly effective in breaking through the stage of denial and minimization that sex offenders often present at the beginning of treatment. The group treatment modality also supports this breaking down of past deviant justifications by providing a common frame of reference within which group members may challenge and assist each other.

The RET component of therapy is implemented in a group format for 20 consecutive weeks. Each session is 1.5 hours long for experimental groups and 2 hours long for comparison groups. This time difference equalizes therapist contact and balances the additional time the experimental group spends in behavior therapy. The RET therapy is guided by a treatment manual written specifically for the project (Lange, 1986). All clinical staff receive extensive training in the use of this manual prior to the initiation of groups. This training program is also videotaped in order to provide the therapists with an ongoing review of the materials. To ensure the integrity of treatment delivery, each session is either videotaped or audiotaped and then reviewed by the clinical director. Segments of the videotapes are also reviewed by the author of the treatment manual at regular intervals in order to provide the therapists with feedback concerning the ongoing integrity of the treatment delivery. The clients report weekly on their progress in reaching goals in RET by completing goal-attainment scales. This form is a 16-item, 5-point Likert Scale, which subjectively measures the client's perception of progress in understanding and applying the principles of RET. In conjunction with this rating scale, therapists also chart each client's progress over the same 16 items after each RET session.

The first 3 weeks of therapy aim at demonstrating the fundamentals of the ABCs of the rational–emotive approach. The clients initially learn that situations in their daily lives (As) neither cause their emotional difficulties nor necessitate their behavioral responses (Cs) of either over- or underreacting to situations. The clients learn that such affective and behavioral responses are mediated through cognitive processes, thoughts, and beliefs about activating events (Bs). The clients are taught in Sessions 2 and 3 to identify the types of irrational thinking that mediate over- and underreactions to situations (e.g., catastrophic and absolutistic thinking and rationalizations). In Session 3 the clients learn to identify underlying irrational beliefs that support past deviant behaviors. In the sessions that follow, the clients are given a systematic way to challenge past deviant cognitions and to restructure their thinking toward accepting responsibility for their actions through a process of cognitive restructuring. The overall focus of sessions is on having the clients challenge their deviant cognitions and replace them with rational thinking. The sessions are delivered in a didactic manner, with the therapist presenting the materials and demonstrating their application to real-life situations. Homework is given for each session in order to provide the clients with practice in applying the methods covered in session. The therapist constantly involves the clients in the presentation by asking them to apply the concepts to actual life experiences.

The first four sessions establish the groundwork for challenging the deviant justifications clients typically use to engage in deviant behaviors and to avoid adult relations. Initially, the topic of sexual deviance is addressed only peripherally, and less sensitive areas of daily functioning are used as examples to demonstrate RET principles. This allows the client to become familiar with the concepts discussed while also building group rapport. After these initial sessions, using the general skills they have learned, the clients are asked to directly challenge their own deviant justifications and to assist other members in so doing. This process of critical self-examination is often difficult at first. Members are keenly aware of the shift toward working on the real problems related to their sexual deviance, which most find unsettling. However, the initial group rapport and the common frame of reference in the RET model built in the first four sessions facilitates the process of mutual challenging and mutual support at this critical stage.

The next six sessions (Sessions 5 through 10) focus on challenging each client's deviant thoughts and justifications by cognitively restructuring his thinking toward rational attitudes, including acceptance of responsibility and commitment to avoiding further relapses to deviant behavior. Initially the clients retrospectively examine the justifications that supported their deviant behaviors or nonacceptance of responsibility. The clients gain insight into their use of rationalizations and irrational beliefs, insight that will serve them later in the prevention of relapse. The focus of the sessions then shifts to utilizing the four-step process of cognitive restructuring to enhance or initiate appropriate adult relationships. This is done by examining the irrational thoughts and beliefs that underlie the clients' difficulties in forming adult relationships (e.g., fear of rejection, fear of failure). These cognitions are challenged in the same manner as are deviant cognitions.

Beginning with Session 11, the focus of the group shifts to building a sense of self-efficacy and social adequacy so that clients can maintain functional and pleasurable adult relationships. Helping the client give up his deviant sexual behavior without building toward an appropriate replacement sets him up for failure. The client would feel frustration from the lack of an appropriate sexual outlet and would continue to have low self-efficacy, both of which may ultimately lead to relapse. The goal of this stage of treatment is to provide a sense of self-control, self-mangement, and, ultimately, self-efficacy.

In Sessions 16 through 18, communication skills are addressed. The focus here is on learning a seven-step model for practicing behavioral rehearsal for changing ineffective verbal and nonverbal communication skills. The clients are then taught assertiveness skills in order to enhance the chances of succeeding in having their needs met in adult relationships.

The final sessions are designed to review the RET model and create individual plans for continued practice of the principles learned.

Behavior Therapy

While undergoing the RET phase of treatment, experimental clients also participate in one of the two primary forms of behavior therapy designed to reduce sexual arousal: verbal satiation and olfactory aversion. In the inpatient setting this procedure is usually carried out three times per week in a laboratory setting. Because it would not be feasible to have outpatient clients attend three sessions per week, they perform this therapy once per week in the laboratory and twice per week at home. The home sessions are recorded on audiotape and are reviewed by the staff to ensure compliance.

Verbal Satiation

Verbal satiation (Laws & Osborn, 1983) is designed to reduce deviant arousal by satiating the client with his own deviant fantasies. Initially the client verbalizes the most highly arousing fantasies that he has developed over the years. But, as he carries out this procedure over and over, the fantasies become boring and lose their arousal value. The client tries to compensate for this by attempting to develop new fantasies. However, because he is forced to verbalize these new fantasies so repetitiously, they, too, quickly lose their arousal value, often before they are even fully developed. In this way, deviant fantasies are paired with boredom and lack of sexual arousal. At the CPCM, the client verbalizes deviant fantasies for concentrated thirty-minute intervals, with no pauses.

The client is escorted to a booth and instructed to put on the penile strain gauge and headphones. He indicates when he has the strain gauge in place and is seated comfortably. When a stable baseline is obtained (less than 20% of full erection for 2 to 5 minutes), the therapist tells him to begin verbalizing deviant fantasies. Unobtrusively and periodically, the therapist listens to the session to make sure that the client is indeed verbalizing deviant fantasies. If the client is not verbalizing deviant fantasies, the therapist interrupts the session and instructs him to carry out the procedure correctly. The therapist then has the client repeat the entire 30-minute session.

The client is issued an audiocassette recorder and an audiocassette and is instructed to perform the verbal satiation procedure two times per week at home on separate days. Sessions must be 30-minutes long, and the client is instructed not to masturbate during them. The client turns in audiotapes of these sessions weekly to be reviewed for compliance with appropriate procedures. Failure to complete home sessions properly is grounds for termination.

Olfactory Aversion

Olfactory aversion (Laws, Meyer, & Holmen, 1978; Maletzky, 1980) is designed to reduce deviant arousal by pairing it with an aversive stimulus. In this way the client learns to associate deviant sexual arousal with negative consequences. The aversive stimulus is ammonia, which the client self-administers by breaking a crushable ammonia capsule and then inhaling the fumes. The agent immediately dissipates the client's erection and associated arousal. The presentation of the aversive stimulus is always paired with the beginning of the deviant fantasies and is periodically repeated throughout the fantasies. The client participates in this procedure once per week in the laboratory and twice per week at home.

The client is given one or two breakable ammonia capsules and escorted to a booth. He is then instructed to put on the penile strain gauge and headphones. After a stable baseline has been obtained, the therapist instructs the client to begin verbalizing deviant fantasies out loud for 15 minutes. The client is instructed to crush the ammonia capsule and inhale a small dose of it as soon as he begins to verbalize the deviant fantasies. The capsule is then stored in a small covered jar, the lid of which is removed only during inhalations. In this way, the ammonia capsule retains its potency. Clients are instructed to inhale the ammonia fumes whenever they feel they are becoming aroused or, at minimum, every 2 minutes during the 15-minute session.

The treatment sessions in the laboratory are closely monitored. The client verbalizes the fantasies into a microphone while wearing the penile transducer.

In this way, laboratory staff can ensure that the client is focusing on deviant fantasies, pausing rarely, and inhaling the ammonia fumes appropriately. The laboratory staff are able to give the client immediate feedback if he fails to comply with the treatment protocol. If the therapist discovers that the client is not carrying out the procedure correctly, the entire session is repeated.

As with the verbal satiation procedure, the client is issued equipment needed to perform the olfactory aversion procedure two times per week at home on separate days. He is instructed to inhale a small dose of ammonia periodically throughout the entire fantasy. The client turns in audiotapes of these sessions to his therapist for review and feedback.

The clients who participate in behavior therapy "successfully complete" it when they produce less than 20% of a full erection to deviant stimuli for 8 consecutive weeks as measured in the biweekly probe sessions. All clients continue to participate in the probe sessions throughout treatment, thus providing an ongoing measure of whether behavior-therapy treatment gains are maintained. If the deviant arousal returns, behavior therapy is reinstigated until this arousal again meets criterion.

TREATMENT COMPONENTS: PHASE 2

Relapse Prevention

Clients assigned to the experimental group undergo RP during the second phase of treatment (Marlatt & Gordon, 1985). Although the relapse prevention model was originally developed for the treatment of other types of addictive behaviors, its principles are easily translated to the treatment of sexual deviance (George & Marlatt, 1986; George & Marlatt, Introduction, this volume; Pithers, Marques, Gibat, & Marlatt, 1983). In general, RP is well suited for the treatment of sex offenders. As a group, sex offenders are known to be at high risk for relapse. Abstinent sex offenders often report strong, seemingly uncontrollable urges to resume deviant sexual activity. They also lack the specific coping skills needed to deal with these deviant urges. RP addresses these issues by teaching specific, adaptive coping strategies. Sex offenders also have well-established behavior patterns of which they are usually unaware. Ongoing monitoring and assessment, which are also critical components of RP, provide the offender insight into his pattern of offending.

In this component of therapy clients learn the importance of identifying cognitive and behavioral precursors to reoffending and intervening at the earliest possible point in the cognitive behavioral chain. They also learn the importance of a balanced daily lifestyle for more adaptive functioning.

RP procedures allow each client to address his specific pattern of sexual offending (including the identification of high-risk situations, lapses, and relapse) and foster the development of individualized strategies for coping at these strategic points.

There are, of course, some necessary modifications to be made in transferring traditional RP concepts to sexual offenders. One obvious modification of the model is in the definition of the terms *lapse* and *relapse*. As explained by George and Marlatt (1986), the usual definition of a lapse as any isolated recurrence of the targeted behavior is unacceptable within the parameters of sexually deviant behaviors. The costly consequences of sexual victimization of a child mandate that these terms be redefined to accommodate social and ethical concerns and, at the same time, salvage the applicability of the model. George and Marlatt (1986) describe the modification of these concepts for treatment purposes as follows:

> The designation of a lapse should coincide with an earlier point in the behavioral chain that precedes commission of an offense [idiosyncratic to the offender's] . . . highly individualized and perhaps even ritualistic sequences of preoffense cognitions and behaviors. The term lapse shall refer to any reoccurrence of willful and elaborate fantasizing about sexual offending or any sources of stimulation associated with offending. (pp. 1–2)

Usually the point in the chain immediately preceding the deviant behavior—most commonly, willful deviant fantasies—is identified as the onset of a lapse. A relapse is the recurrence of a sexual offense, which is perceived as a full-scale reestablishment of the problematic behavior.

The RP phase of treatment as outlined by George and Marlatt (1986) primarily addresses the following treatment goals: (1) to learn specific assessment methods for monitoring motivation and deviant behavior patterns, (2) to develop specific coping skills for dealing with high-risk situations (HRSs), lapses, and relapses; and (3) to develop and/or strengthen social support networks within the community. These goals are addressed through processing and integrating the five basic components of relapse prevention: motivation, assessment, coping skills, balanced daily lifestyles, and social supports.

The treatment program is implemented in weekly sessions of 1.5 hours over a 20-week period. The first therapy session consists of an overview of the RP treatment approach and definitions of terminology. Clients are introduced to the concept of cognitive–behavioral chains and begin developing their own chains during this session. During the second through the sixth week of therapy, the five basic components of the model are introduced independently (Jenkins-Hall & Anderson, 1987).

Session 2 focuses primarily on the principle of motivation. Essentially, the client is encouraged to look at motivation as an entity that waxes and wanes. If motivation is high, he is less likely to reoffend. If it is low, his risk for relapsing is high. The client is given a structured scale for rating his current motivation and engages in several exercises designed to examine this issue.

Session 3 focuses on the importance of assessment and ongoing monitoring in the prevention of relapse. One primary assessment tool is the *record of deviant sexual urges* (George & Marlatt, 1986). The client uses this record sheet to track his deviant sexual urges on a daily basis, including the time; the circumstances; his thoughts and feelings before, during, and after the situation; the intensity of the urge; and the coping skills he used.

Session 4 introduces methods for coping with high-risk situations and lapses. It is emphasized that adaptive coping responses can occur at any point in the cognitive–behavioral chain and that the earlier the client intervenes in the chain, the better.

Session 5 focuses on the importance of the client's having a strong social support system as he undergoes the change process. The client is informed that there will be a period of transition as he changes from a deviant to a nondeviant lifestyle and that supportive friendships help reduce the stress associated with the transition. Clients are given guidelines for asking for support.

Session 6 emphasizes the importance of a balanced daily lifestyle. As stated by George and Marlatt (1986):

> Another important feature of the RP program is learning to develop other sources of gratification. For many offenders, deviant sexual activities became the predominant, if not the only method of self-indulgence. In creating a satisfying life without sexual deviance, you will need to develop alternative indulgences [pleasurable activities]. These alternatives will help to balance out the sense of deprivation that you are likely to feel in giving up your sexual deviancy. (p. 17)

The client is asked to develop a routine of engaging in activities he finds pleasurable.

Sessions 7 through 13 are designed to monitor the client's understanding of the previously introduced concepts as well as his ability to integrate the concepts into a pattern of behavior that promotes a healthy, nondeviant lifestyle. These sessions begin with discussion of any HRSs that occurred during the previous week. Next, homework from the previous session, as well as previously recorded self-monitoring data, is reviewed. The client's motivational level and progress in each of the other major RP areas are also monitored weekly. There is usually one major area of focus for a given session. New skills, concepts, or principles pertinent to the major area of focus are introduced and demonstrated through exercises (e.g., the use of the decision matrix, coping with deviant urges, apparently irrelevant decisions). Finally, homework assignments are made for the following week.

Sessions 14 through 20 are designed to develop a contract for extended implementation of skills learned for the prevention of future relapse. This extended contract is written by the client in a language that he understands. It is highly individualized and based on his specific pattern of relapse, the assessment and coping skills he is most comfortable using, and the pleasurable activities and avenues for social support that he has identified. The client is asked to make multiple copies of the contract and to keep the copies in strategic places so that he is easily reminded of his plan for remaining deviance-free.

As in the RET component, clients in RP complete goal-attainment scales designed to track the areas of motivation, assessment, coping skills, social supports, and daily lifestyle. Integrity ratings are provided by external, expert raters as described above.

Conventional Follow-Up for RET

While clients in the experimental group participate in RP, clients assigned to the comparison group participate in a more conventional follow-up (CF). The intent of follow-up for any psychotherapeutic intervention is to insure that insights, skills, and techniques learned during the regular course of therapy are maintained and applied to appropriate aspects of daily living. Usual follow-up involves less frequent and less intensive contact with clients, with the client assuming a more autonomous, responsible role.

Very few clinicians approach follow-up in a systematic fashion. Follow-up efforts range from casual inquiries about the client's welfare among fellow professionals to sporadic contact with clients on a monthly or less frequent basis. There is usually no objective attempt to measure the maintenance of treatment gains and very little documentation of client contact during the follow-up stage of treatment.

Therapy for sex offenders is not an exception to traditional therapy in this respect. Most sex offender treatment programs, while recognizing the need for some type of long-term follow-up of their clientele, have been unsuccessful in this endeavor. One strength of the CPCM is its focus on long-term follow-up of all clients whether assigned to experimental or comparison groups.

Throughout the CF phase of treatment, clients are expected to be monitored weekly through daily self-reports of their deviant–nondeviant sexual arousal and activity, periodic physiological assessment of arousal patterns, and other self-report measures of community adjustment.

The CF group, which is also guided by a manual (Jenkins-Hall, 1987a), focuses on the maintenance of four basic skills learned during the first 20 weeks of therapy:

1. The ability to distinguish the three types of thinking, (irrational, rational, and rationalization) and to strive to use rational thinking.
2. The ability to identify underlying irrational beliefs that lead to excessive feelings of anxiety, depression, anger, and guilt.
3. The ability to use the four-step process in cognitive restructuring for changing irrational thinking, specifically, those cognitions that support sexual deviance.
4. The ability to engage in assertive behaviors in all aspects of daily living, an ability that enhances adult relationships and increases feelings of self-efficacy.

For the purpose of the research grant, it is very important to differentiate the conventional follow-up procedures from the relapse prevention approach to follow-up. Although there are some commonalities, the CF group differs in many substantial ways from the RP group. This group does not (1) teach a new conceptual model for looking at sexual deviance (i.e., the compulsive behavior model); (2) adopt the basic structure of RP, with its focus on motivation, assessment, coping skills, social interactions, and daily lifestyle; (3) use the language of RP (HRSs, lapses, etc.); or (4) emphasize the importance of anticipating and coping with high-risk situations, the major focus of RP.

This follow-up instead (1) focuses on the avoidance of excessive feelings of depression, anxiety, guilt, and anger (which are often associated with sexual offending) by continuing to assist the client in engaging in rational thinking; (2) deals with daily situations (not necessarily high risk) in which the client has experienced one of the excessive, affective reactions by using RET principles; (3) continues to challenge deviant cognitions that maintain sexual offending; (4) allows the client to further develop hetero- and/or homosocial skills through the use of role-plays and behavioral rehearsal, using the seven-step model outlined by Lange (1986); (5) prepares the client for adjustment within the community by strengthening social support networks; and (6) reinforces coping skills needed to reduce stress and to behave adequately in interpersonal situations.

The CF is conducted for 20 weeks, for 1.5 hours per week. The sessions begin with an overview of the major areas of RET. Clients are instructed to keep journals of those daily activities in three specific areas (work, home, and social) that have led to one of the four excessive feelings. Clients are also instructed to document incidences in which they did not respond assertively in those daily activities.

Subsequent sessions begin by reviewing journal entries, examining the types of thinking and underlying beliefs that have led to the negative experience, and restructuring those cognitions using the four-step process. Where the client has failed to respond assertively, role-playing and behavioral rehearsal are used to practice the situation. In addition, clients process issues related to successful community adjustment, such as complying with conditions of probation and developing appropriate social relationships.

The follow-up outlined here is different from the first 20 weeks of RET treatment. It does not teach new principles but capitalizes on old learning through intensive behavior rehearsal, while at the same time allowing for broader generalizations of the learned materials. It is less structured, providing maximal opportunity for the client to address his own relevant issues for improved psychosocial functioning. It allows for maximal interaction among group members, in this resembling a peer-conducted approach. Additionally, it allows the therapist to adopt the role of facilitator rather than instructor. Any new issues addressed relate to the facilitation of the client's adjustment within the community.

Although what is outlined above is described as conventional follow-up, it is only conventional in that its approaches are not new. The approaches are, in fact, common to cognitive–behavior therapy and therapy in general. The degree to which the manual is structured and the methods for obtaining objective data on maintenance of treatment gains, however, make the conventional unconventional.

TREATMENT COMPONENTS: PHASE 3

Individual Follow-Up

The third phase of the program at the CPCM is an individually tailored treatment component designed to address treatment goals not successfully met, in need of refinement, and/or in need of continuous monitoring. The goals of this follow-up are determined in conjunction with the client and are based on specific skill deficits identified during the prior treatment phases. The follow-up capitalizes only on skills previously learned. For example, a client assigned to the comparison group is not taught RP concepts in the individual follow-up phase. Thus, although a client from the experimental group may have the same basic treatment goals as a client from the comparison group, the methods for achieving the goals will be different for each. In either case, the basic goals of treatment remain applicable, that is, learning and implementing cognitive-restructuring techniques in order to prevent recurrence of the deviant behavior, learning to cope with adult situations more effectively, strengthening a sense of self-efficacy and social efficacy, and developing a healthier lifestyle through self-care and social supports. Some of the most frequently addressed additional treatment goals include developing hetero- and homosocial skills, increasing arousal to adult sexual stimuli, and processing issues of sexual identity.

This phase of treatment is carried out on a one-to-one basis. In the initial stages all sessions are conducted for 1 hour. The frequency of the therapy sessions is determined by the client's ability to control and/or manage deviant sexual urges and cope with daily stressors, as indicated by his RP assessment records or CF journal entries. Initially it may be appropriate to see the client on a weekly basis until such time that his progress in the above-mentioned areas is evaluated and it is determined that he may be seen less frequently. All clients are seen at least monthly. The client's treatment plan is evaluated after every ten contacts or once every 90 days in order to review progress and determine the frequency and duration of the next set of individualized contacts. The client is expected to decrease the frequency of his visits to biweekly meetings over a total active period of at least 6 months; thereafter, visits occur monthly.

PRELIMINARY ANALYSES OF DATA

The research aspect of this project is in its infancy. No client has completed the three treatment phases to date, although several clients in the experimental and comparison groups have completed Phase 1. Therefore, the initial data analyses are based primarily on pretreatment assessment. Pretreatment measures were based on a sample of 50 clients. Between-group measures were based on a sample of 11 clients, because only this number had completed Phase 1 of treatment at the time statistical analyses were conducted. Although this sample size is small, certain trends were revealed.

Pretreatment Measures

Analyses were conducted to evaluate the efficacy of self-report and physiological assessment measures. The physiological assessment measures proved to classify clients correctly into offense categories. Analyses of the pedophile slide assessment revealed that homosexual and heterosexual pedophiles responded highest to slides in the male and female categories, respectively. Bisexual pedophiles responded approximately equally to both. With respect to the audiotape assessment, homosexual and bisexual pedophiles responded more to audiotapes of male children, and heterosexual pedophiles responded more to audiotapes of female children. All pedophiles responded more to descriptions of fondling and mutually consenting intercourse ($M = 42\%$ and 47% of full erection, respectively) and less to physical assault ($M = 16\%$) than to all other categories. Responses to slide and audiotape stimuli were highly intercorrelated.

The Sexual Deviance Card Sort and two gender-preference subscales of the Multiphasic Sex Inventory proved to be excellent instruments for correctly identifying clients by diagnosis (male, female, or mixed pedophilia). The other, more traditional, clinical measures (e.g., SCL-90) revealed that the clients were generally in good mental health, not suffering from depression, anxiety, or other gross pathology.

Between-Group Analyses (Phase 1)

Changes in Sexual Arousal

Based on biweekly measurement, all clients showed more arousal to deviant ($M = 43\%$) than to nondeviant ($M = 31\%$) stimuli at baseline, a pattern that continued across the 20 weeks of Phase 1. Both the experimental and comparison groups showed an equivalent significant decrease in deviant arousal across the phase (from about 48% to about 31%).

Pedophile slide and audiotape assessment measures did not differ between groups in pretreatment assessment versus assessment at the end of Phase 1. Both groups showed a marginal decline in deviant sexual arousal as measured by both slides and audiotapes; however, both groups continued to show more arousal to children ($M = 42\%$) than to adults ($M = 23\%$).

Self-Report Measures

Daily self-report measures proved to differ between groups. Not suprisingly, all clients reported more deviant than nondeviant fantasies, a trend that did not change across phases. The experimental group showed a significant reduction in reported deviant fantasies across the phase ($M = 2.09$/day to $M = 1.16$/day), while no change occurred in the comparison group. The experimental group also showed a significant reduction in total masturbations across the phase ($M = 0.52$/day to $M = 0.31$/day), while the comparison group showed no change. Both groups showed a decline in deviant masturbations and a concurrent, slight increase in nondeviant masturbations.

Client questionnaires revealed only marginal differences between groups. For example, the experimental group continued to rate pedophilic items as attractive on the card-sort measure, while the comparison group rated them as neutral.

The self-efficacy questionnaire revealed that both groups admitted that, when presented with high-risk situations, they would be highly tempted to molest children but felt confident they could resist.

Goal-Attainment Scales

Clients in both groups tended to rate themselves considerably higher on the goal-attainment scales than did the therapists, but both clients and therapists indicated significant improvement across the phase.

PRELIMINARY CONCLUSIONS

Pretreatment Data

The physiological assessment of sexual arousal differentiated homosexual, heterosexual, and bisexual pedophiles; thus it appears to be a powerful diagnostic tool. The Multiphasic Sex Inventory also appears to be a promising instrument for grouping types of offenders, but more research is needed to determine which scales are most predictive. The card sort appears to be the best single self-report instrument for classification purposes.

Between-Group Measures

Although ongoing measures of sexual arousal during therapy indicated a trend toward a greater decline in deviant sexual arousal among the experimental group, the experimental and comparison groups showed no difference on the physiological assessment measures at reassessment. One possible explanation for this finding is that clients may have become habituated to the biweekly measurement stimuli, with this reaction to such frequent measurement clouding the findings. To test this hypothesis, the CPCM is reducing the frequency of ongoing measurement sessions from biweekly to monthly.

We have found that the self-report questionnaires in use are not sensitive to the changes that are the goals of the therapies. For example, the primary goal of RET is to change the client's cognitive distortions and maladaptive thinking patterns. However, this is not directly measured by any of the questionnaires employed. The CPCM is currently in the process of developing competency-based measures that will correspond more directly to the goals of each phase of treatment.

Daily self-report measures revealed that changes did occur in clients' sexual behavior patterns. Clients proved to be highly compliant in completing daily self-reports, and this measure appears to be sensitive to treatment intervention.

Goal-attainment scales also appeared to be sensitive to treatment intervention; however, such scales are often criticized for their tendency to measure clients' optimism about their progress and therapists' self-perceptions of their own ability to impart skills and knowledge to clients. We therefore expect these measures to continue to show the strongest indication of client improvement. A noted advantage in the use of goal-attainment scales, however, is that clients are ever mindful of the goals of the therapy. So, although we are seeking more objective measures of progress, we will continue to use these subjective rating scales.

Clients in both the experimental and comparison groups responded positively to the treatment approaches. Many have commented on their relief at receiving concrete skills that can be readily transferred to their daily lives. Although not all clients are able to use such skills as the four steps of cognitive restructuring in the rigorous format in which they are presented, all come to examine their thinking patterns closely and attempt to challenge those thoughts that they recognize as maladaptive.

Although the preliminary findings are not conclusive, we believe that the clients who have participated in RP will fare better during long-term follow-up. These clients appear to have more coping strategies at their disposal and have learned the value of ongoing monitoring in the prevention of relapse. Although cognitive strategies (e.g., RET) may be useful, the ultimate prevention of relapse requires behavioral coping strategies as well. RP clients have the benefit of both.

ISSUES IN PROVIDING OUTPATIENT TREATMENT SERVICES

Many complex issues arise in the provision of outpatient services to this difficult population. Issues such as the community's response, limited confidentiality, and provision of services to special populations are among the most prominent.

The lay community's response to the treatment of sex offenders at the CPCM has for the most part been negative. Punishment and banishment are more often preferred to treatment. Residents find it difficult to see the relationship between providing treatment to the offender and protecting future victims. The treatment approaches used by the CPCM are complicated and sometimes misunderstood. Many efforts at enlightenment (e.g., lectures, seminars) are necessary to allay the fears of the community.

Therapists are sometimes confronted with the ethical dilemma of protecting client confidentiality versus protecting society at large (Kelly, 1987). With mandatory reporting laws, potential clients who have not been discovered by the criminal justice authorities feel discouraged from seeking help, fearing the consequences of being turned in by their therapists. Consequently, the rate of self-referrals is low.

The majority of sex offenders who are put on probation and/or returned to the community after adjudication are incest offenders. Thus most of the referrals received by the CPCM are for incest cases. Although some of these offenders can be accurately diagnosed as pedophiles, they often require specialized service involving a family-therapy component. The CPCM does not offer these comprehensive services at this time.

Outpatient services require a high level of motivation and compliance from clients if treatment is to be effective. This clientele is generally unmotivated and noncompliant. Much of the treatment staff's energy is invested in maintaining an acceptable level of compliance from clients. We have found that a good working relationship with probation officers or other referral agents is helpful in this regard.

Perhaps most challenging is the issue of providing treatment to low-functioning clients. The CPCM screens out those clients with intellectual levels below the low average range. However, a sufficient number of such referrals are received to warrant some attempt at treatment, especially when one considers that this subpopulation is at greater risk for relapse and is extremely difficult to treat. The CPCM is piloting a special-needs group for those clients who are borderline IQ, functionally illiterate, and/or too emotionally unstable to meet grant criteria. The approaches used are simplified, slowed-down versions of the RET and RP treatment components. Group sessions are less structured and paced according to mastery of the material presented. The therapist uses games, role-play–behavior rehearsal, and visual prompts to teach new skills and concepts. Progress is slow, and effective treatment may require an indeterminantly long period of time.

FUTURE DIRECTIONS

CPCM hopes to address the provision of services to incest offenders and to special-needs populations in the future. Not only will this provide an invaluable service to the community, but it will answer important research questions regarding evaluation and treatment of these types of offenders.

Perhaps the most important contribution of this research project will be the long-term follow-up of clients through monthly face-to-face contact. Many of our clients have been sentenced to 10 to 15 years of probation and will be required to attend monitoring sessions as a condition of probation. Structured support groups are being developed to meet the needs of such clients. It is only through extended follow-up that a true test of the RP model can be accomplished.

ACKNOWLEDGMENTS

Preparation of this chapter was supported in part by National Institute of Mental Health Grant No. MH42035 to D. R. Laws and by the Florida Mental Health Institute.

REFERENCES

Abel, G. G. (1979). *Assessment and treatment of sex offenders.* Grant proposal submitted to the National Institute of Mental Health.

Abel, G. G., & Becker, J. V. (1984). Adult Cognition Scale. (Available from G. G. Abel, Behavioral Medicine Institute, 3193 Howell Mill Rd. NW, Ste. 202, Atlanta, GA)

Abel, G. G., Becker, J. V., Murphy, W. D., & Flanagan, B. (1981). Identifying dangerous child molesters. In R. B. Stuart (Ed.), *Violent behavior* (pp. 116–137). New York: Brunner/Mazel.

Avery-Clark, C. A., & Laws, D. R. (1984). Differential erection response patterns of sexual child abusers to stimuli describing activities with children. *Behavior Therapy, 15,* 71–83.

Bancroft, J., Jones, H. G., & Pullan, B. R. (1966). A simple transducer for measuring penile erection, with comments on its use in the treatment of sexual disorders. *Behaviour Research and Therapy, 4,* 239–241.

Bandura, A. (1977). Self-efficacy: Toward a unifying theory of behavior change. *Psychological Review, 84,* 191–215.

Brownell, K. D., & Barlow, D. H. (1976). Measurement and treatment of two sexual deviations in one person. *Journal of Behavior Therapy and Experimental Psychiatry, 7,* 349–354.

Derogatis, L. R. (1978). Brief Hopkins Psychiatric Rating Scale. (Available from L. R. Derogatis, Johns Hopkins University School of Medicine, Baltimore, MD)

Derogatis, L. R., Lipman, R. S., & Covi, L. (1973). SCL-90: An outpatient psychiatric rating scale—Preliminary report. *Psychopharmacology Bulletin, 9,* 13–27.

Ellis, A., & Grieger, R. (Eds.). (1977). *Handbook of rational-emotive therapy.* New York: Springer.

Ellis, A., & Harper, R. A. (1976). *A new guide to rational living.* Englewood Cliffs, NJ: Prentice-Hall.

George, W. H., & Marlatt, G. A. (1986). *Relapse prevention with sexual offenders: A treatment manual.* Unpublished manuscript, Florida Mental Health Institute, Tampa.

Jenkins-Hall, K. D. (1987a). *Conventional follow-up for rational emotive therapy: A treatment manual.* Unpublished manuscript, Florida Mental Health Institute, Tampa.

Jenkins-Hall, K. D. (1987b). *The Significant Other Rating Scale.* Unpublished manuscript, Florida Mental Health Institute, Tampa.

Jenkins-Hall, K. D., & Anderson, C. S. (1987). *Relapse prevention with sex offenders: Revised.* Unpublished manuscript, Florida Mental Health Institute, Tampa.

Kelly, R. J. (1987). Limited confidentiality and the pedophile. *Hospital and Community Psychiatry, 38,* 1046–1048.

Lange, A. (1986). *Rational emotive therapy: A treatment manual.* Unpublished manuscript, Florida Mental Health Institute, Tampa.

Laws, D. R. (1986a). *Sexual Deviance Card Sort.* Unpublished manuscript, Florida Mental Health Institute, Tampa.

Laws, D. R. (1986b). *Self-efficacy rating scale-revised.* Unpublished manuscript, Florida Mental Health Institute, Tampa.

Laws, D. R., Meyer, J., & Holmen, M. L. (1978). Reduction of sadistic sexual arousal by olfactory aversion: A case study. *Behaviour Research and Therapy, 16,* 281–285.

Laws, D. R., & Osborn, C. A. (1983). How to build and operate a behavioral laboratory to evaluate and treat sexual deviance. In J. G. Greer & I. R. Stuart (Eds.), *The sexual aggressor* (pp. 293–335). New York: Van Nostrand Reinhold.

Maletzky, B. M. (1973). "Assisted" covert sensitization: A preliminary report. *Behavior Therapy, 3,* 381–388.

Maletzky, B. M. (1974). "Assisted" covert sensitization in the treatment of exhibitionism. *Journal of Consulting and Clinical Psychology, 42,* 34–40.

Maletzky, B. M. (1980). "Assisted" covert sensitization. In D. J. Cox & R. J. Daitzman (Eds.), *Exhibitionism: Description, assessment and treatment* (pp. 187–251). New York: Garland.

Marlatt, G. A., & Gordon, J. R. (Eds.). (1985). *Relapse prevention: Maintenance strategies in the treatment of addictive behaviors.* New York: Guilford.

Nichols, H. R., & Molinder, I. (1984). Multiphasic sex inventory. (Available from Nichols & Molinder, 437 Bowes Drive, Tacoma, WA 98466)

Pithers, W. D., & Laws, D. R. (1989). The penile plethysmograph: Uses and abuses in assessment and treatment of sexual aggressors. In B. Schwartz (Ed.), *A practitioner's guide to treatment of the incarcerated male sex offender* (pp. 83–91). Washington, DC: National Institute of Corrections.

Pithers, W. D., Marques, J. K., Gibat, C., & Marlatt, G. A. (1983). Relapse prevention with sexual aggressives: A self-control model of treatment and maintenance of change. In J. G. Greer & I. R. Stuart (Eds.), *The sexual aggressor* (pp. 214–239). New York: Van Nostrand Reinhold.

Tanner, J. M. (1962). *Growth at adolescence with a general consideration of the effects of heredity and environmental factors upon growth and maturation from birth to maturity* (2nd ed.). Oxford, UK: Blackwell.

Walen, S. R., DiGiuseppe, R., & Wessler, R. L. (1980). *A practitioner's guide to rational-emotive therapy.* New York: Oxford University Press.

Wessler, R. A., & Wessler, R. L. (1980). *The principles and practice of rational-emotive therapy.* San Francisco: Jossey-Bass.

24

Vermont Treatment Program for Sexual Aggressors

WILLIAM D. PITHERS
GARY R. MARTIN
GEORGIA F. CUMMING

The Vermont Treatment Program for Sexual Aggressors (VTPSA) was created by a special appropriation from the Vermont legislature in 1982. The initial funds supported treatment for only 16 incarcerated sex offenders. Our program currently encompasses 3 residential and 20 outpatient treatment sites, which provide services to 192 offenders in prison and in the community. Thus the VTPSA represents the first integrated, statewide system of inpatient and outpatient treatment for sex offenders.

The VTPSA was also the first therapy program to employ relapse prevention with sexual offenders. Relapse prevention remains the unifying theme across all of our treatment sites. Our model represents a substantial evolution from the initial publication adapting relapse prevention for sexual offenders (Pithers, Marques, Gibat, & Marlatt, 1983), and these modifications in relapse prevention for sexual offenders are contained in this chapter.

Although assessment and treatment techniques subsumed by relapse prevention are central to our program, sex offenders cannot be treated adequately by those procedures alone. We also employ a comprehensive range of therapeutic modalities, including individual, marital, and group psychotherapy; didactic classes; substance abuse counseling; vocational training; behavioral interventions; and psychohormonal therapies.

GLOBAL TREATMENT PHILOSOPHY

The VTPSA represents a systematic program of wide-ranging assessment and intervention designed to help individuals who have engaged in sexual abuse to learn cognitive and behavioral skills that enable them to reduce the probability of further victimizations.

Many different etiologies culminate in sexual assault. At a superficial level these may appear similar; however, the underlying motivation of each individual is considered unique. Therefore, the initial step in effective treatment is a thorough assessment to identify the specific behavioral excesses and deficits that predisposed each individual's sexual aggression. Assessment is also required to determine whether the offender can be treated effectively with available therapeutic modalities.

Since no single etiology accounts for all instances of sexual aggression, no single treatment applied inflexibly to all sexual aggressors will have a high rate of efficacy. Adequate treatment requires a broad range of relatively specific therapeutic components that may be applied selectively to the narrowly defined problems of each individual. Treatment is then prescribed to meet each individual's needs. To evaluate therapeutic progress, elements of the clinical assessment are repeated periodically. In this manner, treatment is performed effectively, efficiently, and expeditiously.

Since every participant in residential treatment returns to the community on parole, our program emphasizes a carefully monitored, progressive transition from a centralized inpatient unit to a regional outpatient therapy group. Therapeutic and supervisory services are intensified during this transitional period. All residential, transitional, and outpatient services are provided by specially trained therapists and probation or parole officers. In this manner, behavioral changes achieved during a relatively short period of residential or outpatient treatment may become enduring characteristics that enable the aggressor to function safely and productively in society.

RESIDENTIAL TREATMENT PROGRAMS

Admissions Criteria for Residential Treatment

All individuals incarcerated for sex offenses in Vermont are screened for potential evaluation at one of our residential programs. Individuals who adamantly declare disinterest in treatment or consistently deny responsibility for an offense are not permitted to undergo a complete evaluation. Similarly, individuals who have demonstrated a lifelong preference for antisocial acts are excluded from evaluation. Men who murdered or mutilated victims or who are impaired by a major psychiatric disorder are not evaluated for admission to treatment. When uncertain about an individual's appropriateness, we provisionally accept the offender for evaluation.

Individuals who have demonstrated a history of prosocial behaviors, with the exception of their sexually aggressive acts, represent the most acceptable candidates for treatment. Ideally, although involuntarily confined as a consequence of his criminal conviction, the offender voluntarily commits to treatment, since his active participation in the program is necessary. Clients who are initially reluctant may later make a voluntary commitment to treatment if they believe therapy is addressing their problems. Optimally, individuals entering treatment accept responsibility for their actions and have some degree of empathy for their victims. In reality, most offenders entering residential treatment minimize their responsibility and the extent of harm inflicted by their acts.

The following inclusionary and exclusionary criteria are used to screen offenders for the complete assessment required for potential entry to residential therapy within the VTPSA:

1. Candidates must be willing to enter the program.
2. Career criminals, with a history of multiple and varied offenses, are inappropriate candidates.
3. Individuals whose offenses involved sadistic aggression are excluded.
4. Prospective clients must agree to participate in a thorough assessment procedure.
5. The structure of the offender's sentence should provide adequate time for inpatient treatment and parole supervision after his return to the community.

Offenders who meet these screening criteria are referred for thorough psychosexual evaluation.

Psychosexual Evaluation

Psychosexual evaluation is conducted as part of the admission process to select the most appropriate candidates for therapy, during treatment to check progress, and periodically after release to detect signs of a potential return to behavior patterns associated with sexual aggression (i.e., the relapse process). The initial psychosexual evaluation consists of the following procedures: the Minnesota Multiphasic Personality Inventory (MMPI), the Psychosexual Assessment Battery, a structured interview, and a physiological evaluation of sexual arousal patterns.

Upon completion of the psychosexual evaluation, a final decision is made regarding appropriateness of the candidate for entry into the treatment program. If an individual is found inappropriate for entry, a memorandum explaining this finding is forwarded to the candidate's correctional caseworker. If the candidate is appropriate for entry to the VTPSA, an acceptance letter is sent to the client and his correctional caseworker, and the client is scheduled for entry upon availability of bed space.

Once a client has been admitted into a residential program, additional assessment techniques are employed to gain information about specific aspects of that individual's functioning. The additional assessment techniques include:

Attitudes Toward Women (Spence & Helmreich, 1978)
Autobiography (Long, Wuesthoff, & Pithers, Chapter 6, this volume)
Beck Depression Inventory (Beck, 1967)
Buss–Durkee Hostility Inventory (Buss & Durkee, 1957)
Clarke Sexual History Questionnaire (Langevin, 1983)
Cognitive Distortions Scale (Abel et al., 1984)
Fear of Negative Evaluation Scale (Watson & Friend, 1969)
Interpersonal Reactivity Index (Davis, 1980)
Millon Clinical Multiaxial Inventory (Millon, 1977)
Multiphasic Sex Inventory (Nichols & Molinder, 1984)
Novaco Anger Scale (Novaco, 1975)
Rape Myth Acceptance Scale (Burt, 1980)
Relapse Fantasies (Marlatt & Gordon, 1985)
Rotter Locus of Control Scale (Rotter, 1966)
Self-Monitoring (MacDonald & Pithers, Chapter 7, this volume)
Situational Competency Test (Chaney, O'Leary, & Marlatt, 1978)
Social Avoidance and Distress Scale (Watson & Friend, 1969)
State–Trait Anger Scale (Spielberger, Jacobs, Russel, & Crane, 1983)
State–Trait Anxiety Scale (Spielberger, Gorsuch, & Lushene, 1970)
Wechsler Adult Intelligent Scale—Revised (Wechsler, 1981)
Sex Fantasy Questionnaire (Wilson, 1978)

Residential Treatment Components

The assessment process yields a comprehensive analysis of the offender's behavioral excesses and deficits. On the basis of this information, a treatment program is prescribed by selecting an appropriate subset of intervention techniques from the battery of available treatment components. Thus a rapist who has difficulty appropriately expressing anger undergoes a treatment program different from that undergone by a pedophile who experiences sexual arousal exclusively to children.

Treatment Sequence

Treatment techniques selected for each offender are introduced sequentially, rather than simultaneously, to increase the likelihood of the client's mastering each skill. If all treatment components were implemented simultaneously, the client would likely be overwhelmed and fail to acquire important skills, potentially heightening a sense of personal inadequacy. It is also important to note that some skills must be acquired before others can be learned. In order to modulate expression of anger, for example, a client must first be able to recognize the cognitive and visceral changes indicating that he is angry.

Treatment generally begins with either a victim-empathy or arousal-disorder group, since both are directly related to the foundations of the offender's abusive behavior. Beginning in this fashion, clients become convinced that their treatment is relevant to their problems and invest themselves in it. Offenders may then derive greater benefit from therapeutic elements less directly related to sexual aggression (e.g., social skills training). The sequence with which therapeutic components are introduced can have a major impact on treatment outcome.

Although treatment is highly individualized, a general progression of therapeutic interventions and goals exists. The initial goal in treating sexual aggressors entails their accepting responsibility for their offenses and the harm inflicted on their victims. Once the offender acknowledges his problematic behaviors and develops empathy for the plight of victims, treatment moves on to remediate skill deficits. At this point, groups focusing on social skills, sexual knowledge, emotional management skills, and decision-making processes are implemented. Treatment progresses to helping the offender recognize the events, emotions, fantasies, and thoughts signifying the earliest stages of relapse. Strategies for coping with these risk factors and lessening the likelihood of relapse are then devised individually.

Residential Group Therapy Components

Both individual and group therapies are employed in the VTPSA. For reasons of treatment efficiency and efficacy, the treatment program emphasizes group therapy. Individual therapy is generally limited to 1 hour weekly. Marital and family therapy are conducted when appropriate. Separate therapy groups focus on the following areas:

1. *Victim empathy.* To the sexual aggressor, his victim may represent a faceless, impersonal entity. To encourage the abuser to acknowledge the full extent of harm caused by his actions and to recognize the victim as a thinking, feeling person, offenders are required to participate in groups designed to increase victim empathy. The structure of our victim-empathy groups is detailed elsewhere (Hildebran & Pithers, Chapter 21, this volume).

2. *Personal victimization.* Some sexual aggressors have themselves been

victims of such abuse. Providing an opportunity for these victim–offenders to discuss the effects of their own victimizations is essential. Often this experience enhances the offender's ability to empathize with his victims. Personal-victimization groups frequently enable offenders to experience emotions that have been suppressed since the time of their abuse. These are typically emotions that the offenders may have previously considered "weak" or "feminine."

3. *Emotional recognition.* Frequently, sexual aggressors report difficulties differentiating affective states. Among offenders harboring doubts about their masculinity, for example, every "nonmasculine" emotion is transformed into anger in order to confirm their masculinity. Emotional-recognition groups focus on the visceral changes accompanying various emotional states and the interrelationship between thought and emotion.

4. *Anger management.* Modulated expression of anger represents a major difficulty for many sexual aggressors. Expression of anger may be (1) inhibited, leading to a welling-up of emotion that gains expression explosively, (2) released indirectly through passive–aggressive behaviors that frustrate interactions with others, or (3) manifested continually as sullen withdrawal. The anger-management group demonstrates that anger can be expressed constructively and used to energize coping responses. Strategies for dealing with chronic, insidious anger are presented.

5. *Communication skills.* Inability to achieve satisfactory interpersonal relationships may play a role in the etiology of sexual aggression. Some offenders possess adequate communication skills but are inhibited by anxiety or belief systems; others simply lack these skills. The intent of this group is to enable expression of thoughts and feelings with regard for the rights of others. Continual role-playing of interpersonal situations is a major group element.

6. *Knowledge of sex.* Some sexual aggressors lack accurate information regarding sexual anatomy and functioning. In some instances, a strong sense of personal inadequacy results. In some cases, anticipation of a loving, intimate relationship is a source of anxiety, since the individual fears that sexual expression will lead to embarrassment rather than pleasure. The influence of attitudes toward sexuality is explored.

7. *Cognitive distortions.* Offenders frequently display thinking errors that justify sexual aggression. For example, an incestuous father may maintain that he was attempting to sexually educate a daughter, claiming that "it would be better for her to have her first sexual experience with somebody who loves her, rather than some teenager who just wants to use her." The cognitive-distortions group challenges thinking errors and presents an opportunity for offenders to acquire more realistic beliefs.

8. *Behavior therapy for sexual arousal disorders.* Excessive arousal to socially unacceptable sexual acts (e.g., rape) or victims (e.g., children) is logically related to sexual aggression. Individuals who reveal disordered sexual arousal

patterns participate in behavioral therapies to alter these patterns. Among the behavioral therapies employed are covert sensitization, masturbatory or verbal satiation, orgasmic reconditioning, and olfactory aversion. Descriptions of these behavior therapy procedures are widely available (see Greer & Stuart, 1983).

9. *Relapse prevention.* Our modification of relapse prevention is discussed in detail later in this chapter.

10. *Transition.* Movement from residential treatment to outpatient therapy poses special difficulties for offenders. To adjust more successfully during this phase of treatment, clients attend a transition group in which difficulties inherent in establishing an independent life and meeting the demands of community living are discussed. This group is attended both by residents about to leave the program and by former clients. Thus, clients on the verge of release from residential treatment benefit from the experiences of former residents.

11. *Problem-solving techniques.* Since it is impossible to anticipate every high-risk situation that an offender will encounter, it is necessary to enable him to devise coping responses to novel risk situations. A problem-solving strategy is employed to accomplish this goal. This strategy entails carefully defining risk situations, brainstorming to generate the maximum number of potential coping responses, evaluating the likelihood that each coping response will lead to the desired goal, and role-playing of the selected response.

Adjunctive Treatment Components

Individual psychotherapy is offered to support clients who are exploring difficult issues in group therapy and to confront clients who are reluctant to do so. Offenders planning to return to their families participate in marital and family therapy. If compulsive fantasies of sexual aggression are evident, antiandrogenic treatment is administered by a consulting psychiatrist or endocrinologist on receipt of the offender's informed consent. Substance abuse counseling is employed when relevant. These individual treatment components further increase the flexibility of our treatment program in addressing the client's specific needs.

Treatment Probation for Lack of Progress

Any individual who is making insufficient progress in treatment is alerted to this fact by staff and placed on 1-month probation within the treatment program. A contract specifying behavioral changes required to regain good standing is given to the client. At the end of this probationary period, the client may be reinstated to good standing, continued on program probation, or transferred from the treatment program to another correctional setting. Any individual who exited unfavorably has the option to apply for reentry.

Criteria for Transition from Residential to Outpatient Treatment

To gain release from the VTPSA, clients must demonstrate consistent and enduring behavioral changes. The precise pattern of changes necessary depends on the individual client. Each offender begins treatment with a unique constellation of behavioral excesses and deficits; the changes in functioning that must be observed prior to release from the residential program are specific to each individual.

The following general objectives must be met prior to recommending release from residential treatment:

1. The offender must be able to describe his high-risk situations in detail.
2. For each high-risk situation, the resident must be able, without hesitation, to verbalize or role-play coping responses to reduce the potential of sexual aggression.
3. The offender is required to anticipate new risk situations that may be encountered and devise effective coping responses for each circumstance.
4. Each offender is expected to perceive and modulate an adequate range of emotions, and an ability to express anger verbally and appropriately, rather than through sexualized aggression, is mandatory.
5. Every offender must demonstrate his understanding that every person in society has a right to define his/her own sex role, providing that role is not illegal.
6. If he has shown a disordered pattern of sexual arousal (i.e., arousal to children or sexual aggression), the offender must demonstrate decreased arousal to such stimuli and increased arousal to consensual sex between adults.

Transitional Release Process

At an appropriate stage of treatment and under adequate supervision, each offender practices his newly acquired behaviors in the community on time-limited passes. When an individual demonstrates continued progress in residential therapy and appropriate behavior during furloughs, he is placed on work release. This enables the offender to obtain employment in the community but requires him to return to the correctional facility during nonwork hours. After a period of successful work release, the offender receives extended furloughs. During this phase of treatment, the client resides in the community, but his freedom of movement is restricted to approved locations at designated hours. During the work-release and extended-furlough phases of treatment, the client continues to participate in treatment at the facility. He also begins to attend outpatient therapy groups, which will be the sole source of treatment once he is released on parole. If the offender demonstrates highly appropriate behaviors throughout the extended-furlough phase of treatment, he is recommended for parole. Upon receiving parole, the client is mandated to attend outpatient therapy groups facilitated by specially trained treatment providers. In this manner, the transition from residential to outpatient treatment is accomplished in a carefully controlled, progressive manner. Since family members and probation and parole officers represent important resources in monitoring the behaviors of sex offenders, clients are required to sign confidentiality waivers and to inform these individuals about their risk factors and offense patterns. By following this structured and collaborative approach to treatment and maintenance of change, the probability of therapeutic success and community safety may be enhanced.

OUTPATIENT TREATMENT

The VTPSA provides outpatient therapy for individuals receiving probationary sentences from the court and for the long-term follow-up of offenders discharged from residential treatment. Attendance at outpatient therapy is mandated as a condition of probation or parole.

In 1983, the first outpatient sex offender treatment group affiliated with the VTPSA was established. The target population was pedophiles who either had been released to the community after incarceration or had been convicted and placed on probation. Currently, comprehensive outpatient services for most paraphilias exist in each of Vermont's 14 counties, with rapists and pedophiles representing the vast majority of our clientele. Specialized group therapy is the primary treatment modality, although adjunctive individual, conjoint, family, and psychohormonal treatment are also available.

Pedophiles and rapists were initially placed in separate outpatient groups. While many of these early outpatient groups continue to be offense-specific, more recently we have mixed offender subtypes and believe that this yields greater therapeutic impact. Rapists tend to be more confrontational than pedophiles, energizing the group; pedophiles tend to be more empathetic than rapists, lending the group some compassion. Groups are generally cofacilitated by a male and female therapist. Probation officers serve as cofacilitators in some groups—but never in a group containing an offender whom they must also supervise.

Funding and Quality Assurance of Outpatient Therapy

The Vermont Department of Corrections subsidizes all outpatient treatment of sexual offenders through contracts with vendors in the public and private sectors. These contracts guarantee providers a minimum annual income from each therapy group. Thus, even if offenders fail to pay for their services according to a sliding fee scale (a violation of probation conditions), treatment providers are supported. Over time, the contractually guaranteed funds supplement offender payments during the first year of a group's existence. Most outpatient groups are entirely self-supporting after the first year, and thereafter the contractually guaranteed funds are rarely expended.

The unique characteristics of sexually aggressive males require that treatment personnel maintain specialized skills. Therefore, all outpatient treatment providers are contractually required to participate in specialized training and ongoing consultation. Probation and parole personnel, trained in the relapse prevention model of client supervision, coordinate their efforts with those of treatment providers. By maintaining frequent contact, the functioning of both the mental health practitioner and probation and parole officer is enhanced.

Admission Criteria for Outpatient Treatment

Recommendations for outpatient versus inpatient treatment are made on a case-by-case basis. However, guidelines are employed in making recommendations about treatment placement to the court. Generally, incest offenders and many extrafamilial child abusers are considered appropriate candidates for outpatient treatment. With these offender subtypes, probation conditions may be implemented to prohibit access to high-risk situations. In contrast, inpatient treatment is recommended most frequently for rapists and for pedophiles who demonstrate preference for sexual acts with children rather than adults (i.e., fixated pedophiles). High-risk situations for fixated pedophiles are simply too numerous to be dealt with in outpatient therapy or through restrictive probation conditions. The interpersonal violence of the rapist, as well as the short warning period prior to rapes, mandate residential treatment.

The court (or parole board) may be requested to impose special conditions of probation (or parole) to prohibit involvement in high-risk situations. Through special conditions of probation the offender may be required to:

1. Participate in offender treatment as directed by the probation officer and to assume the costs of treatment
2. Pay for therapy required by his victims
3. Make restitution to victims for out-of-pocket expenses incurred as a result of the offense

4. Refrain from purchase, possession, or consumption of alcoholic beverages and regulated drugs
5. Submit to alcosensor and/or urinalysis testing as requested by the probation officer
6. Engage in alcohol and/or drug counseling as directed by the probation officer
7. Abstain from purchase or possession of pornographic materials
8. Avoid operating a motor vehicle after dark (or during specified hours when children are going to and leaving school), except for purposes of verified employment, unless in the company of another adult deemed responsible by the probation officer
9. Adhere to a curfew specified by the probation officer
10. Refrain from hitchhiking or picking up hitchhikers
11. Agree not to establish or maintain contact with any minor child or to reside in the same residence with minor children without permission of the probation officer
12. Reside where the probation officer directs
13. Refrain from purchase, possession, and use of firearms

Offenders referred for outpatient therapy are required to sign a treatment contract at the time of sentencing that is entered into the probation document as a special condition. The treatment contract specifies that the offender is, or may be, required to:

1. Assume full responsibility for his offense and behavior
2. Apologize to his victim and acknowledge his responsibility
3. Sign a waiver of confidentiality
4. Attend all sessions and pay for them in a timely fashion
5. Refrain from disclosing information about other clients to anyone outside of the treatment program
6. Participate actively in treatment and demonstrate progress
7. Complete special assignments (e.g., autobiography, victim-empathy readings, behavioral therapies to alter disordered sexual arousal patterns)
8. Encourage significant others to participate in the treatment process
9. Participate in plethysmographic assessment of sexual arousal pattern
10. Refrain from possessing pornography
11. Discuss in treatment any contact with other clients occurring outside of treatment
12. Adhere to any additional contractual requirements that may be invoked to restrict access to the offender's high-risk situations

Clients who fail to adhere to requirements delineated in the probation and treatment contracts may be returned to court for a violation hearing, which may result in the offender's spending his full sentence in prison. Expeditious processing of probation violations enhances participation of remaining group members.

Group Candidacy and Membership

Outpatient group involvement follows a three-level, hierarchical structure: candidacy, membership, and aftercare. Each level in the hierarchy entails greater responsibility and independence (Ballantyne & Petty, 1988).

Offenders entering outpatient groups are initially considered treatment candidates for a month or more. A treatment candidate must request to be elevated to membership status in the group and present a rationale as to why he has earned that status. The group then discusses the candidate's therapeutic involvement and his assistance to other group participants. At the end of this discussion, the candidate stands and is encircled by group members. The candidate must ask each member for his vote and the reasons for his vote. If a member gives a negative response, he must specify what the candidate can do to change his perception. To gain membership, consensus of group members and the cotherapists is necessary. Group members are entitled to give input regarding changes in group structure and development of the group's weekly agenda. However, the cotherapists possess final authority in all decisions.

Group members rotate in filling the role of group scribe. The scribe maintains a notebook that records the date, the people present, the agenda, and the issues covered in group that week. The scribe is responsible for insuring that the meeting runs efficiently, obtaining involvement of more passive participants by seeking their input on issues if necessary, and monitoring the adequacy of each offender's opening statement.

Groups generally consist of six to eight members and one to two candidates. Each group meets weekly for 1.5 to 2 hours. Both candidates and members must pay their group fee to one of the two cotherapists prior to the group.

After fees have been paid and recorded, group members engage in an opening ritual. Each member stands, recites his name, paraphilias, victims' names, and risk factors. He then details any fantasies, urges, lapses, high-risk situations, and sexual behaviors that he engaged in during the past week. If clients consistently raise issues that are unrelated to their sexual offending, they are referred to individual or conjoint therapy to address these problems. Group candidates follow members in completing the opening ritual.

Issues raised during the opening ritual are handled through the standard relapse prevention treatment strategies discussed in Part III of this volume. After these concerns have been addressed, participants present their homework assignments. Homework assignments include audiotapes of covert-sensitization sessions, reports on selected books intended to promote victim empathy, apology letters to victims, sexual autobiographies, victim-impact essays, or any of the therapeutic tasks subsumed by relapse prevention (e.g., decision matrices). Particularly in new groups, clients will have worked on the same assignment. However, as groups age, homework assignments grow less uniform. Some individuals may not have completed an assignment to the satisfaction of the cotherapists and been required to resubmit the task. New members will need to begin homework that older members have completed. The cofacilitators ultimately decide whether an assignment is accepted, but group members are responsible for critiquing assignments. When offenders are unable to read or write, assignments are completed via audiotape. At the same time, illiterate individuals are referred to remedial programs, since functional impediments often affect self-esteem.

As in our residential treatment programs, whenever participation of a group candidate or member lags, he is placed on program probation. The offender receives a document specifying the behaviors that have led to his placement on program probation and the changes that must be manifested within 30 days in order to regain good standing in treatment. If the client does not demonstrate adequate change within the probation period, he is demoted in group status. Members become candidates, while candidates are referred to court for a probation-violation hearing and possible imprisonment.

TWO DIMENSIONS OF RELAPSE PREVENTION: INTERNAL AND EXTERNAL CONTROL

Internal, Self-Management Dimension

Relapse prevention was originally developed as a method of enhancing maintenance of change by clients who were in treatment for compulsive behavioral disorders (e.g., substance abuse, compulsive gambling). As originally articulated by Marlatt and his colleagues (Chaney et al., 1978; Marlatt, 1982; Marlatt & Gordon, 1980, 1985), relapse prevention was designed to strengthen self-control by providing clients with methods for identifying problematic situations; analyzing decisions that precipitated situations enabling a return to the compulsive behavior; and developing strategies to avoid, or cope more effectively with, these risky circumstances. Thus, as originally proposed, relapse prevention represented a method of enhancing self-management skills.

When first modified for application to sexual aggressors (Pithers et al., 1983), relapse prevention remained solely a means of enhancing offenders' self-control. The initial application of relapse prevention in the VTPSA (Pithers, 1982) demonstrated that the maintenance model appeared effective in aiding self-management. A statewide network of outpatient group therapists who participated in relapse prevention training was established to assist client maintenance. Relapse prevention successfully accomplished the goals of increasing the client's awareness and range of choices concerning his behavior, developing specific coping skills and self-control capacities, and creating a general sense of mastery over life. This aspect of the modified relapse prevention model is now referred to as the internal, self-management dimension (Pithers, Cumming, Beal, Young, & Turner, 1989).

Unfortunately, while the internal, self-management dimension of relapse prevention often worked well, sexual aggressors frequently neglected to employ their new skills at certain critical moments. Although the importance of acknowledging lapses to therapists and probation and parole officers was repeatedly stressed during therapy, and the mythical goal of attaining behavioral perfection was dismissed frequently, clients leaving the inpatient treatment unit sometimes neglected to inform us of their lapses. Occasionally lapses were reported to our treatment team by a released offender's spouse, friends, or coworkers but not by the client himself. Even when offenders recognized that other clients who self-reported lapses were reinforced by receiving therapeutic intervention and maintaining access to the community, while those whose lapses were reported by third parties received punitive consequences, the trend toward secrecy at critical moments remained.

Generally, relapse prevention appeared to enhance sex offenders' self-management skills by decreasing the frequency of lapses. However, when lapses occurred, offenders often did their best to deny them to individuals involved in their treatment and supervision, and possibly to themselves. At critical moments determining the difference between lapse and relapse, the internal, self-management dimension of relapse prevention sometimes proved inadequate. Offenders either believed that acknowledging lapses would lead to their being returned to prison for parole violations or that their problems would go away if they just did not think about them. Thus, although the internal, self-management dimension of relapse prevention was beneficial in enhancing self-control, it did not prove adequate.

External, Supervisory Dimension

Since offenders are at times unreliable informants regarding lapses, creating other methods of gaining access to information about their functioning was considered essential. In order to enhance community safety, an external, supervisory dimension of the relapse prevention model was developed (Pithers, Kashima, Cumming, Beal, & Buell, 1987, 1988). The external, supervisory dimension serves three functions: (1) enhancing efficacy of probation or parole supervision by monitoring of specific offense precursors, (2) increasing efficiency of supervision by creating an informed network of collateral contacts to assist the probation officer in monitoring the offender's behaviors, and

(3) creating a collaborative relationship between the probation officer and mental health professionals conducting therapy with the offender.

Traditionally, probation or parole supervision of sexual offenders was a challenging enterprise. Gaining information essential to adequate supervision of a sexual offender was considered a nearly impossible feat. Parole violations noted frequently among many offenders (e.g., intoxication, neglect of supervision appointments, failure to pay restitution) were rarely noted among sex offenders. Often the lack of detailed information about the offender's behaviors produced a sense of attempting to conduct supervision within a vacuum, a disquieting feeling in an age of heightened professional liability.

In contrast, specification of an offender's apparently irrelevant decisions, high-risk situations, and offense precursors provides probation and parole officers with identifiable indicators of impending danger of relapse. Since probation and parole officers monitor specific risk factors that are related to the client's sexual offenses (rather than attempting to keep an eye on all his behaviors, many of which have no bearing on his reoffending), efficiency of the probation and parole officer's functioning is increased. Whenever the probation or parole officer detects the presence of an offense precursor, he/she has determined that the sexual offender is involved in his relapse process. Since offense precursors appear most commonly in a distinct sequence, that is, emotion–fantasy–cognitive distortion–plan–act (Pithers et al., 1983), the type of precursor exhibited provides an indication of the imminence of potential relapse. With this information, the parole officer may determine the type of intervention required by an offender's lapse (e.g., additional condition of parole, consultation with offender's therapist, parole revocation).

A second element of the external, supervisory dimension of relapse prevention entails the instruction of collateral contacts on the principles of relapse prevention. All members of the collateral network (e.g., spouse, employer, coworkers, friends) are informed about apparently irrelevant decisions, high-risk situations, lapses, the abstinence violation effect, and offense precursors. They learn that assisting the offender's identification of factors involved in his relapse process will increase the likelihood of his avoiding a reoffense. In the offender's presence, network members are encouraged to report lapses to the parole officer or therapist.

Care must be exercised in evaluating the ability of collateral contacts to serve this function. A fearful spouse who has been battered into submissiveness is unlikely to disclose information about her husband if she fears additional abuse. Similarly, wives who are overdependent on their husbands may be reticent to risk providing any information that could potentially get their husbands into trouble. Employers who treasure the compulsive work habits of some sexual offenders may be reluctant to mention information that they fear could lead to loss of good employees. Certain religiously devout individuals, who believe they can show their love for others by forgiving them their misdeeds, may do so rather than tell others. Community members who express hatred for offenders may fabricate reports of their misbehaviors in an effort to damage them. Management of the collateral network demands good judgment.

By eliciting cooperation from the collateral network, and training them in the intricacies of relapse prevention, efficacy of probation and parole supervision is enhanced. Rather than attempting to monitor the offender's behaviors alone, individuals who have more contact with the offender can help. This process creates an extended supervisory network.

We require the offender to inform network members about his offense precursors. The probation and parole officer later requests each network member to summarize what he/she was told. By following this procedure, two goals are accomplished. First, the accuracy and completeness of information presented by the offender can be evaluated, enabling the parole officer to estimate how well the offender understands his offense precursors and the importance others have to his behavioral maintenance. Second, informing the offender's extended network about his offense precursors destroys the secrecy necessary for commission of sexual aggression. Behaviors that once may have seemed unimportant to others, but that were centrally involved in the relapse process, can then be recognized as signs for concern.

The final element of the external, supervisory dimension of relapse prevention is the liaison between the probation officer and mental health professional. Regularly scheduled meetings between these professionals are essential. By reviewing case-specific information, the probation officer and mental health clinician may discern aspects of the offender's behaviors that were previously unknown. Early in outpatient treatment, it is not unusual to discover that the offender has discussed an important issue with only one of the two (or more) professionals involved in his care. In other instances, the offender may depict an event differently to each professional in his treatment and supervision network.

During regular meetings between the probation officer and mental health professional, the extent and consistency of the offender's disclosures may be compared. In addition to insuring that each professional possesses all available information, these meetings also enable detection of the client's efforts to split his supervisory team. Since scheduled meetings allow the routine exchange of information, telephone calls and messages between meetings are regarded as indications of critical events to be dealt with immediately rather than as needlessly annoying disruptions in an overburdened schedule.

The combined functions of collateral contacts and specially trained probation professionals, along with the collaborative relationship between probation and mental health professionals, are referred to as the external, supervisory dimension of the relapse prevention model. Since offenders are not consistently reliable informants regarding their own relapse processes, establishing these additional resources is vital to adequate treatment and supervision and, therefore, to the safety of potential victims. Taken together, the internal and external dimensions of relapse prevention offer improvements over traditional treatment approaches to sexual offenders.

Criteria for Exiting Outpatient Groups

Group members are required to meet stringent criteria prior to gaining approval to exit outpatient therapy. The client must demonstrate acceptable scores on all psychometric inventories and the penile plethysmograph. The ability to recognize, and respond adaptively to, apparently irrelevant decisions and high-risk situations must have been demonstrated by the client's involvement in treatment and his behaviors in the community. He is required to have completed all probation conditions (e.g., payment for victim's treatment). Completion of all homework assignments is mandatory. Adequate use of recreational time is necessary. The client must also agree to participate once a month in an aftercare group until expiration of probation or parole. Aftercare groups are essentially support groups that meet without involvement of treatment professionals. In addition, an offender may be maintained under probation or parole supervision even though he has progressed out of formal therapy.

Once a group member believes he has met all the exit criteria, he must request a vote of group members. The procedure employed to vote on group membership is also employed to decide group exits. An unanimous vote, including those of group cofacilitators, is required for approval.

CONCLUSION

Mental health and correctional professionals working with sexual aggressors bear a tremendous social responsibility. The ultimate goal of sex offender treatment is increasing the safety of the community. Therefore, the need to provide intensive supervision and therapy for sexual aggressors cannot be stressed too empathically. Only through the combined efforts of mental health and probation or parole professionals can we enhance the probability that changes induced by treatment will be maintained after formal therapy has ended. In this fashion, the number of people who must face the trauma of sexual abuse will be reduced.

REFERENCES

Abel, G. G., Becker, J. V., Cunningham-Rathner, J., Rouleau, J., Kaplan, M., & Reich, J. (1984). *The treatment of child molesters.* (Available from SBC-TM, 722 West 168th Street, Box 17, NY, NY 10032)

Ballantyne, W., & Petty, J. (1988). A *hierarchical model of group membership.* (Available from William Ballantyne, West Central Mental Health Services, West Lebanon, NH 03784)

Beck, A. T. (1967). *Depression: Causes and treatment.* Philadelphia: University of Pennsylvania Press.

Burt, M. R. (1980). Cultural myths and supports for rape. *Journal of Personality and Social Psychology, 38,* 217–230.

Buss, A. H., & Durkee, A. (1957). An inventory for assessing different kinds of hostility. *Journal of Consulting Psychology, 21,* 343–349.

Chaney, E. F., O'Leary, M. R., & Marlatt, G. A. (1978). Skill training with alcoholics. *Journal of Consulting and Clinical Psychology, 46,* 1092–1104.

Davis, M. H. (1980). A multidimensional approach to individual differences in empathy. *JSAS Catalog of Selected Documents in Psychology, 10,* 85.

Greer, J. G., & Stuart, I. R. (Eds.). (1983). *The sexual aggressor: Current perspectives on treatment.* New York: Van Nostrand Reinhold.

Langevin, R. (1983). *Sexual strands: Understanding and treating sex anomalies in men.* Hillsdale, NJ: Erlbaum.

Marlatt, G. A. (1982). Relapse prevention: A self-control program for the treatment of addictive behaviors. In R. B. Stuart (Ed.). *Adherence, compliance, and generalization in behavioral medicine.* New York: Brunner/Mazel.

Marlatt, G. A., & Gordon, J. (1980). Determinants of relapse: Implications for the maintenance of change. In P. O. Davidson & S. M. Davidson (Eds.), *Behavioral medicine: Changing health lifestyles.* New York: Brunner/Mazel.

Marlatt, G. A., & Gordon, J. R. (Eds.). (1985). *Relapse prevention: Maintenance strategies in the treatment of addictive behaviors.* New York: Guilford.

Millon, T. (1977). *Millon Clinical Multiaxial Inventory: Manual.* Minneapolis: NCS Interpretive Scoring Systems.

Nichols, H. R., & Molinder, I. (1984). *Multiphasic Sex Inventory.* (Available from Nichols & Molinder, 437 Bowes Drive, Tacoma, WA 98466)

Novaco, R. W. (1975). *Anger control: The development and evaluation of an experimental treatment.* Lexington, MA: Lexington Books.

Pithers, W. D. (1982). *The Vermont Treatment Program for Sexual Aggressors: A program description.* Waterbury: Vermont Department of Corrections.

Pithers, W. D., Cumming, G. F., Beal, L. S., Young, W., & Turner, R. (1989). Relapse prevention: A method for enhancing behavioral self-management and external supervision of the sexual aggressor. In B. Schwartz (Ed.), *A practitioner's guide to the treatment of the incarcerated male sex offender* (pp. 121–135). Washington, DC: National Institute of Corrections.

Pithers, W. D., Kashima, K., Cumming, G. F., Beal, L. S., & Buell, M. (1987, January). *Sexual aggression: An addictive process?* Paper presented at the New York Academy of Sciences, New York, NY.

Pithers, W. D., Kashima, K., Cumming, G. F., Beal, L. S., & Buell, M. (1988). Relapse prevention of sexual aggression. In R. Prentky & V. Quinsey (Eds.), *Human sexual aggression: Current perspectives* (pp. 244–260). New York: New York Academy of Sciences.

Pithers, W. D., Marques, J. K., Gibat, C. C., & Marlatt, G. A. (1983). Relapse prevention with sexual aggressives: A self-control model of treatment and maintenance of change. In J. G. Greer & I. R. Stuart (Eds.), *The sexual aggressor: Current perspectives on treatment* (pp. 214–239). New York: Van Nostrand Reinhold.

Rotter, J. B. (1966). Generalized expectancies for internal versus external control of reinforcement. *Psychological Monographs, 80* (1).

Spence, J. T., & Helmreich, R. L. (1978). *Masculinity and femininity: Their psychological dimensions, correlates and antecedents.* Austin: University of Texas Press.

Spielberger, C. D., Gorsuch, R. L., & Lushene, R. E. (1970). *Manual for the State–Trait Anxiety Inventory.* Palo Alto, CA: Consulting Psychologists Press.

Spielberger, C. D., Jacobs, G., Russel, S., & Crane, R. S. (1983). Assessment of anger: The State–Trait Anger Scale. In J. N. Butcher & C. D. Spielberger (Eds.), *Advances in personality assessment* (Vol. 2, pp. 159–187). Hillsdale, NJ: Erlbaum.

Watson, D., & Friend, R. (1969). Measurement of social-evaluative anxiety. *Journal of Consulting and Clinical Psychology, 33,* 448–457.

Weshsler, D. (1981). *Manual for the Wechsler Adult Intelligence Scale—Revised.* New York: Psychological Corporation.

Wilson, G. (1978). *The secrets of sexual fantasy.* London: Dent.

V

CAN RELAPSES BE PREVENTED?

In this final section Pithers and Cumming present some initial outcome data from the Vermont Treatment Program for Sexual Aggressors. This program was selected for this task because it has the largest number of offenders in long-term follow-up, the critical test of RP efficacy.

They begin their discussion with a consideration of the ways in which RP offers distinct advantages over traditional treatment models. Examination of these factors provides some clarification of why the recidivism statistics on sex offender treatment programs have been so uniformly dismal over the years.

They next compare outcome data from the Vermont RP program with data from the former program for Mentally Disordered Sex Offenders at Atascadero State Hospital in California, in its day one of the largest of the traditional programs. The data are clearly in favor of the RP approach.

Importantly, and this bears continuing attention, RP was significantly more effective with pedophiles than with rapists. This finding, which was touched on earlier in this volume, suggests different psychological dynamics in these two offender classes. Further consideration of these issues is beyond the scope of the current work.

25

Can Relapses Be Prevented?
Initial Outcome Data from the Vermont
Treatment Program for Sexual Aggressors

WILLIAM D. PITHERS
GEORGIA F. CUMMING

RELAPSE PREVENTION OR RELAPSE REDUCTION?

When one works with clients whose acts are as socially and personally distressing as those of sexual aggressors, the promise inherent in a treatment approach called "relapse prevention" (RP) can be enticing. An intervention nominally proposing to *prevent relapse* of sexual offenders holds appeal, since such crimes traumatize victims, damage families, threaten members of society who might prefer to deny existence of such danger to their personal safety, and frequently are repeated by individuals who had been previously apprehended and incarcerated for sexual violence. A maintenance model known as relapse prevention appears to offer an implicit promise: Follow these procedures and the problem will not recur.

Considered from this perspective, relapse prevention clearly is misnamed. No existing therapeutic intervention can prevent relapses. Referring to any treatment model as relapse prevention implicitly, if not explicitly, purveys a false assurance of effectiveness.

A central premise of the relapse prevention model, that people make decisions that influence the probability of problematic behaviors recurring, alludes to the reason that no intervention can prevent relapses. All clients, including sexual aggressors, make their own decisions. Despite the best efforts of mental health providers to provide sexual aggressors with enhanced decision-making skills and greater empathy for abuse victims, some sex offenders will choose to continue their pattern of interpersonal violence. Rather than concluding that relapses signify that treatment is ineffective and ending all efforts to deter victimization, awareness of the potential for reoffenses should make treatment providers and society eager to take every possible measure to enhance therapeutic efficacy and community safety.

ADVANTAGES OF RELAPSE PREVENTION OVER TRADITIONAL TREATMENT MODELS

While no constellation of interventions prevents relapse, the procedures deline-ated in this text may enable reduction of relapse rates. Comparing various approaches to treatment and maintenance of change in sexual offenders, Pith-ers, Cumming, Beal, Young, and Turner (1989) found that modified relapse prevention offers several advantages: (1) a more realistic therapeutic goal of control versus cure, (2) progressive transition versus abrupt discontinuation of treatment, (3) reliance on multiple versus single sources of information about client maintenance, (4) integration versus disaffiliation of mental health and probation or parole professionals, and (5) definition of behavioral maintenance as a continuum rather than an abstinence–relapse dichotomy.

Therapeutic Control as a Treatment Goal

Historically, sex offender treatment programs operated solely within total insti-tutions (e.g., prisons or maximum security state hospitals). Such programs were founded on the notion that sex offenses were performed by individuals afflicted with "sexual psychopathy." Between 1938 and 1966, 31 states enacted sexual psychopath statutes. Typically, if found to be a "sexually dangerous person" after a psychiatric interview, the offender was civilly committed to institutional treatment for an indeterminate period. Typically, no aftercare was provided once a client was discharged from the treatment institution.

Although the creation of sexual psychopath statutes and institutional treatment programs were well intended, recent meta-analyses of outcome data from these early efforts have demonstrated that the enterprise was a failure (Furby, Weinrott, & Blackshaw, 1989). Recidivism data from these early institu-tional programs have been used to argue that the efficacy of sex offender treatment has not been proved (Brecher, 1978). Citing these data, a group representing the psychiatric profession has advocated incarceration, rather than treatment, of sexual aggressors (Group for the Advancement of Psychiatry, 1977).

Nearly all of the initial programs for sex offenders adopted the central premise of the medical model: Treatment enables cure. Within this framework, if a disorder is sufficiently severe, therapeutic intervention might necessitate hospitalization. In many disorders, the medical model functions quite well, but in regard to sex offenders, treatment programs adopting the medical model concept of "cure" have generally been eliminated rather than the disorder they attempted to address. Treatment programs based on sexual psychopath statutes remain active in only five states. Thus, abundant evidence converges to the conclusion that treatment programs conducted solely within institutions are ineffective in lessening the probability of future sexual abuse.

For some disorders, within our current state of technology, cure is not possible. Sexual aggressors cannot be cured. They are not afflicted by a disease. Providing offenders with the hope of an irreversible elimination of their disorder establishes an expectation that assures failure. Encouraging offenders to believe that behavioral perfection is attainable insures a sense of personal inadequacy when lapses in self-management are inevitably encountered.

Many forms of therapy fail to prepare clients for lapses (i.e., the moods, fantasies, and thoughts associated with the relapse process). This neglect appears to have two sources: a belief that treatment can cure sex offenders or a fear that predicting recurrence of lapses licenses the offender to have them freely.

Anyone who believes that discussing the likelihood of lapses encourages their occurrence should forbid their children to participate in fire drills at school, neglect to inform them about the existence of child abusers, and refrain from telling them about methods to avoid contracting Acquired Immune Deficiency Syndrome. Obviously, it is better to instruct people in how to identify and deal with risky situations so that they can avert disastrous experiences, rather than pretending such dangers do not exist.

Progressive Transitions in Treatment

Most institutional treatment programs for sex offenders do not provide specialized care during the offender's transition from prison to the community. Typically, outpatient therapy begins only after inpatient therapy ends. In our approach to relapse prevention, therapeutic change cascades. That is, the next step in the client's therapy always begins before the existing stage of treatment is phased out.

A highly structured exit sequence is employed within the Vermont Treatment Program for Sexual Aggressors (VTPSA). When an offender in inpatient treatment is ready to progress to the next stage of therapy, he enters a special transition group containing men who are leaving, or have recently left, inpatient therapy. If behavioral maintenance continues during this phase, the offender receives unsupervised furloughs and enters a regional, outpatient treatment group while also continuing his involvement in the transition group. When the offender demonstrates self-management under conditions of greater freedom, he is placed on extended furlough in the community, continuing his participation in the outpatient and transition groups. Given prolonged behavioral maintenance, the offender is recommended for parole and progresses into solely outpatient treatment. If the offender demonstrates maintenance in outpatient therapy for several years, he may enter a self-help group. Thus a slow progression of overlapping treatment stages is provided to assist the offender's reentry into the community.

Treatment within the relapse prevention model never ends. Offenders who believe they have successfully completed treatment are making an "apparently irrelevant decision" (AID) predisposing their own relapse. Sexual aggressors must continually monitor their moods, thoughts, and behaviors in an effort to discern the earliest possible sign of their relapse process. Those who neglect to do so are primed for relapse.

Reliance on Multiple Sources of Information

Exclusive reliance on a sex offender's self-report to assess maintenance of change simply is not a good idea. Sex offenders have numerous incentives to misrepresent their progress in treatment. To the extent that the offender likes and wishes to please his therapist, he may be tempted to propose that he has made great progress when he actually has not. Individuals paying their way through outpatient treatment may need to justify (or attempt to end) the expenditure by making a fictitious claim of attitudinal and behavioral change.

Traditional treatment relies almost exclusively on the client's self-reports and the therapist's intuitions to evaluate improvement. Since sex offenders have strong incentives to misrepresent their progress, and therapists' intuitions have never been empirically validated, additional sources of information must be sought. Modified relapse prevention within the VTPSA formalizes mechanisms for acquiring information from others who have the opportunity to observe the offender's behaviors. In this fashion, the offender's behavioral maintenance and therapeutic compliance are examined more thoroughly, and important decisions are less often made on the basis of misinformation.

Integration of Parole and Mental Health Professionals

Profound disaffiliation often exists between mental health practitioners and correctional professionals. This distrust appears to develop because the two professional groups seldom work in an integrated fashion. Typically, both groups work independently with the same difficult clients, feel frustrated at their own perceived lack of efficacy in helping the clients change (clinicians' perspective) or in monitoring their criminal behaviors (parole officers' perspective), and blame the other profession for undermining their efforts.

The notion of working together appears alien because the goals of the professionals often seem divergent and little trust exists between the two. Each group makes different assumptions about the client. Mental health providers traditionally are thought to regard clients with genuineness, empathy, and warmth, while correctional workers are believed to consider clients manipulative, callous, and immoral.

The structure of relapse prevention helps to mend this professional chasm. By working together with a common goal of deterring sexual victimization of others, each profession learns how the other can facilitate its own effectiveness. Mental health clinicians discover that parole officers can acquire information that is essential to evaluating efficacy of treatment. Parole officers find that mental health professionals can provide detailed information about the offender's moods, cognitive distortions, and fantasies that is normally unavailable to them. By sharing information under a full waiver of client confidentiality, collaborating professionals are vastly more effective than competing ones.

Relapse prevention offers professionally neutral language and concepts. Rather than attempting to collaborate with someone who seems to be speaking a foreign language, members of both professions can easily adopt the concepts of relapse prevention. Since neither profession can lay exclusive claim to knowledge of AIDs, high-risk situations, lapses, offense precursors, and relapse processes, each group can employ the concepts with equal levels of understanding and ownership.

Maintenance Viewed as a Continuum

Although one might assume that sex offender treatment models based on therapeutic approaches to addictive behaviors would be similar to their progenitors, comparison of relapse prevention and "12-steps" programs reveals major differences in orientation and implication.

Carnes (1983) provides superb insight into the phenomenology of sexual "addicts." However, he proposes that sexual addicts may be treated through adaptation of the "12-steps" of Alcoholics Anonymous (AA). Under Carnes's treatment model, participants attend self-help groups, with ancillary therapy for "co-addicts" (i.e., spouses). Following the 12-steps model, sex addicts subscribe to tenets advocating that troubled individuals must be in total control of their problematic behavior at all times. The addict is considered to be either absolutely in control or absolutely out of control. No intermediate stages exist. As long as an addict maintains perfect behavioral control, 12-steps tenets represent useful concepts. However, anything less than total control is considered total failure.

Unfortunately, human beings never maintain absolute control over their behaviors across time and situations. Rather than being in either absolute control or absolute dyscontrol, most of us find that, at any moment, our behavioral management falls somewhere on a continuum between the two extremes. Our ability to exert behavioral control is affected by many internal and external variables. Thus encouraging individuals to accept beliefs that hold them totally responsible for maintaining absolute behavioral control is an unrealistic, and possibly dangerous, goal.

Additional difficulties exist with the 12-steps approach to behavioral abstinence. Although this model provides information about indicators that may alert participants to an impending relapse, it does not offer any specific procedures that may be invoked to cope with lapses, other than calling another group member. Specific procedures that encourage "learning from experience" are not offered within the AA approach. Thus participants learn to recognize signs of impending trouble but do not develop skills that enable them to lessen the likelihood of encountering problems in the first place.

The 12-steps model, as applied to sex offenders, advocates beliefs that appear contradictory and that may pose a countertherapeutic double-bind. At the same time that the goal of absolute behavioral control is advanced, the premise that "addicts are powerless over their behavior" (Carnes, 1983, p. 12) is espoused. Thus, although sexual addicts are encouraged to seek perfection, they are informed that they are powerless to attain that goal. However, this tenet is doubtlessly appealing to the sexually aggressive client who would like to convince the court, his therapist, his friends, and his victims that he was "powerless" to refrain from the victimization.

The dilemma of demanding that a powerless offender maintain behavioral perfection is supposedly resolved by "ask[ing] addicts to rely totally on their Higher Power for their recovery" (Carnes, 1983, p. 151). Although reliance on a Higher Power is a noble goal that may benefit a select group of people, countless sex offenders have purportedly discovered religious dedication in prison, only to find that total reliance on religion was shortsighted. Total reliance on a Higher Power neglects the adage that "God helps those who help themselves." One might equally well propose that, for some offenders, the pattern of "being forgiven" and "sinning anew" could be considered a phase of their relapse process.

Relapse prevention offers a more realistic approach to enhancing maintenance of behavioral change. Contrary to the 12-steps model, relapse prevention proposes that individuals always exist somewhere along a continuum of behavioral control. Relapse prevention provides individuals with specific skills that may be employed to enhance self-control in problematic situations. In addition, rather than offering a single approach that is applied uniformly to all, relapse prevention offers a wide range of therapeutic activities that may be instituted prescriptively to meet the unique behavioral assets and deficits of each individual.

EFFICACY OF TREATMENT
OF SEXUAL AGGRESSORS

Considerable conflict exists among researchers regarding operational definitions of *recidivism*. The criterion for relapse (e.g., self-reported offenses, police suspicion, arrest, reconviction) varies across research studies. As with any treatment outcome research, duration of the follow-up period holds major implications for the apparent efficacy of an intervention. Universally, longer follow-up entails greater recidivism rates. Finally, the different offense characteristics of subject samples in various studies are reflected in recidivism data. Lifelong, preferential pedophiles generally have high relapse rates, while incestuous fathers relapse infrequently. With these caveats, the following outcome data are presented.

In a thorough review of controlled outcome investigations, Furby, Weinrott, and Blackshaw (in press) have concluded that little evidence exists to support the efficacy of sex offender treatment. However, these authors acknowledge that the outcome studies included in their review came from treatment programs that did not employ specialized therapeutic procedures for sexual offenders. They believe outcome data from specialized treatment programs will demonstrate therapeutic efficacy (M. R. Weinrott, personal communication, May 9, 1988).

Outcome Data from Vermont Treatment Program
for Sexual Aggressors

The initial application of relapse prevention with sexual offenders occurred in the VTPSA in 1982. Since that time, relapse prevention has served as the common thread of our 3 inpatient treatment units and 24 outpatient therapy groups. As detailed in Chapter 24 of this volume, Vermont's application of relapse prevention involves the collaborative efforts of mental health and probation or parole professionals. Every professional involved in our treatment program has attended specialized training programs we have developed. In most districts of the state, specialized teams of parole officers have been formed to supervise sex offenders. To ensure adequate collaboration of mental health and probation or parole professionals, all individuals working with sex offenders attend a regional, monthly meeting. Given this framework, the VTPSA represents a unified body of highly trained professionals.

Our model of relapse prevention remains extremely vigilant of the offenders' behaviors. Program participants are supervised intensively by probation or parole officers, in accordance with the external, supervisory dimension (Pithers, Martin, & Cumming, Chapter 24, this volume) of the relapse prevention model, until expiration of their sentence. Special conditions of probation or parole prohibit the offender from engaging in specific high-risk situations. Offenders are required, as a probation or parole condition, to attend specialized sex offender therapy groups weekly. Given this level of community supervision and therapeutic involvement, the probability of undetected relapse appears low relative to most existing treatment programs.

In the past 6 years, the VTPSA has provided services to 167 clients (147 pedophiles and 20 rapists), all of whom were convicted for their crimes. During this time span, 6 offenders have relapsed; a seventh stands accused of reoffending and awaits trial. Thus the relapse rate for 167 offenders over 6 years is 4%. This stands in sharp contrast to most sex offender recidivism data previously reported for similar time periods (Furby et al., in press). Relapse prevention appears to effectively diminish reoffense rates.

Different Effects of Relapse Prevention on Rapists and Pedophiles

Examining the recidivism rates of pedophiles and rapists who have participated in the VTPSA may yield important information. That is, relapse prevention may possess differential efficacy with rapists and pedophiles. Of the 20 rapists in our follow-up sample, 3 (15%) performed an additional sexual assault during the 6-year follow-up period. In comparison, of the 147 pedophiles, 4 (3%) have reoffended. Of the 4 relapses by pedophiles, 2 occurred within 5 months of the initiation of our outpatient therapy network; a third took place 3 weeks after the offender's parole officer permitted him to discontinue participation in treatment against the co-therapist's advice.

Statistical comparison of the proportion of relapses relative to sample size of each of the two offender subtypes (i.e., pedophile and rapist) revealed a significant difference $[\chi^2 (1, N = 167) = 3.91, p < .05$ (statistic corrected for continuity due to low expected frequency of relapses)]. In comparison to their overall representation within our treatment program, rapists have greater than expected frequency of relapse, while fewer pedophiles than expected have relapsed.

Perhaps similar relapse rates are identified by research from programs that have not used relapse prevention. Should this be the case, relapse prevention might be considered ineffective in the treatment and maintenance of sexual offenders. Alternately, if research reveals differences in recidivism data for rapists and pedophiles after several years of follow-up, the discrepancy identified in outcome data from the VTPSA may be attributed to the impact of relapse prevention.

Sturgeon and Taylor (1980) examined, in 1978, the recidivism status o. every sex offender released in 1973 from treatment at California's Atascadero State Hospital, an institution that employed a standard peer-group "milieu" therapy at that time. Their data revealed that rapists' highest risk of relapse occurred within the first year after release from institutional treatment. In contrast, pedophiles recidivated with the greatest frequency 2 to 3 years after discharge.

Our reanalysis of Sturgeon and Taylor's data revealed that the proportion of rapists reoffending during the first year after release was statistically significantly greater than the proportion of pedophiles relapsing during that period [χ^2 (1, N = 200) = 4.71, $p < .05$]. Thus rapists appeared to reoffend more quickly after discharge from treatment than pedophiles. However, one might question whether these short-term differences in treatment outcome faded with prolonged exposure to risk factors and potential victims.

Our reanalysis of Sturgeon and Taylor's report demonstrated that, at the conclusion of the 5-year follow-up, rapists and pedophiles had reoffended at nearly the same rate. Statistical comparison of the proportion of the two offense groups that reoffended revealed no significant difference in relapse rates [χ^2 (1, N = 133) = 0.62, $p < .80$]. Thus, when relapse prevention was not utilized, rapists and pedophiles had similar reoffense rates by the end of the fifth year after their institutional release. Since differential reoffense rates were discovered for rapists and pedophiles within the VTPSA after a 6-year follow-up, with pedophiles reoffending at a significantly lower rate than rapists, the discrepancy in these rates appears attributable to relapse prevention.

Additional evidence of the differential impact of relapse prevention may be ascertained by comparing the actual proportions of rapists and pedophiles who reoffended after discharge from Atascadero State Hospital or the VTPSA. As indicated, Atascadero State Hospital did not offer relapse prevention as a treatment component at the time of the Sturgeon and Taylor report, while the VTPSA has employed relapse prevention since its inception. Since, with the exception of relapse prevention, these two programs are similar, differences identified in these comparisons represent the influence of relapse prevention as a method for assisting clients' maintenance of behavioral change.

Statistical comparison of the proportions of reoffenses of rapists from Atascadero State Hospital and the VTPSA was not significant [χ^2 (1, N = 54) = 0.41, $p < .50$]. Inspection of these proportions reveals that, while a smaller percentage of the Vermont rapists than the Atascadero rapists relapsed (15% versus 26%), the difference was not statistically significant. However, the social significance of this difference should not be ignored.

Comparing the proportions of pedophiles from the two programs who reoffended, a highly significant statistical difference emerged [χ^2 (1, N = 246) = 15.52, $p < .001$]. While 18% of the pedophiles from Atascadero relapsed, only 3% of those from the VTPSA have repeated an offense. Thus several lines of evidence suggest that relapse prevention significantly decreases the proportion of pedophiles who reoffend. In contrast, relapse prevention did not, at a statistically significant level, diminish the proportion of rapists who reoffended. Given the existing data, one may speculate that these differences in efficacy of relapse prevention have emerged as a reflection of the underlying dynamics of men who rape or engage in child sexual abuse (see Hall, Chapter 17, this volume, for a detailed consideration of this issue).

Theoretical Basis for Differential Effect of Relapse Prevention

Differences in the dynamics and precursors of rapists and pedophiles may possibly explain both the greater frequency of relapses for rapists than pedophiles during the first year after release from treatment (Sturgeon & Taylor, 1980) and the discrepancy in impact of relapse prevention on the two offender subtypes.

The discovery that the first year after release sees the highest frequency of rape relapses may reveal the influence of anger and power as the predominant motivations for sexual violence. Eruptions of anger and feelings of disempowerment have precipitous, explosive onsets, which often represent exacerbation of chronic states. In individuals for whom these issues are problematic, loss of behavioral control can take place rapidly. Rapists manifest few precursive risk factors prior to their offenses. They move from periods of adequate self-management to relapse within a relatively short time. Few opportunities to observe signs of anger exist prior to relapse.

The finding that pedophiles relapse with the highest frequency several years after discharge may reflect their misguided efforts to obtain "intimacy" and "relationships." Many pedophiles groom victims, gaining the familiarity that enables prolonged sexual access. Development of any human relationship, even the profoundly disturbing, coercive interaction of a pedophile and victim, takes time. Pedophiles are more likely than rapists to display precursive risk factors over a relatively lengthy period of time. These characteristics afford greater opportunity for identification of precursors, therapeutic intervention, and restoration of self-control.

CASE EXAMPLES OF THE RELAPSE
PREVENTION PROCESS

Case Example One: Dennis M

Dennis M, a 22-year-old rapist who had been in residential treatment for 2 years, had recently received approval to obtain a job in the community as part of his release process. After an extended and frustrating search, Dennis gained employment pumping gas at night for a notoriously difficult boss who refused to grant him time off work to attend treatment activities (e.g., outpatient therapy,

AA). His employer's abrasive nature created increased levels of frustration and anger, which were risk factors that challenged Dennis's ability to cope.

While returning to the correctional center from his workplace one evening, Dennis noticed an illuminated window in a small house near the sidewalk. Dennis felt tempted to peep in the window, lapsing into a fantasy about whom he might see beyond it. He paused momentarily in this high-risk situation, acknowledged his fantasy and the accompanying urge, and then ran the entire way back to the correctional center.

Dennis waited 2 weeks to describe his lapse in transition group. He later indicated he had waited so long because he felt ashamed, suggesting that he may have experienced a mild abstinence violation effect. After discussing the event in group, Dennis decided to seek a daytime job and resume his outpatient therapies.

Shortly after assuming a new job in a corner store, Dennis was assigned the duty of unpacking and displaying newspapers and magazines. When the first shipment arrived, Dennis was surprised to note that it contained a number of pornographic magazines. Realizing pornography to be a risk factor, Dennis asked a female salesperson if she would trade him this chore for one of her choosing. She readily agreed. Dennis discussed the episode the following day in outpatient therapy.

Dennis took less time to report his second high-risk situation than his initial lapse, suggesting that he had experienced the processing of the first lapse to be relatively constructive. In the second high-risk situation, he had the option of coping by requesting his coworker to change job duties since he had previously informed his employer and coworkers about his offense and risk factors. In two instances, lapses in high-risk situations had been stopped from evolving into potential relapses.

Case Example Two: Leonard C

Leonard C, convicted for a sexual assault on a 24-year-old female, had been working in a restaurant for several months while on work release. In individual therapy, Leonard reported a lapse that had occurred at his workplace. While rearranging supplies stored in the basement of the restaurant, Leonard heard the door to the waitresses' changing room squeaking open. Turning toward the sound, he noticed an attractive woman clad only in brief underwear. He thought of asking her for a date, decided she would probably decline, and imagined that the rejection would immediately precipitate a rape fantasy. He reportedly dealt with the immediate high-risk situation and lapse by leaving the basement and resuming other work.

After disclosing his lapse, Leonard was asked to develop a strategy that might enable him to avoid a repetition of that situation. He proudly announced that he had decided to purchase a Yale lock, which the waitresses could use to protect themselves from him.

Leonard's proposed avoidance strategy was clearly inappropriate, placing responsibility on the waitresses to protect themselves from becoming his victims. His response did not affect his own beliefs or behaviors, doing little to enhance his self-management. In light of Leonard's response, the treatment team was sufficiently concerned about his behaviors to call his employer to check on his recent work performance. The boss enthusiastically commented that Leonard was his most hard-working employee, volunteering that Leonard had spent several hours of his own time rearranging supplies in the basement over the past week. Since Leonard had not been entirely honest in reporting his exposure to high-risk situations and lapses, he was removed from work-release status and returned to the residential treatment program for a refresher course in relapse prevention.

Case Example Three: Vincent S

Vincent S, whose 29-year history of abusing children had led to arrests in nine states, had established his first intimate relationship with a female peer soon after his release from residential treatment. During conjoint therapy, the potential risks of having children, and thereby creating potential victims, were discussed. A year after his release from residential treatment, Vincent proudly announced in an outpatient group that his partner might be pregnant. Other group members confronted Vincent about his apparently irrelevant decision of engaging in intercourse without birth control, a high-risk situation for a lifelong pedophile. Two weeks later, after informing the group that his partner was not pregnant, Vincent reported that he had scheduled an appointment to have a vasectomy. He decided having children would represent a high-risk situation and that birth control should be his responsibility.

CONCLUSION

No therapeutic intervention can promise that sexual offenders will not victimize again. However, initial outcome data derived from application of relapse prevention within the VTPSA suggest that this approach represents an effective method for decreasing recidivism, particularly with pedophiles. The model may be less applicable to rapists, although additional data may demonstrate this early conclusion to have been premature.

REFERENCES

Brecher, E. M. (1978). *Treatment programs for sex offenders*. Washington, DC: U.S. Government Printing Office.

Carnes, P. (1983). *The sexual addiction*. Minneapolis, MN: CompCare Publications.

Furby, L., Weinrott, M. R., & Blackshaw, L. (1989). Sex offender recidivism: A review. *Psychological Bulletin, 105,* 3–30.

Group for the Advancement of Psychiatry. (1977). *Psychiatry and sex psychopath legislation*. New York: The Group for the Advancement of Psychiatry.

Pithers, W. D., Cumming, G. F., Beal, L. S., Young, W., & Turner, R. (1989). Relapse prevention: A method for enhancing behavioral self-management and external supervision of the sexual aggressor. In B. Schwartz (Ed.), *A practitioner's guide to the treatment of the incarcerated male sex offender* (pp. 121–135). Washington, DC: National Institute of Corrections.

Sturgeon, V. H., & Taylor, J. (1980). Report of a five-year follow-up study of mentally disordered sex offenders released from Atascadero State Hospital in 1973. *Criminal justice journal, 4,* 31–63.

Conclusion

Although the title of this book is *Relapse Prevention with Sex Offenders*, it should be considered an interim statement, not an ordered set of conclusions that the treatment is definitively effective in this application. As most readers are aware, RP has become highly visible in the past decade, and it appears that it might well be an effective treatment for most, if not all, disorders of impulse control.

That assertion, however, is far from proven, even in its original applications to alcoholism and drug abuse. In those applications it appears to be the best, but not the only, game in town. In recent years a sort of bandwagon effect has been observed, a rush to apply the concept to sex offenders. I, and many of my colleagues, have contributed to this effect. Upon reflection, after making my contribution, I decided that this was highly premature. The idea behind this book, then, was not to contribute further to the phenomenon but rather to slow it down a bit and make a determination of how far we had come.

Looking back over this work now, at the end of this labor, I can see that we have come a very long way in the past 6 or 7 years. More importantly, careful reading of all the contributions will clearly show you how far we have yet to go. The optimism of our contributions notwithstanding, there remains *no* definitive evidence that RP or any other treatment for sex offenders diminishes relapse rates over the long run. You will be wise to consider this book not as a set of statements about treatment efficacy but rather as a set of marching orders. Here we show you some of the things that have been done. If those statements have heuristic value, if they stimulate the reader to disprove, replicate, extend, or otherwise continue this important work, we will have done our job.

Index